Complementary Therapies and Wellness

Practice Essentials for Holistic Health Care

Jodi L. Carlson, M.S., O.T.R./L.

Putnam Hospital Center
Carmel, New York

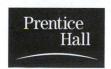
Prentice Hall

Upper Saddle River, New Jersey 07458

Library of Congress Cataloging-in-Publication Data
Carlson, Jodi L.
   Complementary therapies and wellness : practice essentials
for holistic health care / Jodi Carlson.
      p. cm.
   Includes bibliographical references and index.
   ISBN 0-13-031936-8
   1. Holistic medicine.   2. Alternative medicine.

R733 .C367 2002
615.5—dc21
                                        2002020574

Publisher: Julie Levin Alexander
Publisher's Assistant: Regina Bruno
Senior Acquisitions Editor: Mark Cohen
Assistant Editor: Melissa Kerian
Editorial Assistant: Mary Ellen Ruitenberg
Director of Production and Manufacturing:
   Bruce Johnson
Managing Editor for Production: Patrick Walsh
Production Liaison: Alexander Ivchenko
Production Editor: Karen Berry
Manufacturing Manager: Ilene Sanford

Manufacturing Buyer: Pat Brown
Creative Director: Cheryl Asherman
Cover Design Coordinator: Maria Guglielmo Walsh
Formatting: Pine Tree Composition, Inc.
Marketing Manager: Nicole Benson
Product Information Manager: Rachele Strober
Printer/Binder: Courier Westford
Copy Editor: Carol Lallier
Cover Design: Joseph DePinho
Cover Printer: Phoenix Color

Pearson Education Ltd., London
Pearson Education Australia Pty, Limited, Sydney
Pearson Education Singapore, Pte. Ltd.
Pearson Education North Asia Ltd., Hong Kong
Pearson Education Canada, Ltd., Toronto
Pearson Educación de Mexico, S.A. de C.V.
Pearson Education—Japan, Tokyo
Pearson Education Malaysia, Pte. Ltd.
Pearson Education, Upper Saddle River, New Jersey

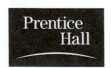

10 9 8 7 6 5 4 3 2 1
ISBN 0-13-031936-8

To Cheryl Gherardini and Nancy Baker,
two very special teachers who communicated a profound level of acceptance.

Contents

Preface

One of the interesting aspects of interacting with people who practice holistically is determining how each practitioner became interested in such practice. I came to the study of holistic practice and complementary therapies through my interest in spirituality, relaxation, and imagery. As an undergraduate, I studied all of the theology I could get my hands on, searching, I now realize, for a spiritual practice. I wanted to feel centered and whole. Carolyn Myss, author of *Energy Anatomy* (Boulder, CO: Sounds True, 1996), laughs when she speaks of trying to find God by studying. I don't think that this is so uncommon for some academic types. And at the very least I value the impulse.

When I became an occupational therapist, I channeled some of this search into learning therapeutic techniques such as relaxation and imagery, which helped me access a feeling of being centered and whole. Regular practice of such methods has enhanced both my personal life and clinical skills. Personally, these methods have enhanced my development, or emotional maturity, as I have been able to focus more on what is truly important and gradually leave behind the "blocks" (sometimes they feel like pieces of granite) I carry from childhood and develop day to day. Clinically, these methods have allowed me to better "walk the talk" of a therapist—doing what I ask of my clients—and to be as fully "present" as possible in therapeutic interactions.

It seems fitting to continue my involvement in integrative practices by editing this text. The audience—students and practitioners of physical and occupational therapy—is diverse. Some of you might be wondering why you are even reading this book, having been assigned readings for a course. Others may already practice alternative therapies or have an integrative practice and seek more knowledge so that you can better integrate the therapies into your practice. Whomever you are, I hope that you will come away from this book with an expanded awareness of what is possible in the realms of health care practice.

Acknowledgments

This book was created through the hard work and dedication of many people.

The authors, Ellen Anderson, Stacey Austin, John Barnes, Sherry Borcherding, Jennifer Bottomley, Ann Burkhardt, Ron Caplan, Elicia Dunn Cruz, Irene DeMasi, Judith Deutsch, Mary Lou Galantino, Scott Gold, Phyllis Gordon, Ken Harrison, Patricia Judd, Larry Kopelman, Susan Laeng, Sandy Matsuda, Ann Marie McClintock, Guy McCormack, Maureen McKenna, Rob Ofir, Judith Parker, Gretchen Schaff, Ron Scott, Suzanne Scurlock-Durana, and Frank Stein, are all generous and valuable resources to laypeople and health professionals alike. Thank you for sharing your expertise and time.

Ellen Taira has been a fantastic teacher of editing and a true support. Ann Marie McClintock, Ann Scott, Judith Parker, and others helped tremendously in identifying talented therapists and writers. Ann Marie McClintock, Suzanne Scurlock-Durana, and my sister, Amy Carlson, supported me and my family energetically at great times of need. Mark Cohen and Melissa Kerian of Prentice Hall offered help and encouragement whenever needed. And our reviewers, Liane Hewitt, MPH, OTR, Department Chair, Occupational Therapy Program, Loma Linda University; Susan Ramsey, PT, MA, Assistant Program Director, Physical Therapist Assistant Program, Harcum College; Becky Rodda, PT, MHS, OCS, Clinical Assistant Professor, University of Michigan–Flint; Marjorie E. Scaffa, Ph.D., OTR, FAOTA, Chairperson and Associate Professor, Department of Occupational Therapy, University of South Alabama; Gale D. Seefeld, MA, OTR, Program Director, Maric College; and Jodi L. Teitelman, Ph.D., Associate Professor, Department of Occupational Therapy, Virginia Commonwealth University, provided relevant and valuable criticism which shaped this text for the better. It is inevitable to forget acknowledging someone. Be assured that you who go unmentioned are appreciated as well.

Most importantly, I want to thank my husband, Yoni, my parents, Ken and Nancy Carlson, and my sister, Cheryl Hallock. I really could not have done my part of this project without you.

Jodi L. Carlson

About the Authors

Ellen Zambo Anderson, P.T., M.A., G.C.S., Assistant Professor, University of Medicine and Dentistry of New Jersey, School of Health-Related Professions, Program in Physical Therapy. (Chapter 9, "Introduction to Energy Therapies" and Chapter 5, "Researching Complementary Therapies")

Stacey Austin, O.T.R., Certified yoga instructor. (Chapter 24, "Yoga")

John F. Barnes, P.T., Developer, John F. Barnes approach to myofascial release; Founder, Myofascial Release Treatment Centers of Pennsylvania and Arizona. (Chapter 16, "Myofascial Release")

Sherry Borcherding, M.A., O.T.R./L., C.S.T., Associate Professor, University of Missouri–Columbia; certified craniosacral therapist and Reiki master. (Chapter 14, "Craniosacral Therapy")

Jennifer M. Bottomley, Ph.D., M.S., P.T., President, Section on Geriatrics of the APTA and Rehabilitation Consultant. (Chapter 4, "Utilization, Reimbursement, Legislative, Fraud and Abuse, and Documentation Issues" and Appendix 1, "NIH Definitions of CAM Therapies")

Ann Burkhardt, M.A., O.T.R./L., F.A.O.T.A., B.C.N., Director of Occupational Therapy, New York Presbyterian Hospital-Columbia Presbyterian Center, Associate Professor of Clinical Occupational Therapy, Columbia University, and Clinical Associate, Mercy College, Dobbs Ferry, New York. (Chapter 28, "Smoking Cessation")

Ron Caplan, Ph.D., Associate Professor of Public Health, Richard Stockton College of New Jersey. (Chapter 2, "The Evolution of Complementary and Alternative Medicine in the United States")

Jodi L. Carlson, M.S., O.T.R./L., Associate Editor, *Physical and Occupational Therapy in Geriatrics;* home health care therapist. (Chapter 1, "Basic Concepts," and Chapter 11, "Introduction to Mind-Body Interventions")

Elicia Dunn Cruz, M.S., O.T.R., Assistant Professor, Department of Occupational Therapy, University of Texas Medical Branch (UTMB), Galveston, Texas; active in community-based health promotion. (Chapter 12, "Introduction to Health Promotion")

Irene De Masi, M.A., P.T., Vice President of the Onsite Rehabilitation Service Division for Kessler Rehabilitation Corporation; Clinical Assistant Professor, University of Medicine and Dentistry of New Jersey School of Physical Therapy; certified Structural Integration practitioner. (Chapter 22, "Structural Integration [Rolfing]")

Judith Deutsch, Ph.D., P.T., Associate Professor of Physical Therapy, University of Medicine and Dentistry of New Jersey; editor of *Neurology Report.* (Chapter 22, "Structural Integration [Rolfing]" and Chapter 5, "Researching Complementary Therapies")

Mary Lou Galantino, Ph.D., P.T., Founder of L.I.F.E. Physical Therapy in Houston, Texas; Associate Professor of Physical Therapy, Richard Stockton College of New Jersey. (Chapter 2, "The Evolution of Complementary and Alternative Medicine in the United States" and Chapter 27, "Chronic HIV Disease")

Scott Gold, O.T.R./L., Staff therapist with Heartland Rehabilitation; certified Shiatsu practitioner. (Chapter 21, "Shiatsu")

Phyllis Gordon, M.S., O.T.R., Private practitioner specializing in manual therapy. (Appendix 2, "Other Therapies")

Ken Harrison, Ph.D., Professor of Economics, Richard Stockton College of New Jersey. (Chapter 2, "The Evolution of Complementary and Alternative Medicine in the United States")

Patricia Judd, M.S., P.T., Regional Vice President of Operations, Kessler Rehabilitation Centers in West Orange, New Jersey. (Chapter 22, "Structural Integration [Rolfing]")

Larry Kopelman, P.T., N.D., Ph.D., President of Healthworks of Staten Island; Professor of Integrative Medicine at Capital University; editorial board member for practical pain management; board certified in pain management, naturopathy, and forensics. (Chapter 13, "Biofeedback" and Chapter 6, "Creating an Integrative Clinic")

Susan Laeng, B.S., P.T., M.S., Doctor of Oriental Medicine; combines a practice of physical therapy, acupuncture and hatha yoga. (Chapter 24, "Yoga")

Sandy Matsuda, O.T.R./L., Ph.D., Assistant Professor of Occupational Therapy, University of Missouri–Columbia; T'ai Chi practitioner for 27 years. (Chapter 23, "T'ai Chi")

Ann Marie McClintock, O.T.R./L., Cofounder and Director, Wellness Workers of Gibbsboro, New Jersey; Reiki master. (Chapter 19, "Reiki")

Guy McCormack, O.T.R., Professor and Chair, Master of Occupational Therapy Program, Samuel Merritt College; therapeutic touch practitioner for over 20 years. (Chapter 17, "Noncontact Therapeutic Touch" and Chapter 26, "Pain Control")

Maureen McKenna, Ph.D., Assistant Professor of Physical Therapy, Wheeling Jesuit University. (Chapter 8, "Introduction to Asian Medical Systems")

Reuven Ofir, B.S., M.A., Ph.D., Assistant trainer of the Feldenkrais Method®. (Chapter 15, "The Feldenkrais Method®")

Judith A. Parker, M.S., O.T.R./L., Director, OTA Program, Mercy College, Dobbs Ferry, New York; private practitioner blending CAM and occupational therapy. (Chapter 20, "Relaxation, Meditation, and Breath")

Gretchen Schaff, P.T., Private practitioner and reflexology teacher. (Chapter 18, "Reflexology")

Ron Scott, J.D., L.L.M., M.S.P.T., O.C.S., Associate Professor and Chair, Department of Physical Therapy, Lebanon Valley College, Annville, Pennsylvania. (Chapter 3, "Legal Issues")

Suzanne Scurlock-Durana, C.M.T., C.S.T-D., Developer, *Healing from the Core,* a program for conscious awareness and healing; senior instructor, craniosacral therapy and somato-emotional release training with the Upledger Institute. (Chapter 7, "Developing Therapeutic Presence")

Franklin Stein, Ph.D., O.T.R./L., F.A.O.T.A., Professor of Occupational Therapy, University of South Dakota; founding editor, *Occupational Therapy International.* (Chapter 25, "Stress Management")

1

Basic Concepts

Jodi L. Carlson

- Define major concepts related to complementary and alternative medicine (CAM).
- Discuss paradigms of health and their influence on expectations for therapy.
- Discuss options for using CAM in therapy.
- Discuss issues related to therapeutic etiquette.

This book is designed to provide practical information about complementary care in addition to specific information about many complementary therapeutic approaches that therapists use. Part 1, "Essentials," covers the "nuts and bolts" of complementary practice, such as history, legal implications, documentation, and how to create an integrative clinic. Part 2, "Foundation Principles," includes chapters on major areas relevant to therapies covered by the book, such as Chapter 11, "Introduction to Mind-Body Interventions." Part 3, "Specific Therapies," focuses on many of the methods or modalities that physical and occupational therapists use in practice. It may be necessary to read more than one introductory chapter to understand basic principles of certain therapies. For example, yoga is classified as a mind-body method, but concepts such as Asian medical systems, energy therapies, body-based approaches, as well as mind-body therapies, are all germaine to understanding it. Finally, Part 4, "Wellness and Special Applications," covers holistic and complementary practice with different groups of people and problems.

Note that there are several chapters on health promotion and illness prevention (e.g., smoking cessation). Physical and occupational therapists typically see clients in the context of rehabilitation, and infrequently address such areas. There are, however, compelling reasons to address the topics in this text. Health promotion and illness prevention is classified by the National Center for Complementary and Alternative Medicine (NCCAM) as a major area of alternative and complementary health (see Appendix 1). Many of the medicine systems on which alternative approaches are based, such as Traditional Chinese Medicine, focus on

It is necessary for the therapist seeking a greater understanding of topics in this text to know basic terms and develop an appreciation for alternative models of health, illness, and the notion of curing. Concepts (such as alternative, complementary, integrative, holistic, and wellness) all have specific meanings that should be appreciated so that therapists understand each other and accurately communicate with other health professionals. Paradigms of health, both traditional and alternative, help the therapist understand the different contexts in which health, healing, and curing can occur. Understanding how therapy approaches can be used and understanding therapeutic etiquette will enhance therapy practice as well.

health promotion and illness prevention. That therapists do not traditionally incorporate these components into therapy makes these topics "alternative," by definition, to therapy practice. Therefore, in the spirit of addressing clients holistically, factors such as prevention, models of health belief, and even smoking cessation are covered. It is impossible to comprehensively cover all of the topics vital to holistic practice. However, the intent is to describe best practice in specific areas and stimulate readers to search out further knowledge and develop comprehensive, holistic practice in areas pertinent to their own practice.

Definitions

The National Center for Complementary and Alternative Medicine (NCCAM) defines *complementary and alternative medicine (CAM)* as ". . . those treatments and healthcare practices not taught widely in medical schools, not generally used in hospitals, and not usually reimbursed by medical insurance companies" (NCCAM, 2000). When these therapies are used alone (NCCAM, 2000), replacing or instead of traditional health care (Cohen, 1998), they are called *alternative therapies.* This is a somewhat limited term defined by its relationship not only to other health care practices but also to standards of practice in medicine, which sometimes differ from standards of practice for therapists. This means, for example, that Traditional Chinese Medicine, despite being the primary medicine of a large group of people, is considered alternative in the United States and other parts of the world. It also means that approaches that therapists might consider traditional, such as biofeedback or hydrotherapy (see Appendix 1), are defined as alternative when viewed from a wider scope of health care practice as a whole.

Therapies that are defined as alternative sometimes become accepted by the mainstream and are then considered *traditional* or *conventional.* An example of a medical practice that was once considered alternative (although it is not clear if the term applied at that time) but is now considered traditional is radiation therapy for cancer (Federal Register, 1992). Thus, we can expect that some of the therapies discussed in this book may be considered (by a majority of health care practitioners) traditional in the future, as research demonstrates positive outcomes and practice acceptance becomes widespread. On the other hand, practices once considered traditional, such as bloodletting, can fall out of favor as knowledge and health care evolve (Cohen, 1998).

Complementary therapies or medicine refer to alternative health care approaches that are used in conjunction with traditional practice (NCCAM, 2000). The term *integrative,* often used interchangeably with complementary in reference to medicine or therapies, seems to be developing into a term that refers to a comprehensive mix of traditional and complementary therapies without allegiance to a particular school or school of thought (Ali, 1998).

The term *holistic* is defined as "relating to or concerned with wholes or with complete systems rather than with the analysis of, treatment of, or dissection into parts" (*Merriam-Webster's Collegiate Dictionary,* 10th ed., s.v. "holistic"). In health care, holistic refers to a focus on the whole being, and holistic providers view people and illness as multifaceted. Illness is addressed through an understanding of not only biological but also social, behavioral, and spiritual factors, and with a variety of interventions (Cohen, 1998). Of course, many clients seek out symptom relief, and it is necessary for the therapist to address symptoms or sometimes the client will not come back to therapy. However, practicing holistically would also address the "system" of the client—the person and environment in which the symptom takes place.

Cruz defines *wellness* in this text as referring ". . . to social, emotional, and spiritual aspects of health that extend beyond the absence of disease and disability. Wellness includes movement toward a greater awareness of and satisfaction from all aspects of life . . ." (2003, p. 114). This definition includes both the population at large, which therapists traditionally do not treat, and the population of rehabilitation participants known to therapists as patients.

Paradigms of Health

The prevailing belief about health and disease in Western society is that health is an optimum state and disease or illness are states to be avoided. Inherent in this notion are value judgments people may place on sick and healthy people, and society's sometimes "idolatrous" value of health (Newman, 1986). The Western medical model typically promotes disease cures as the ultimate goal, and focuses infrequently on prevention and overall balance.

Not everyone views health and illness as dichotomous. Traditional Chinese Medicine, for example, emphasizes balance. Illness is viewed as imbalance, which can be addressed via energy pathways (Ziyin & Zelin, 1996). Perhaps the most eloquent writer on the subject of Western alternative views of health is Margaret A. Newman, a nursing theorist. Newman (1986), drawing from the theories of such notables as Teilhard de Chardin, David Bohm, and Martha Rogers, proposed that health and illness are not a continuum but are a single process, with peaks and troughs. In this conceptualization, illness becomes a display of health (Newman, 1986). How could this be? Illness in this context is an expression of the body seeking greater health: "Most of us prefer harmony, but we may need the repatterning that disharmony can stimulate" (Newman, p. 21).

Who has not known a person who, upon receiving a diagnosis of an illness, radically changed his or her life, possibly changing diet, beginning an exercise regime, or quitting a hated job? The end result is promotion of a lifestyle that the person "knew" intuitively was important to live. Newman proposes that when people see patterns in their lives and ". . . relate to them in an authentic way . . ." (p. 17), they evolve to a higher plane of consciousness. (A simpler way to think of this is to say that when people know intuitively that something is or isn't right for them and their behavior follows this, they evolve.) In the context of what Newman is describing, illness stimulates life changes that promote evolution: "We evolve by having our own equilibrium thrown off balance and then discovering how to attain a new state of balance, temporarily, and then move on to another phase of disequilibrium" (p. 27).

Ideally, people should not require illness to evolve and change: "If we understood the pattern of our lives, then perhaps we would be in a position to maintain harmonious relationships without the necessity of a shock" (pp. 20, 21). Sometimes, however, people need to make changes but will not or cannot unless forced. Illness can be a big impetus to change. In Newman's model, this *does not* imply blame. It is simply a pattern that occurs to facilitate balance. What a different way of looking at clients and oneself!

Epstein and Altman (1994) propose concepts of health and healing that are similar to Newman's. They describe healing as the development of consciousness, occurring through a sequence of 12 interconnected and interdependent stages. The authors envision these stages as a spiral path of both ascent and descent, and suggest that people proceed, "developing up" or "slipping down" the healing path. These stages (see Table 1.1) can be thought of as explicit descriptions of the general evolution of consciousness that Newman describes.

Stages of Change

An important aspect of Epstein and Altman's theories for therapists is the notion that the action or lack thereof required in each stage varies considerably from stage to stage, and that the helpfulness of specific therapy approaches or interventions will vary depending on which stage a person is in. For example, asking someone to take responsibility for a problem or using alternative methods of healing will probably not be effective if a person is in a stage such as Stage 1, when a person's developmental "task" is to simply acknowledge that suffering is occurring.

Prochaska and DiClemente's (1982) transtheoretical model supports the notion that therapists must tailor interventions to the developmental stage of the client. These authors have found that people go through different stages in changing health behaviors. Miller and Rollnick (1991), writing about the use of Prochaska and DiClemente's model in treatment of many conditions, have noted that therapists need to use different approaches with clients, depending on which stage the client is in, in the change process. An example is smoking cessation efforts: A client who has not begun to contemplate quitting smoking will not be ready to quit smoking. Instead, this person should be approached from a psychoeducation perspective and be provided with resources for future smoking cessation efforts. These authors note, "We believe that problems of clients' being 'unmotivated' or 'resistant' occur when a counselor is using strategies inappropriate for a client's current stage of change" (1991, pp. 15, 16). Such notions certainly call for therapists to expand knowledge beyond rehabilitation protocols.

Healing and Curing

Epstein also points to the profound difference between *healing*—". . . involving the harmonious alignment of the physical, emotional, mental, and spiritual aspects of our being and how we relate to the world" (p. 1) and *curing*—the elimination of diseases, symptoms, or crises. Yet, he does not necessarily consider healing and curing dichotomous. To the contrary, Epstein points out that curing can be important to healing when it offers time and increased comfort, acting as a "rest stop" to healing.

Table 1–1 Stages of Healing*

Stage/Title	Characteristics
1. Suffering	Understanding that something is amiss; accepting that nothing is working to address the problem and that one is helpless.
2. Polarities and Rhythms	Becoming aware that problems occur in cycles or patterns, attempting to control the situation through external means, and discovering that one is responsible for one's distress.
3. Stuck in a Perspective	Developing the awareness that being "stuck" has created the distress.
4. Reclaiming Our Power	Choosing to stop dishonoring oneself.
5. Merging with the Illusion	Developing a strong sense of self and beginning to integrate parts of oneself that were previously alienated, disliked, or ignored.
6. Preparation for Resolution	Continuing to integrate parts of oneself.
7. Resolution	Experiencing resolution so that parts of oneself are integrated.
8. Emptiness in Connectedness	"Opening" and experiencing a profound connection with external events.
9. Light Behind the Form	Becoming aware of one's energetic connection to the life force and other people.
10. Ascent	Awareness of the oneness of creation.
11. Descent	Living in the world with the awareness of the previous stages.
12. Community	Recognizing that further integration stems from bringing ones own "gifts" to the community, and experiencing the earlier stages to develop further wholeness.

**Aside from "New Age" language, there is a paucity of terms to describe such concepts. The reader is asked to appreciate the concepts by suspending judgment based on such language.*

Adapted from Epstein and Altman (1994).

Using Alternative and Complementary Therapies

The therapies presented in this text have a number of general uses: as preparatory activities, as therapeutic exercises, as meaningful activities (Burkhardt, 2001) and as self-care. As preparatory activities, such therapies would be used in the same way as physical agent modalities

(PAMs)—to prepare clients for therapeutic activities or exercises. For example, Shiatsu could be used to decrease muscle tone in preparation for functional activities. Therapies can be used as therapeutic exercises. For example, yoga poses can be performed to enhance many areas of therapeutic intervention, including strength, coordination, and relaxation. Therapies can be used as meaningful activities. For example, meditation can be taught to a client not only to address therapy goals, such as increased relaxation and attention, but also for the purpose of pleasurable and meaningful engagement. Finally, therapies can be used as self-care approaches for therapists themselves.

Therapeutic Etiquette

Therapeutic etiquette refers to the respect therapists must have for the point of view of their clients. Pushing new or different ideas on people may result in refusal to receive or participate in services that could be helpful. This is unfortunate because therapies can often be presented in ways that both accurately represent the method (which is necessary for informed consent) and fit within the person's views and beliefs.

All therapists need to become experienced at explaining what they do in layman's terms that do not frighten or repel people. It is even more crucial to become practiced in this skill as a complementary therapist. It is necessary to develop an understanding of when someone is open or not open to language that could be considered "way out" (e.g., energetic interpretations of an illness or phenomenon) and to develop alternative ways of speaking about the same intervention so that it can be accepted and used by everyone it could possibly help. For example, some clients might be put off if a therapist talked about their chakras being out of balance, but might accept language such as "it seems that you are somewhat out of balance."

Sometimes, describing methods or effects can be differentiated into a Western and Eastern approach. An example of two different interpretations of a complementary therapy is provided in Scott Gold's chapter on Shiatsu. The Eastern presentation of the therapy describes chi, the energy that flows throughout people's bodies, and manipulation of chi flowing in meridians for balance. The Western presentation of the therapy describes how Shiatsu (or acupressure—sometimes a more accessible term) relaxes the body, helping clients maximize therapy, and of the release of points that get constrained, like muscles that get tense.

One way to become better at reading people for their openness to complementary therapy language and speaking to people in different ways about complementary therapy techniques is to practice with friends, family, and colleagues. One must become skillful at reading body language, being able to note when someone is uncomfortable with a topic (e.g., looks away, appears angry or anxious, refuses to continue the conversation) versus open to a line of conversation (e.g., comments enthusiastically about the topic, offers his or her own knowledge on the subject, asks for more information). The author has successfully broached the idea of auras with ultra-conservative physicians by noting that in the past scientists did not know that X rays or electromagnetic energy existed, and suggesting that the possibility of such energy that is perceived by few people may just be that—not perceived by them but there, nonetheless.

The American Psychological Association (APA, 1990) has issued guidelines on how a therapist can avoid conflict with clients about religious convictions. These guidelines, such as not imposing ideological systems on the client, are useful when thinking about complementary practice as well. Dossey's (2001) adaptation of Edgley and Brissett's (1998) guidelines address similar points in layman's terms:

- Be more polite. . . . In health care, this means according dignity to everyone we serve, addressing patients respectfully and listening patiently to what they have to say, and respecting their choices no matter what they may be.
- Be tolerant of those whose moral judgments differ from our own.
- Stop being self-righteous. . . . People should not be badgered, whether they choose synthetic chemicals or natural products. Individualism and eccentricity should be respected. (p. 16).

Language Choices

Physical and occupational therapy practitioners are referred to as therapists in this text, unless a more specific term is required. And, because this book is guided by holistic practice notions, recipients of therapy services are called clients.

> *I just want to let everyone know that it is a miracle to be here. It is a wonder to be able to help people. The knowledge available in the alternative medical field can transform health in this country and the world—if only healthcare providers will open their minds and develop their skills. (Abromovitz, cited in Horrigan, B., 2000, p. 85)*

STUDY QUESTIONS

1. Define traditional, alternative, and complementary therapy, providing examples of each with rationales.
2. Think about where your beliefs about health and disease fall on the different health paradigms. Describe how these beliefs can affect, both positively and negatively, your clients.
3. Trace your interest in the health professions. Are you interested in learning an alternative therapy or practicing complementary therapy? Why, or why not?
4. What are the implications of beliefs about healing and curing for clients?
5. Describe important aspects of therapeutic etiquette.

REFERENCES

Ali, M. Seven care principles of integrative medicine. *Journal of Integrative Medicine, 2*(2), 77–81.

American Psychological Association. (1990). Guidelines regarding possible conflict between psychiatrist's religious commitments and psychiatric practice. *American Journal of Psychiatry, 147*(4), 542.

Burkhardt, A. (2001). Introduction. In A. Burkhardt & J. L. Carlson (Eds.), *Complementary Therapies in Geriatric Practice: Selected Topics*. Binghamton, NY: Haworth Press.

Cohen, M. H. (1998). *Complementary and Alternative Medicine: Legal Boundaries and Regulatory Perspectives*. Baltimore, MD: Johns Hopkins University Press.

Cruz, E. D. (2003). Introduction to wellness and health promotion. In J. L. Carlson (Ed.), *Complementary Therapies and Wellness: Practice Essentials for Holistic Health Care*. Upper Saddle River, NJ: Prentice Hall.

Dossey, L. (2001). The nag factor. *Alternative Therapies in Health and Medicine, 7*(1), 12–16, 90–91.

Edgely, C., & D. Brissett. (1998). *A Nation of Meddlers*. Boulder, CO: Westview Press.

Epstein, D. M., & N. Altman. (1994). *The 12 Stages of Healing*. San Rafael, CA: Amber-Allen Publishing.

Federal Register. (1992). Congressional Directive by the Senate Appropriations Committee to the National Institutes of Health for Fiscal Year 1992. No. 104, 102nd Congress, 1st Session.

Horrigan, B. (2000). Conversations: Alan Abromovitz, MD: Integrated Patient Care: One Physician's Success Story. *Alternative Therapies in Health and Medicine, 6*(4), 79–85.

Miller, W. R., & S. Rollnick. (1991). *Motivational Interviewing: Preparing People to Change Addictive Behavior*. New York: The Guilford Press.

National Center for Complementary and Alternative Medicine (NCCAM). (2000). [online]. Available: www.nccam.nih.gov.

Newman, M. A. (1986). *Health as Expanding Consciousness*. St. Louis, MO: C. V. Mosby.

Prochaska, J., & C. DiClemente. (1982). Transtheoretical therapy: Toward a more integrative model of change. *Psychotherapy: Theory, Research, and Practice, 19*, 276–288.

Ziyin, S., & C. Zelin. (1996). *The Basis of Traditional Chinese Medicine*. Boston: Shambhala Publications.

2

The Evolution of Complementary and Alternative Medicine in the United States: The Push and Pull of Holistic Health Care into the Medical Mainstream*

Ronald Caplan, Kenneth Harrison, and Mary Lou Galantino

CHAPTER OBJECTIVES

- Understand the political and economic forces "pushing" and "pulling" holistic health are into mainstream American healthcare.
- Understand the effect of managed health care on the growth of holistic health care.

Health care in the United States is currently undergoing a radical and rare reorganization. In addition to changes in its financing (from fee-for-service to capitated payments, salaries, and diagnostic-related groups) and delivery (from solo practices and small community hospitals to group practices, managed care, and integrated hospital systems), there is now a fundamental change in its very content. The last paradigmatic shift in the content of American health care occurred nearly 100 years ago. Between 1890 and 1920, biomedicine, or "scientific medicine," which accepts a machine model of the human body, defines health as the absence of debilitating symptoms, disease as the onset of debilitating symptoms, and employs drugs and surgery to reduce or eliminate these symptoms, came to dominate American health care (Caplan, 1989).

*Portions of this article previously appeared in *Orthopaedic Physical Therapy Clinics of North America,* 9(3), 275–289. Reprinted with permission.

According to the biomedical paradigm, disease is a biological and/or chemical break-down of the human machine, and doctors are the highly trained "mechanics" who intervene to restore proper function (i.e., health) (LeShan, 1982). Most Americans accepted this approach to health care without question. Other holistic forms of health care, which had different understandings of the human body, different definitions of health and disease, and consequently utilized different healing practices, were labeled "medical quackery" and bitterly opposed by the biomedical community, especially the American Medical Association (AMA) (Caplan, 1987). Eventually, these "irregular practitioners" were pushed to the fringes of American health care, and there they have stayed until quite recently.

During the past 100 years, specific theories and practices of biomedicine have significantly changed; however, the biomedical paradigm has always dominated American health care. In fact, it largely became synonymous with American health care. But the supporters of biomedicine have never been able to achieve at least one of their long sought goals: a complete monopoly over American health care. Dominance, yes. Monopoly, no. Instead, a form of "apartheid medicine" was established—two separate and unequal health care paradigms. The dominant one was the biomedical paradigm, which was firmly grounded in the germ theory of disease and the machine model of the human body. Its principal practitioners are conventionally trained health care providers.

The other, the holistic paradigm, is part of the Vitalist tradition and comprises a more eclectic group of practices, which range from A to Z—from acupuncture to Zen meditation and nearly everything in between (Micozzi, 1996a). While no widely agreed upon definition of holism exists, most of its practitioners believe that the human body contains some form of vital energy and hence has the ability to heal itself. Chiropractors refer to this energy as innate intelligence. Acupuncturists call it Chi.

Most holistic practitioners also believe that health is a dynamic and harmonious relationship between the body's internal and external environments. In other words, health is the proper balance among mind, body, and spirit, along with one's surrounding physical and social environments. According to this paradigm, health is not the absence of debilitating symptoms, and the principal role of the practitioner is to help the body heal itself. In short, the practitioner acts more like a gardener helping plants to grow than a mechanic fixing a machine (LeShan, 1982).

Until the early 1970s, the biomedical community paid little attention to these "other healers" (Gervitz, 1988). And when they did, their intentions were quite hostile. For example, during the 1960s, the AMA established its Committee on Quackery, which had as its prime mission "the containment of chiropractic and, ultimately, the elimination of chiropractic" (Lisa, 1994, p. 270). During these "glorious decades of American medicine," most biomedical practitioners were quite content to reap the considerable benefits of their dominant position (Schwartz, 1972). American health care, which they largely controlled, was growing at unprecedented rates, along with their own personal wealth, power, and prestige (Coulter, 1975). Alternative health care practitioners, such as chiropractors, homeopaths, and naturopaths, had been successfully banished to the health care hinterland and represented little, if any, real threat.

As noted earlier, these practitioners were largely separate from and unequal to their biomedical counterparts. With respect to their separation, there was little or no interaction between them, such as patient referrals or even conversations at professional meetings. For example, in 1967 the AMA told its members that it was unethical for a physician to associate professionally with chiropractors (Lisa, 1994). According to the AMA's Judicial Council, this

Therapy Focus

Many forces have impacted the evolution of CAM, including public disillusionment with traditional treatment and biomedical suppression of alternative health care practices, some forms of which were ultimately ruled illegal. Therapists interested in CAM should understand the political and economic forces "pushing" and "pulling" holistic health care into the medical mainstream. This knowledge, and the historical perspective it provides, will help them successfully meet the obstacles and opportunities of the continuing evolution of CAM in the United States.

prohibition included the playing of a game of golf with a chiropractor, accepting patients from a chiropractor, or referring patients to a chiropractor. In fact, it was considered unethical for a physician to associate with any "unscientific practitioner" (Lisa, 1994, p. 207).

Hence, during these years, the biomedical and holistic paradigms developed largely independent of each other. However, holistic practitioners, including chiropractors (who were the largest and best organized), could not come near the political power, wealth, prestige, paradigm-building research, and professional cohesiveness of the biomedical community. However, their situation was about to improve.

The 1970s: The Onset of the Health Care Crisis

In 1969, President Nixon officially declared a "massive crisis" in the nation's health care system. A medical establishment long above reproach was now very much on the defensive. The chief complaint was that medical care was too expensive. A closely related problem was the safety and efficacy of many conventional medical practices. For example, in the early 1970s, the public was shocked to learn of the life-threatening side effects of many commonly prescribed medications and the inherent dangers of many routine medical procedures.

As a result, many consumers ended their unquestioning acceptance of biomedicine and embraced two major reform movements: the holistic health care and the self-care movements. Both stressed the potential hazards and limitations of conventional medicine and urged the public to seek alternatives (Salmon & Berliner, 1980). Therapy practices such as biofeedback, which provided clients with self-care alternatives to learn to regulate their own bodies, became popular at this time. Many federal and state policies, such as the 1973 inclusion of chiropractic in Medicare and Nevada's establishment of a separate licensing board for Chinese Medicine, also helped holistic health care providers.

Throughout the 1970s, consumer demand for and confidence in a wide assortment of holistic therapies, none of which involved hospitalization, drugs, or surgery, significantly and steadily increased (Lappe, 1979). Chiropractic (Nordstrom, 1980), naturopathy, and homeopathy became the preferred choice of millions of consumers and enjoyed a well-satisfied and loyal constituency (Caplan, 1984). These phenomena represented small yet widening cracks in the medical establishment's hegemony over American health care.

The Increasing Hostilities of the 1980s

The economic and political environments, both inside and outside of American health care, dramatically changed in the 1980s. By 1980, Americans had suffered nearly a decade of high inflation (12.6 percent), interest rates (11.5 percent), and unemployment (7.2 percent). On the health care scene, total spending was nearly $250 billion, about 9.5 percent of Gross National Product. At a time when most could ill afford it, corporations were spending $60 billion a year for the health care benefits of their employees. Moreover, medical costs were rising at an annual rate of over 10 percent. Reducing these costs became the Reagan administration's primary health care objective.

Health care reformers employed the analytical tools of economics and the philosophical doctrines of modern conservatism. Instead of stressing the many inefficiencies of medical markets, as their predecessors had done, they pointed out the many regulatory failures of government intervention (Schelling, 1976). The Reagan administration's staunch faith in the marketplace had profound policy implications, especially in health care. On the consumer side of the market, most reform measures tried to decrease, relatively speaking, the public's demand for medical care. For example, cutbacks in Medicare and Medicaid took the form of reduced levels of funding, increased out-of-pocket expenditures for beneficiaries, stricter eligibility standards, and fewer covered services. The administration also urged significant increases in the deductibles and co-insurance rates for private health insurance. It believed that such changes would force consumers to use less medical care (i.e., lower the demand for medical care), shop around for the lowest-priced provider, and reduce pathogenic behaviors, such as cigarette smoking. In other words, these policies were designed to make consumers healthier while easing inflationary pressures. On the supply side, the Reagan administration sought to increase the number and diversity of medical providers, as well as the competition among them.

The administration also wanted to reduce the federal government's role in the medical marketplace while encouraging greater participation by the private sector. As a result, prepaid groups (PPGs) such as health maintenance organizations (HMOs) and preferred provider organizations (PPOs) spread rapidly (McClure, 1983). A variety of private delivery systems that emphasized competition and the profit motive, ranging from investor-owned hospitals to free-standing ambulatory care units, also proliferated (Wohl, 1984).

These policies helped create a social environment more hostile to the practice of holistic health care than that of the 1970s. Unconventional forms of health care became the first candidates for cutbacks. Alternative health care providers, who depended most upon this source of payment, such as chiropractors, were especially vulnerable to insurance cutbacks (Caplan & Scarpaci, 1989). Furthermore, in this era of tight-fisted health care budgets, few insurance companies were willing to extend their coverage to any new group of providers. They believed, perhaps wrongly, that new services would not replace existing ones but be used in addition to them (Caplan, 1999). And finally, affordable malpractice insurance became a concern for providers such as midwives (Caplan & Scarpaci, 1989).

Developments on the supply side were also harming the holistic community. For example, most HMOs and PPOs excluded alternative practitioners from their prepaid package of health care. Enrollees wishing to utilize such practitioners had to pay the entire cost themselves. This financial barrier usually prevented them from going outside the group for their health care, as it was intended to do. Consequently, as more people enrolled in these group plans, the pool of prospective patients for alternative practitioners became smaller.

Some Powerful Countervailing Forces

Throughout the 1980s, procompetition health care reforms generally hurt the holistic health care community and further marginalized it. However, during this same period, there were some powerful countervailing forces pushing and pulling some holistic practitioners closer toward the mainstream of American health care (Alster, 1989). For example, federal and state governments were actively pushing for greater acceptance of some forms of holistic health care.

At the federal level, the United States Court of Appeals was one of the principal pushers. In 1987, 11 years after five chiropractors filed an antitrust suit against the AMA and nine other medical organizations, a federal judge ruled that the defendants had illegally conspired to destroy the chiropractic profession (Caplan, 1991b). This ruling, coupled with the 1984 decision of the Joint Commission in Accreditation of Hospitals to allow hospitals more leeway in granting medical staff membership to nonphysicians and nondentists, added legitimacy to some holistic health care providers and helped certain providers such as chiropractors and midwives move into hospitals and managed care plans (Richards, 1984).

During this period, many states also helped to enhance the legitimacy of holistic health care. For example, in 1980 Arizona became the first state to license homeopaths (Caplan, 1984). In 1985, California required all group health insurance plans to include acupuncture as a benefit and extended this requirement to include all Workers' Compensation insurance in 1989.

During the 1980s, the two principal integrating forces pulling holistic health care toward the mainstream were a steadily growing number of frustrated consumers and practitioners of conventional medicine. By 1990, about one-third of Americans (34 percent) were using at least one alternative health therapy and spent approximately $13.7 billion on alternative health care, three-quarters of which ($10.3 billion) was out-of-pocket. This latter figure was reasonably close to the country's annual out-of-pocket expenditure for all hospitalizations, which was $12.8 billion (Einsenberg et al., 1993).

As the public's demand for alternative therapies steadily increased, a growing number of biomedical practitioners were also becoming more interested in holistic concepts. For example, in 1977 several thousand physicians attended the Association for Holistic Health Conference in San Diego. The following year the American Holistic Medical Association (AHMA) was founded by "a group of physicians who felt the need for an organized forum to explore and promote holistic health care" (Caplan & Gesler, 1998, p. 190). By 1988, approximately 200 self-described holistic medical and osteopathic physicians belonged to the AHMA. Dentists in 1980 and nurses in 1981 founded similar organizations, the Holistic Dental Association and the American Holistic Nurses' Association respectively. As the number of physicians, dentists, and nurses trained in biomedicine but practicing holism increased, the boundary between holistic health care and mainstream medicine began to break down.

The Mainstreaming of Holistic Health Care in the 1990s

In 1992 alternative health care gained some important respectability with the establishment of the Office of Alternative Medicine (OAM) as part of the National Institutes of Health (NIH). OAM's mission was to scientifically evaluate alternative medicine and disseminate its findings to the public (Nienstedt, 1998). In 1998 OAM became the National Center for Complementary and Alternative Medicine (NCCAM). It had a similar mission, but its budget had jumped to $50 million. NCCAM actively encourages collaborative research between the biomedical community and practitioners of holistic health care and, as of press time, NCCAM funded 11 specialty research centers with average funding of $850,000 over three years (Hazzard, 1999).

Many state and local governments continued to officially sanction holistic health care in the 1990s. For example, 41 state governments now require chiropractic coverage of some form. Some states, like Washington and Connecticut, now mandate that insurers cover all licensed alternative health care practitioners (Muir, 1999). Many states have also adopted provider practice acts, which define the legitimate scope of holistic health care, and have licensed many of its practitioners (Baer & Good, 1998). With respect to support by local governments, the city of Seattle recently established the country's first naturopathic health clinic. Supported by tax revenues, it employs both naturopaths and medical physicians (Weber, 1996).

As noted earlier, throughout the 1980s and much of the 1990s, holistic health care was not covered by health insurance. Believing that added services would cost them more money, few insurance companies or managed care plans were willing to extend their coverage to any new group of providers, such as acupuncturists or massage therapists. It was thought that only if these practitioners could demonstrate that a significant number of consumers would actually prefer their services and would substitute them for more expensive conventional care could this particular obstacle be overcome.

By the latter half of the 1990s, these types of long-standing obstacles to coverage were in fact being overcome. An increasing number of insurance companies and managed care plans had become convinced that some of the leading alternatives to biomedicine were safer, cheaper, and in many cases customer preferred (Weber, 1996). For example, the Mutual of Omaha reported saving $6.50 for every dollar spent on Dr. Dean Ornish's diet and wellness plan for preventing and reversing heart disease (Gordon & Silverstein, 1998). Managed care plans began making similar moves and for similar reasons. Oxford Health Plans, one of the nation's largest managed care companies, led the way. In 1996 Oxford was the first managed care company to develop an alternative health care network for its over 2 million enrollees (Oxford Breaks Ground, 1996).

Holistic health care has also received some helpful coverage from the popular media. In 1996 *Life* magazine's cover story proclaimed a "healing revolution," in which more and more medical doctors are "mixing ancient medicine and new science to treat everything from the common cold to heart disease" (Colt, 1996, p. 35). In May 1997, Dr. Andrew Weil, a Harvard educated physician and one of the principal leaders of the holistic health care movement in the United States, appeared on the cover of *Time* magazine next to the question "Can This Guy Make You Healthy?" (Kluger, 1997).

The following year *Time*'s cover story concerned the "herbal medicine boom" (Greenwald, 1998). With respect to television coverage, clearly the most influential so far was the 1993 PBS production entitled "Healing and the Mind," hosted by Bill Moyers. In this six-part series, Moyers traveled to China and around the United States conducting fascinating and provocative interviews with physicians, scientists, and patients about their understandings of the mind-body connection and its impact on health. The accompanying book containing these interviews became an immediate best-seller (Moyers, 1993). No doubt, this kind of print and television coverage has helped bring holistic health care into the mainstream of America's discourse about health and healing.

During the 1990s, consumers, hospitals, physicians, medical schools, and leading medical journals continued to pull holistic health care toward the medical mainstream. By 1997, more than 4 out of 10 adults in the United States (42 percent) reported using some form of alternative health care in the previous year (Landmark Report, 1998). In 1997 Americans spent approximately $21.2 billion on alternative health care, 50 percent more than in 1990. However, unlike 1990, more than half of this expenditure (58.3 percent) was paid out-of-pocket (Eisenberg et al., 1998).

By the late 1990s, a significant and growing proportion of the country's adult population used, preferred, and were willing to pay for a wide variety of holistic health care practices. Nearly one-half of adults in the United States (45 percent) reported that they would be willing to pay more for their health care in order to have access to these practitioners (Landmark Report, 1998).

The public's increasing demand for holistic health care is affecting the biomedical community as well. For example, reminiscent of the women's movement in the 1970s when the hospitals responded with birthing centers, a growing number of hospitals in the 1990s began to establish some type of holistic health care center or program, such as hospital-based massage therapy (Koch, 1999). Even the AMA recognized the need for its profession to respond to the public's growing interest in alternative health care practices. For example, it supported the teaching of courses on alternative health care in medical schools (Wetzel, Eisenberg, & Kaptchuk, 1998). Medical professionals such as Dr. Marc Micozzi, executive director of the College of Physicians of Philadelphia, recognized the increasing need to teach medical students in the United States about holistic health care. Micozzi explained, "More and more people are using alternative medicine as dissatisfaction with conventional medicine grows. . . . Those who train health care workers can no longer afford to ignore [it]" (Micozzi, 1996a). By 1997, more than one-half of the nation's medical schools (64 percent) offered courses on alternative health care (Wetzel, Eisenberg, & Kaptchuk, 1998).

In November 1998, the *Journal of the American Medical Association (JAMA)* dedicated an entire issue to alternative medicine. In the words of Dr. George Lundberg, the editor of *JAMA,* "It is the beginning of the beginning of acceptance of some forms of 1998 alternative medicine into mainstream medicine" (Okie, 1998, p. 1). Other medical journals, most notably the *New England Journal of Medicine,* have also reported on the growth and practice of alternative health care in the United States (Angell & Kassirer, 1998)

While it appears that these members of the biomedical community are seeking to widen health care to accommodate some holistic health care providers, other members of the medical community want to radically transform American health care. They seek to change not only its geography but its methodology as well. They want a fundamental rethinking of not only where various practitioners practice (i.e., along side each other in a hospital or as part of a managed care network), but also what they practice (i.e., the dominant paradigm of conventional health care). In other words, they are pulling holistic practitioners into the mainstream in order to establish a totally new paradigm in American health care.

Throughout the 1990s, self-described holistic medical doctors and doctors of osteopathy became steadily stronger, in terms both of numbers and influence. For example, by 1996, over 600 of them belonged to the AHMA, representing a threefold increase in membership in just 8 years (Caplan & Gesler, 1998). During this period, the Association's best known president was Dr. Bernie Siegel, a surgeon and best-selling author of *Love, Medicine and Miracles* and *Peace, Love and Healing*. The growing influence of these doctors, at least clinically, has been in the area of chronic conditions, which currently affect over 100 million Americans (Hoffman, Rice, & Sung, 1996).

Other well-known physician advocates of integrating holistic health care practices into biomedicine are Drs. Mehmet Oz, Dean Ornish, and Deepak Chopra (Brown, 1995). And hospitals are often their most important allies. For example, Columbia-Presbyterian Medical Center in New York City allowed Dr. Oz to establish a Cardiac Complementary Care Center to test the efficacy of different holistic health care practices, such as therapeutic touch and guided imagery, during the treatment of his heart patients (Brown, 1995).

Nonphysician Holistic Practitioners

During the 1990s, the number and influence of holistic nurses, dentists, and a wide variety of therapists also increased. In addition to their holistic practices, what they all have in common is a desire to "integrate" this holism into conventional medicine.

Dr. Jon Kabat-Zinn, with a Ph.D. in molecular biology, also successfully integrated some forms of holistic health care into conventional medicine. Like Dr. Oz, Dr. Kabat-Zinn is based in a large urban teaching hospital. In 1992, he founded the Stress Reduction Clinic at the University of Massachusetts Medical Center in Worcester, Massachusetts. This clinic is an out-patient facility and over 4,000 people participated in its program by 1994 (Kabat-Zinn, 1994). Most are referred by their doctors for a wide range of illnesses, such as cardiac and respiratory conditions, diabetes and panic attacks (Strawn, 1999, p. 430). The clinic's principal program consists of 8 weeks of intensive training in mindfulness meditation and other relaxation techniques. To reach the inpatient population, Dr. Kabat-Zinn developed a video program called "The World of Relaxation," which is played on his hospital's inhouse cable channel seven times a day (Kabat-Zinn, 1990). It is also being used by hospitals around the country for in-patient education.

The use of CAM by therapists has not been adequately tracked. While the use of alternative and complementary approaches by occupational and physical therapists has not resulted in the establishment of holistic organizations or groups for each profession, certainly not all therapists have ignored these approaches. For example, physical therapists have been teaching self-regulation via biofeedback for decades, and occupational therapists have a rich history of holistic treatments. Such treatments are classified by NCCAM as CAM, depending on what they are used to treat. However, these treatments are so ingrained in their respective disciplines that they are not considered alternative.

There are a number of factors that complicate the tracking of CAM use by therapists. CAM tracking has traditionally been method- or practitioner-specific. Since occupational and physical therapists are often accepted members of health care teams, they are by definition traditional, and may not be identified on surveys. Such surveys may also not identify therapists as CAM providers, because CAM might be so highly integrated into therapy that clients participating cannot distinguish it from traditional treatment.

Since the mid-1990s the literature has documented a growing use of a wide variety of CAMs by therapists. Alternative health care techniques, such as myofascial release, massage, and acupuncture, are becoming increasingly popular among physical therapists and being integrated into their practices (McLaughlin, 1995; Galantino et al., 1999). Among techniques used by occupational therapists are guided imagery, manual therapies, aromatherapy, therapeutic touch, meditation, conscious breath work, acupressure, and lifestyle coaching (AOTA, 1998). Finally, the publication of *Complementary Therapies in Rehabilitation* (Davis, 1997) was seen by many therapists as public endorsement of therapist's use of CAM. Anecdotally, this publication encouraged therapists to talk more openly about their use of CAM and to document its use.

In short, there are many excellent opportunities for rehabilitation specialists to incorporate CAM into their healing practices and few good reasons not to (Umphred, Galantino, & Campbell, 2000).

A New Paradigm

In the 21st century, apartheid medicine in America—biomedical and holistic practitioners, separate and unequal—is being abolished (Institute for Alternative Futures, 1998). In its place a new health care paradigm is developing that incorporates the principles and practices of biomedicine and holistic health care. Dr. Andrew Weil refers to this new, more comprehensive paradigm as "integrative medicine." Systems theory is also used to describe the holistic health paradigm.

Regardless of the term—integrated medicine or systems theory—a problem exists. The former does not convey at all what is being "integrated," and the latter suffers a similar vagueness with the word *system*. Consequently, the authors have coined two new terms— *biolistic* and *biolism*—to describe this new health care paradigm. These terms clearly identify biomedicine and holistic health care as this paradigm' s two key constituent elements.

Whatever one calls it, this new emerging paradigm will synthesize the best of biomedicine and holism, and will come to dominate American health care in the 21st century.

Recommendations

With respect to holistic practitioners (both inside and outside of biomedicine), our recommendations fall into four main categories: research, education, alliance-building and politics (REAP) (Caplan, 1991b).

In the area of **research,** the most important task is establishing the legitimacy of the new biolistic paradigm in American health care. This emerging paradigm must be shown to be compatible with biomedicine and no less scientific, effective, or economical. All members of the holistic health care community should support this type of paradigm-building research (Kuhn, 1970). All holistic practitioners should undertake a large-scale campaign to better **educate** the public, including the medical professions, about their approach to health and healing. The campaign should also continually update the public about the latest research findings regarding holism in health. The degree to which the public is convinced of, or at least familiar with, their viewpoint on these key issues will be a critical factor in determining the future course of the biolistic paradigm. Moreover, at a time when most patients do not pay the full cost of their health care, the need to educate third-party payers, especially the federal government, should not be overlooked.

All holistic practitioners and their supporters should join together in the common defense of this new health care paradigm. These **alliance-building** activities should take place at both the micro level (among individual practitioners) and the macro level (among national and state organizations). For example, at the micro level, holistic practitioners should cooperate with medical doctors in some type of group setting designed to deliver the best possible care. Such groups have three important advantages: First, patients get the benefit of a wide range of integrated therapies. Second, practitioners benefit from the cross-fertilization that takes place in such an environment (Studdert et al., 1998). And finally, by having such a diverse group of practitioners working together, age-old prejudices, mistrust, and misunderstandings may eventually give way to greater mutual respect and cooperation. While a relatively small number of such multidisciplinary clinics, or team centers, do exist, their numbers should be greatly increased (Miles, 1999).

At the macro level, organizations, such as the American Holistic Nurses' Association and the American Holistic Medical Association, should work more closely together to firmly establish holism in American health care. All would benefit from such a development, but none can accomplish it alone.

Finally, holistic practitioners (and their supporters) need to join together to politically protect and promote their approach to health and health care. **Political activities** should target all three levels of government—federal, state and local. At the federal level, three key areas to watch are antiquackery legislation, Medicare and Medicaid, and any efforts at national health care reform. At the state and local levels, biomedicine is much better organized and dominates most health-related agencies, such as the powerful medical licensure boards. Consequently, the issues most important to holistic practitioners tend to center around medical licensure and the definition of medical practice. For example, in 1990 the Supreme Court of North Carolina outlawed homeopathy in the state. After a huge outcry from supporters of homeopathy, the state legalized it 3 years later (Baer & Good, 1998). All such attempts to monopolize health care or unduly limit the practice of holistic practitioners through government intervention should be rigorously and collectively resisted.

Members of the biomedical community should neither fight nor ignore this new emerging health care paradigm. They should embrace it and see it as a relatively rare and rather unique marketing opportunity to increase their customer base (Featherstone & Forsyth, 1997). Those who successfully do this will have a competitive advantage over those who do not. For example, hospitals should be establishing some type of holistic health care program within their facilities. Although there are some obstacles, such as the credentialing of the practitioners, intake and treatment protocols, and data management, they would not be insurmountable (Miles, 1999). And, more importantly, clients as well as the hospital would greatly benefit.

There are compelling reasons for hospitals to establish holistic health care programs. Most hospitals have been able to keep profit margins relatively high by cutting costs, expanding outpatient services, and diversifying into postdischarge care (Iglehart, 1999). However, as managed care advances, Medicare cuts back, utilization rates decline, and competition intensifies, it will become increasingly difficult for many hospitals to remain profitable (Zuckerman, 1999). By establishing some type of hospital-based holistic health care program, hospitals could solve many of their financial problems. They would be building on past successes, like expanding outpatient services, while securing new opportunities for enhanced revenues. Such programs would bring into the hospital relatively wealthy, healthy, and better-informed consumers, who could one day become profitable patients (Astin, 1998). As noted earlier, since nearly half of this spending is paid directly by the patient at the time of delivery, billing and collecting costs are relatively low.

Also, because a holistic health care program allows a hospital to provide services that are both valued and preferred by growing portion of the public, public perceptions of and confidence in their local hospital can be enhanced. In addition, the hospital would be well positioned to exploit the continuing shift toward the new health care paradigm, such as growing third-party coverage and research dollars (Berman & Swyers, 1997). And finally, the per capita supply of holistic health care practitioners is expected to increase by 124 percent by the year 2010. The comparable growth rate for conventional doctors is only 16 percent (Cooper & Stoflet, 1996). This growth in the supply of holistic providers should help keep their future wage or income demands relatively low, at least compared to their medical counterparts (Cooper, Laud, & Dietrich, 1998).

For similar reasons, other members of the biomedical community, such as traditionally practicing physical and occupational therapists, should follow a similar strategy. The growing popularity of holism in American health care may signal areas where biomedicine is failing to adequately meet people's health care needs (for example, people with AIDS [Standish, Calabrese, & Galantino, 2002]). Those in the biomedical community who choose to ignore these signals may be doing so at their own peril, especially in the highly consumer-driven medical markets of the 21st century.

Summary

A revolution is occurring in American health care; not only in its financing and delivery, but its very content as well. While a number of different forces have suppressed holistic health care in the United States, such as professional medical groups and government health care reform, other forces have encouraged the development of holistic health care in the United States, including government at the federal, state, and local levels, and consumer demand. This shift in medical thinking is occurring at a rapid rate. According to John Weeks, the editor and publisher of *The Integrator,* a Seattle-based trade journal, "It's astonishing how rapidly a system which used to look at alternative health care as fraud and quackery is now exploring it" (Muir, 1999, p. 1). Therapists educated about the history of holistic health care in the United States will be better prepared to address future obstacles and capitalize on trends to enhance practice and meet client needs.

STUDY QUESTIONS

1. Explain the political and economic forces pushing and pulling holistic health care into the mainstream of United States health care.
2. What is the biolistic approach to health care?
3. How is managed care helping and hurting the growth of holistic health care in the United States?

REFERENCES

Alster, K. B. (1989). *Holistic Health Movement*. Tuscaloosa, AL: University of Alabama Press.

Angell, M., & J. P. Kassirer. (1998). Alternative medicines—The risks of untested and unregulated remedies. *New England Journal of Medicine, 339,* 839–841.

AOTA. (1998). Complementary care survey results. *OT Week, 12*(48), 4.

Astin, J. A. (1998). Why patients use alternative medicine: Results of a national study. *Journal of the American Medical Association, 279,* 1548–1553.

Baer, L. D., & C. M. Good. (1998). The power of the state. In R. J. Gordon, B. C. Nienstedt, & W. M. Gesler (Eds.), *Alternative Therapies: Expanding Options in Health Care*. New York: Springer.

Berman, B. M., & J. P. Swyers. (1997). Establishing a research agenda for investigating alternative medical interventions for chronic pain. *Primary Care: Clinics-in-Office-Practice, 24,* 743–758.

Brown, C. (1995, July 30). The experiments of Dr. Oz. *The New York Times Magazine*, pp. 21–23.

Caplan, R. (1987). The clash over quackery: Protecting alternative care. *Health/Pac Bulletin,* 22–26.

Caplan, R. (1989). The commodification of American health care. *Social Science and Medicine, 28,* 1139–1148.

Caplan, R. (1991b). Chiropractic in the United States and the changing health care environment: A view from outside the profession. *Journal of Manipulative and Physiological Therapeutics, 14,* 46–50.

Caplan, R. (1999). The economics of complementary health practices. In C. C. Clark (Ed.), *Encyclopedia of Complementary Health Practice*. New York: Springer.

Caplan, R. L., & W. M. Gesler. (1998). Biomedical physicians practicing holistic medicine. In R. J. Gordon, B. C. Nienstedt, & W. M. Gesler (Eds.), *Alternative Therapies: Expanding Options in Health Care*. New York: Springer.

Caplan, R. L., & J. L. Scarpaci. (1989). The consequences of increased competition on alternative health care practitioners in the United States. *Holistic Medicine, 4,* 125–135.

Caplan, R. L. (1984). Chiropractic. In J. W. Salmon (Ed.), *Alternative Medicines: Popular and Policy Perspectives*. New York: Travistock.

Colt, G. H. (1996, Sept.). See Me, Feel Me, Touch Me, Heal Me. *Life*, pp. 35–50.

Cooper, R. A., & S. Stoflet. (1996). Trends in the education and practice of alternative medicine clinicians. *Health Affairs, 15,* 226–238.

Cooper, R. A., P. Laud, & C. L. Dietrich. (1998). Current and projected workforce on nonphysician clinicians. *Journal of the American Medical Association, 280,* 788–794.

Coulter, H. L. (1975). *Divided Legacy: A History of the Schism in Medical Thought*. 3 vols. Washington, DC: Weehawken Book Company.

Davis, C. M. (1997). *Complementary Therapies in Rehabilitation*. Thoroughfare, NJ: SLACK.

Einsenberg, D., R. Kessler, C. Foster, et al. (1993). Unconventional medicine in the United States. *New England Journal of Medicine, 328,* 246–252.

Eisenberg, D. M., R. B. Davis, S. L. Ettner, et al. (1998). Trends in alternative medicine use in the United States, 1990–1997. *Journal of the American Medical Association, 280,* 1569–1575.

Featherstone, C., & L. Forsyth. (1997). *The New Partnership Between Orthodox and Complementary Medicine*. Forres, Scotland: Findhorn Press.

Galantino, M. L., S. T. Eke-Okoro, T. W. Findley, & D. Condoluci. (1999). Use of noninvasive electroacupuncture for the treatment of HIV-related peripheral neuropathy: A pilot study. *The Journal of Alternative and Complementary Medicine, 5,* 135–142.

Gervitz, N. (Ed). (1988). *Other Healers: Unorthodox Medicine in America*. Baltimore: Johns Hopkins University Press.

Gordon, R. J., & G. Silverstein. (1998). Marketing channels for alternative health care. In R. J. Gordon, B. C. Nienstedt, & W. M. Gesler (Eds), *Alternative Therapies: Expanding Options in Health Care*. New York: Springer.

Greenwald, J. (1998, Nov. 23). Herbal healing. *Time*, pp. 59–69.

Hazzard, M. (1999). National Center for Complementary and Alternative Medicine. In C. C. Clark (Ed), *Encyclopedia of Complementary Health Practice*. New York: Springer.

Hoffman, C., D. Rice, & H. Y. Sung. (1996). Persons with chronic conditions. *Journal of the American Medical Association, 276*, 1473–1479.

Iglehart, J. K. (1999). The American health care system. *New England Journal of Medicine, 340*, 70–75.

Institute for Alternative Futures. (1998, July). The future of complementary and alternative approaches (CAAs) in U.S. health care. Alexandria, VA.

Kabat-Zinn, J. (1994). *Wherever You Go, There You Are: Mindfulness & Meditation in Everyday Life*. New York: Hyperion.

Kabat-Zinn, J. (1990). *Full Catastrophe Living: Using the Wisdom of Your Body and Mind to Face Stress, Pain and Illness*. New York: Dell.

Kluger, J. (1997, May 12). Mr. Natural. *Time*, pp. 68–75.

Koch, L. (1999). Hospital-based massage therapy. In C. C. Clark (Ed.), *Encyclopedia of Complementary Health Practice*. New York: Springer.

Kuhn, T. S. (1970). The Structure of Scientific Revolutions. Chicago: University of Chicago Press.

Landmark Report on Public Perceptions of Alternative Care. (1998, Jan.). Sacramento, CA, Landmark Healthcare, Inc.

Lappe, M. (1979). Holistic health: A valuable approach to medical care. *Western Journal of Medicine, 131*, 475–478.

LeShan, L. (1982). *The Mechanic and the Gardener: Making the Most of the Holistic Revolution in Medicine*. New York: Holt, Rinehart, and Winston.

Lisa, P. J. (1994). *The Assault on Medical Freedom*. Norfolk, VA: Hampton Roads Publishing Company.

McClure, W. (1983). The competition strategy for medical care. *Annuals: American Academy of Political and Social Science, 468*, 30–47.

McLaughlin, C. (1995). Alternative therapies: Gaining acceptance in mainstream medicine. *ADVANCE for Physical Therapists, 6*, 10–11, 62.

Micozzi, M. S. (Ed.). (1996a). *Fundamentals of Complementary and Alternative Medicine*. New York: Churchill Livingston.

Miles, R. (1999). Complementary health centers and networks. In C. C. Clark (Ed.), *Encyclopedia of Complementary Health Practice*. New York: Springer.

Moyers, B. (1993). *Healing and the Mind*. New York: Doubleday.

Muir, J. (1999). How alternative are we? Boom of alternative health care in Portland, Oregon. *Business Journal–Portland, 16*, 19.

Nienstedt, B. C. (1998). The federal approach to alternative medicine: Co-opting, quackbusting, or complementing? In R. J. Gordon, B. C. Nienstedt, & W. M. Gesler (Eds.), *Alternative Therapies: Expanding Options in Health Care*. New York: Springer.

Nordstrom, B. (1980). Chiropractic Health Care: A National Study of the Cost of Education, Service Utilization, Number of Practicing Doctors of Chiropractic and Other Key Policy Issues. Washington, DC, FACTS.

Okie, S. (1998, Nov. 11). Widening the medical mainstream. *The Washington Post*, pp. 1, 6.

Oxford Breaks Ground with Alternative Health Network. (1996). *Primary Care Weekly, 2*, 1.

Richards, G. (1984). Nonphysicians make slow headway on staff privileges. *Hospitals, 58*, 82–86.

Salmon, J., & H. Berliner. (1980). Health policy implications of the holistic health movement. *Journal of Health Politics, Policy and Law, 5*, 535–553.

Schelling, T. C. (1976). Government and health. In C. M. Lindsay (Ed.), *New Directions in Public Health Care: A Prescription for the 1980s*. San Francisco: Institute for Contemporary Studies.

Schwartz, H. (1972). *The Case for American Medicine: A Realistic Look at Our Health Care System*. New York: David McKay Company.

Standish, C. J., Calabrese, C., & Galantino, M. L. (2002). *AIDS and Complementary and Alternative Medicine: Current Science and Practice*. New York: Churchill Livingston.

Strawn, J. (1999). Mindfulness. In R. J. Gordon, B. C. Nienstedt, & W. M. Gesler (Eds.), *Alternative Therapies: Expanding Options in Health Care*. New York: Springer.

Studdert, D. M., D. M. Eisenberg, F. H. Miller, et al. (1998). Medical malpractice implications of alternative medicine. *Journal of the American Medical Association, 280,* 1610–1615.

Umphred, D. A., Galantino, M. L., & Campbell, B. R. (2000). Establishing a model for the use of complementary medicine and research in orthopaedic practice. *Orthopaedic Physical Therapy Clinics of North America, 9*(3), 443–460.

Weber, D. (1996, Nov./Dec.). The mainstreaming of alternative medicine. *Healthcare Forum Journal,* 16–27.

Wetzel, M. S., D. M. Eisenberg, & T. J. Kaptchuk. (1998). Courses involving complementary and alternative medicine at U.S. medical schools. *Journal of the American Medical Association, 280,* 784–787.

Whol, S. (1984). *The Medical Industrial Complex*. New York: Harmony Books.

Zuckerman, A. M. (1999, Mar./Apr.). Will the bottom drop out? *Spectrum,* pp. 1–2.

3

Legal Issues

Ron Scott

CHAPTER OBJECTIVES

- Understand issues relating to the legal climate within which therapists practice.
- Understand liability issues affecting therapy practice.
- Understand basic risk management strategies designed to minimize exposure to legal challenges.

The legal environment within which clinical health care professionals practice is complex, ever-changing, and only moderately predictable. An entire body of health law has emerged since World War II, covering issues ranging from health care malpractice to informed consent to medical research, among a myriad of other concerns. Providers engaged in nontraditional therapeutic interventions may face even greater liability exposure than their colleagues based in traditional therapies for a variety of reasons, including, among others, a relative dearth of support for their practices in the scientific literature and an unwillingness of peers and others to testify favorably in litigation about such practices.

The United States is far and away the most litigious nation-state on the face of the planet and in world history. The reasons for Americans' litigiousness are many, and include a sense of powerlessness against a large bureaucratic system; greed; ease of litigation and related limited sanctions for bringing frivolous actions; and the legions of attorneys readily available to help clients pursue their legal actions against fellow citizens and entities. Health care malpractice legal actions constitute only a small percentage of the estimated 2 million total civil cases filed each year; however, the consequences of being named a health care malpractice defendant in such an action are devastating to the reputations and well-being of these health care professionals, irrespective of the outcome of litigation (i.e., win or lose, such defendants always lose something, particularly peace of mind).

The aforementioned commentary is not intended in any way to give short shrift to the many meritorious patient lawsuits brought against providers each year or to disparage personal injury attorneys who often (as attorneys do generally) undertake meritorious cases *pro*

This chapter discusses legal aspects of holistic practice and complementary therapy. The same legal principles that apply to health care clinical practice generally apply to holistic and complementary therapy. A therapist decreases his or her liability exposure by providing clients with competent, compassionate care in accordance with acceptable practices and procedures.

Informed consent to examination and intervention for holistic practice and complementary therapy includes, in addition to all other required disclosure elements, disclosure of the nature of the procedure in detail in lay language, including the philosophy underlying the proposed care, where appropriate. Nothing in this chapter is intended to constitute legal advice. Such advice can only be imparted by an individual's personal counsel, based on differing state and federal law, as applicable. Therapists are encouraged to proactively consult with counsel regarding potential legal issues.

bono, or without expectation of payment for services. The analysis in this section merely points out that all parties to health care malpractice litigation are victims, suffer stress and (at least transitory) diminution of esteem, and expend a great deal of time in pursuit of vindication of their positions. Authorities have urged in the recent past that perhaps a no-fault systems of medical error adjudication would be a better model for client complaint resolution than the current litigation model. Clients and providers may also take otherwise litigible disputes to alternative dispute resolution fora, such as mediation and binding arbitration, by mutual agreement.

This chapter explores generally liability issues associated with health care delivery—both traditional and nontraditional. By way of required disclaimer, the information presented herein is intended solely as general information and not dispositive of the law of any particular state nor as specific legal advice for any individual or discipline. Such specific advice can only legally and ethically be rendered by one's personal, state-licensed attorney, based on federal and state-specific law, as applicable.

For individuals or groups not having a personal attorney, one can easily be engaged via the county bar association lawyer referral service, in place in every jurisdiction in the United States. The lawyer referral service offers initial consultation at no- or low-cost as a public service, whose monetary receipts are used to fund legal services for socioeconomically disadvantaged legal clientele.

Liability Issues in Client Management

It is a truism to state that every individual possessing mental capacity is legally responsible for his or her conduct vis-à-vis others who may be harmed by that conduct. A special legal duty applies to health care professionals—especially those privileged under state licensure to interact within clients' intimate zones of physical contact and learn their deepest confidences.

Health professionals are legal fiduciaries—that is, persons in a legally recognized special position of trust in relation to clients they serve. Health professionals promise under their fiduciary duty to place clients' best interests above all other competing interests, including their own and those of employers and other entities. It is this fact that makes practice under the managed care delivery paradigm so problematic, in that this system is fraught with competing interests. Regrettably, the United States Supreme Court, on June 12, 2000 in the appellate case of *Pegram v. Herdrich* (2000), ruled that managed care organizations do not violate a fiduciary duty owed to clients by paying primary care providers monetary incentives to minimize care-related cost outlays. Who knows when or if the public will compel their congressional representatives to legislatively reverse this decision?

Bases for Health Care Malpractice Liability Exposure

Whether practicing in traditional or nontraditional health care settings and practices, providers face health care malpractice liability exposure incident to their interaction with clients. Such liability exposure is based on client injury (physical, psychological, or both) and a legally recognized basis for imposing monetary liability for such injury. The legal basis for health care malpractice liability exposure include

◆ Professional negligence, or substandard care delivery;
◆ Intentional conduct resulting in client injury;
◆ Breach of a therapeutic promise made to a client incident to the professional relationship; and
◆ Strict or absolute liability (without regard to fault) for client injury from (1) dangerously defective care-related products and (2) abnormally dangerous clinical activities.

The legal case law literature confirms that the overwhelming majority of health care malpractice cases are based on allegations of professional negligence, or substandard care delivery. Every health care provider is charged under law to provide at least minimally acceptable care delivery to clients. That translates to providing care that professional colleagues and other third parties would deem to be minimally acceptable practice for the provider's discipline.

In order to prove that professional negligence has occurred, a client must prove four fundamental elements by a preponderance or greater weight of evidence at trial:

◆ That the defendant-health professional had a legal duty to care for the client. Such a special legal duty arises only when a provider accepts a client for care or when the client presents with a life-threatening emergency.
◆ That the defendant-health care professional violated the special legal duty owed by practicing in a way that peers and other authorities would consider substandard. For holistic and complementary therapy professionals, "other authorities" might include providers from within the same discipline (e.g., physical or occupational therapy) or from related health care disciplines.
◆ That as a direct result of the defendant-health care professional's substandard care delivery, the plaintiff-client suffered physical and/or psychological injury ("causation").
◆ That the client-plaintiff is entitled to monetary "damages" in order to remedy her or his loss.

The benchmark for the legal standard of care is minimally acceptable practice, not average or optimal practice. If the legal standard were average practice, then by definition, half of providers would be providing substandard or negligent care. If the standard were optimal quality care (as is the aspiration for quality improvement processes), then virtually no one would be practicing within legal standards—especially under managed care, which emphasizes minimal (cost) care.

How is the legal standard of care established in legal proceedings? Normally, the legal standard of care is proven in court through the introduction of expert witnesses who, after being qualified through an open credentials review, testify as to their opinion of whether a health care professional-defendant's conduct vis-à-vis a client met or fell below minimally acceptable practice standards. In order to qualify as an expert witness, the purported expert must have sufficient knowledge, through formal and informal education, training, and experience, to assist the jury or judge in determining liability or nonliability and must have knowledge of the therapist's practice standards in his or her state of practice. In the face of competing expert testimony, a lay jury or a judge weighs their relative credibility and makes a decision based on that analysis and other evidence presented at trial.

In the case of holistic or complementary therapists, experts from nontraditional disciplines may or may not be allowed to testify as experts, based not so much on the credentials of the purported experts, but on whether the domain of practice itself falls within the ambit of general scientific acceptability. There are two principal standards for admission of scientific evidence in legal proceedings. Under the traditional *Frye* standard (*Frye v. United States,* 1923), for scientific evidence to be admissible, it has to be generally acceptable in the scientific community. Under the emerging *Daubert* standard (*Daubert v. Merrill Dow Pharmaceuticals,* 1993), such evidence may be admissible at a judge's discretion, even if not generally accepted by the scientific community, if it may be helpful to the trier of fact (i.e., decision maker: judge or jury) and it is based on scientifically valid principles.

In addition to expert witness testimony, the legal standard of care (for traditional and nontraditional health disciplines) may be established through the introduction into evidence of learned treatises (i.e., authoritative or reference texts) and noteworthy (normally peer-reviewed) journals. Holistic, complementary, and nontraditional providers and professional organizations should strive to ensure that their research is published in such texts and journals in order to be admissible as evidence-based practice in support of the standard of care for their disciplines.

Readers should also note that the illegal boycott of complementary, holistic, or nontraditional health care disciplines and providers by "mainstream" providers and organizations may be legally actionable, as it was in *Wilk v. American Medical Association* (1990). In this 1990 case, the appellate court ruled that the American Medical Association's attempted boycott of the chiropractic profession constituted an illegal antitrust law violation; that is, it unduly restrained the ability of chiropractors to freely practice their profession.

In addition to professional negligence, there are several other potential bases of health care malpractice liability exposure. Intentional misconduct is a basis of liability that may expose the provider simultaneously to adverse civil, criminal, and administrative legal action. Of particular concern is alleged sexual battery, or impermissible intimate physical contact with a patient or client. This area of liability exposure may be growing faster than any other, making its prevention all the more important for individual providers and professional groups. Preventive risk management measures are discussed in the section "Risk Management Tactics and Strategies" in this chapter.

Failure to achieve a promised therapeutic result, which is a legally actionable breach of contract, occurs when a health care professional makes an explicit promise to a patient or client to effect a cure or specific level of recovery, and fails to achieve the promised result. The law does not favor the imposition of breach of contract liability incident to health care delivery, because the law views the health care professional–client relationship as a special status relationship akin to attorney–client, minister–parishioner, or parent–child relationships, and not as an ordinary, arm's-length business relationship. In many cases, courts require the payment of special consideration (money) to support contractual duties incident to the provider–client relationship and may also require a written contractual agreement in order to enforce one.

Holistic and complementary therapists, like health care professionals generally, are urged not to make express promises to clients, guaranteeing specific results. Keep in mind, however, that the formation and documentation of care-related goals do not equate to making contractual promises to clients. Care-related client goals are merely the manifestations of clinicians' professional judgment, reflecting aspirations for care outcomes, and not contractual promises. (As an aside, though, clients or their surrogate decision makers should always be active participants in care-related goal-setting, since such goals are the clients' goals, and not those of the provider.)

Health care malpractice liability may also attach when clients are injured by dangerously defectively manufactured or designed care-related products. In such cases, clients' legal burden of proof in malpractice litigation may be short-circuited, so that the client may only have to prove the existence of such a defect and resultant injury, without the need for expert testimony or proof of a breach of the legal standard of care. As with breach of contract liability, the legal system is loathe to allow health care professionals to face strict liability (without regard to fault) for care-related products, under the theory that health care delivery is a professional service, and not the sale of a product. To the extent, however, that providers do sell products to clients in the course of business, they may face the same product liability exposure that other commercial vendors or product manufacturers do.

The final potential basis for health care malpractice liability exposure arises when clients are injured as a result of abnormally dangerous clinical care activities. Although authorities debate whether such liability exposure in fact exists for health care providers, holistic and complementary therapy professionals are again urged to ensure that their care-related activities are evidence-based, carried out only with legally sufficient client informed consent, and carried out reasonably and safely.

Informed Consent in Health Care Delivery

In all clinical health care delivery settings, client informed consent to examination and intervention are legal prerequisites to care delivery. The law of client informed consent is based on preeminent respect for client autonomy over care-related decision making. Such respect for client autonomy may operate at the expense of another professional ethical duty, that being beneficence (i.e., acting in a client's best interests). Even still, the principle of nonmaleficence, or "do no intentional malicious harm" to clients, applies with full force to all provider–client relationships.

By definition, client informed consent is a process within which a health care professional makes sufficient disclosure of care-related information so as to empower a client to make a knowing, intelligent, voluntary, and unequivocal decision to accept or reject a recommended therapeutic intervention.

The disclosure elements for legally sufficient client informed consent to therapeutic intervention include

- The client's diagnosis;
- A summary of examination and evaluative findings
- A description of and justification for the recommended intervention(s);
- A description of the expected benefits of the recommended intervention (goals of intervention);
- A description of material (client decisional) risks of possible serious harm or complication; and
- Disclosure of reasonable alternative interventions, if any, to the one(s) recommended, including their relative benefits and risks.

Such disclosure of information by providers to clients must be made in lay person's language and in a language that a client understands. For clients lacking mental capacity to make decisions, the information disclosure must be made to legally recognized surrogate decision makers.

Abbreviated client informed consent must also be obtained prior to carrying out a client examination. Information disclosure for client consent to examination includes the nature of and procedures incident to the examination, as well as any expected risk of harm or complication associated therewith.

Documentation of client informed consent to care may be accomplished through publication and dissemination of a client informed consent clinic policy, which clients may review. Such documentation may also be placed in clients' health records, in short or long form.

Holistic or complementary therapists should also ensure that clients fully understand the nature of the holistic or complementary therapy practice, especially including the philosophy and nature of the proposed care. Informational brochures describing the practice may be particularly helpful in avoiding misunderstandings about the nature of the interventions in general.

Risk Management Tactics and Strategies

In any clinical health care delivery practice or setting, special attention must be paid by providers and managers to quality improvement. A key component of any quality management program is liability risk management. Health care risk management is defined as processes designed to minimize providers' and the organization's exposure to liability for injury to clients and others.

In a group practice, clinical risk management activities should be coordinated by an appointed risk manager. In solo practices, either the practitioner or a consultant devises the risk management program, and the solo practitioner implements it.

Risk management, or self-protection from liability exposure, does not in any way derogate from the fiduciary duty owed by providers and health care organizations to clients. It is a program merely designed to augment quality improvement processes with self-protective measures that benefit providers and the organization—but not at the clients' expense.

Systematic clinical liability risk management measures range from the simple to the complex. They include, for traditional and nontraditional providers, among a myriad of other possibilities

- Facility safety management and safety vigilance by all employees to prevent client, staff, or visitor injury;
- Equipment calibration in accordance with manufacturer recommended schedules and/or customary practice;
- Universal client informed consent to examination and intervention;
- Appropriate respect for client autonomy, confidentiality, and modesty;
- A comprehensive policies and procedures manual, binding upon all professional and support staff, as applicable;
- Appropriate consultation and referral to complementary health and related professionals, as needed for client special needs;
- Avoidance of client or significant other misunderstanding of the nature of therapeutic intervention or touch so as to prevent unwarranted allegations of sexual harassment or misconduct;
- True empathy for the status of clients under care; and
- Regular consultations with, and in-service presentations by, legal counsel on issues such as health care malpractice case law pronouncements; antitrust, business, employment, and sexual harassment and misconduct law; and encroachment and licensure issues, especially including avoidance of the unlicensed practice of another health discipline.

Summary

Holistic and complementary therapies offer expanded and important therapeutic options to clients seeking relief of pain and cure from disease or dysfunction. Such therapies, to the extent that they are evidence-based (i.e., supported in the professional literature) and safe, are potential valuable adjuncts to (or substitutes for) traditional therapies that may be less efficacious alone. If all clinical health care professionals realize that all disciplines, including medicine, are allied health professions—that is, allied in support of clients served—then it becomes more facile to accept seemingly nontraditional validated approaches to client care.

The common law (case-based) legal system is flexible and willing to support legitimate new approaches to health care delivery. As traditional providers, third-party payers, and relevant others, we should be willing to do the same. That is part of our fiduciary duty to the clients we serve.

STUDY QUESTIONS

Consider the following two hypothetical examples, discuss them, and brainstorm over possible solutions in individual or clinical group settings.

1. A therapist is engaged in a limited-scope women's health practice within which she provides pelvic floor examinations and interventions for soft tissue dysfunction. A client sues

the therapist, claiming professional negligence—that the therapist was unable to care for pelvic floor muscle dysfunction. Who can testify against the therapist on behalf of the client? What other legal issues are presented in this scenario?

2. A therapist utilizes craniosacral therapy techniques that he recently learned in a series of professional continuing education courses in the care of clients with physical dysfunction. He uses these techniques pursuant to referring physician "evaluate and treat" orders. A therapist from the same discipline practicing in the same small town lodges a complaint with the applicable licensing board, claiming encroachment and unlicensed practice. What is the resolution of this complaint?

SUGGESTED READING

Furrow, B. R., T. L. Greaney, S. H. Johnson, T. S. Jost, & R. L. Schwartz. (2000). *Health Law,* 2nd ed. St. Paul, MN: West Group.

Rozovsky, F. A. (1990). *Consent to Treatment: A Practical Guide,* 2nd ed. Boston: Little, Brown.

Scott, R. W. (2000). *Legal Aspects of Documenting Patient Care,* 2nd ed. Gaithersburg, MD: Aspen Publishers.

Scott, R. W. (2000). *Health Care Malpractice,* 2nd ed. New York: McGraw-Hill.

Scott, R. W. (1998). *Professional Ethics: A Guide for Rehabilitation Professionals.* St. Louis, MO: Mosby.

Scott, R. W. (1997). *Promoting Legal Awareness in Physical and Occupational Therapy.* St. Louis, MO: Mosby.

REFERENCES

Daubert v. Merrill Dow Pharmaceuticals, Inc. 509 U.S. 579 (1993).

Frye v. United States. 293 F 1013 (D.C. Cir. 1923).

Pegram v. Herdrich. No. 98-1949 (U.S. Supreme Court, June 12, 2000).

Wilk v. American Medical Association. 895 F.2d 352 (7th Cir. 1990).

4

Utilization, Reimbursement, Legislative, Fraud and Abuse, and Documentation Issues

Jennifer M. Bottomley

CHAPTER OBJECTIVES

- Develop an understanding of reimbursement issues affecting CAM.
- Describe current utilization trends of CAM.
- Describe legislative initiatives related to CAM utilization.
- Discuss fraud and abuse concerns related to CAM.
- Understand documentation concerns about CAM.

Complementary and alternative medicine (CAM) approaches are increasingly finding their way into mainstream traditional medical practices. Undeniably, the demand for alternative, holistic health care among consumers is growing, as evidenced by several recent reports on the use of alternative medicine among the general public (Astin et al., 1998; Astin et al., 2000; Daily, 1999; Ernst, 2000). As a result, health insurance issues have evolved related to reimbursement of these services by health maintenance organizations (HMOs), federal health insurance programs such as Medicare and Medicaid, and other private third-party insurers. Many legislative initiatives have also surfaced that address the potential of insurance coverage for holistic health care services.

This chapter explores the current state of reimbursement for nonphysician-prescribed alternative and complementary interventions for disease management and preventive and health maintenance approaches to healthcare. Additionally, legislative initiatives that are currently being sought by alternative practitioner groups in a quest for legislative recognition and support related to reimbursement issues will also be presented. A brief discussion related to federal and private insurers' concern of fraud and abuse will be included. Lastly, documentation, research and the need for evidence-based, outcomes-oriented utilization of holistic

The topics presented in this chapter are important to the past and future of CAM. Knowledge of utilization trends will help therapists understand growth patterns and attempt to anticipate future growth. Knowledge of reimbursement is important for the solvency of any therapy practice. The history of legislation related to this topic is important because it indicates support at the national level for CAM. Issues such as fraud, abuse, and documentation, while important to the traditional therapist, may be even more crucial to complementary providers as the credibility of complementary approaches is being established.

services will be addressed. Because reimbursement and legislation are constantly changing, the reader is urged to update this information periodically. One resource for such updates is *Alternative Therapies in Health and Medicine* (see "Resources" at the end of this chapter).

Utilization of Complementary and Alternative Medicine

Utilization of complementary and alternative therapies by consumers has been increasing over the past decade (Astin, 1998; Astin et al., 2000; Eisenberg et al., 1993; Eisenberg et al., 1998; Pelletier, 1997, 1998). It has been hypothesized that the increasing interest in and utilization of CAM services is related in part to the establishment in 1992 of the Office of Alternative Medicine (OAM), recently renamed the National Center for Complementary and Alternative Medicine (NCCAM) by the National Institutes of Health (NIH). Congressional legislature mandated that the NIH investigate the "safety and efficacy" of CAM therapies, bringing these unconventional forms of therapies into the political and public spotlight. This legislation was prompted by consumer (voter) interest and an apparent push by CAM disciplines for recognition as a less costly alternative to traditional health care practices.

A survey of elderly Medicare eligible persons enrolled in a supplement plan provided by Blue Shield of California revealed that 41 percent reported use of CAM (Astin et al., 2000). In this survey, the most frequently cited therapies of the respondents indicated that 24 percent sought care from herbalists, 20 percent from chiropractic, 15 percent from massage therapists, and 14 percent from acupuncturists. It was an interesting finding in this study that CAM users tended to be the younger segments of the Medicare population surveyed, suggesting a possible cohort effect. Characteristically, those who chose CAM interventions tended to be more educated, reported the presence of arthritis or depression (or both), were not hypertensive, engaged in regular exercise, practiced meditation, and made more frequent physician visits (Astin et al., 2000). The utilization of CAM was not associated with any observed changes in health status. It was suggested by the authors that a significant portion of CAM use is for prevention and health promotion and maintenance rather than for the treatment of disease and illness. Respondents expressed considerable interest in receiving third-party coverage for CAM and were willing to pay an additional premium for supplemental coverage of CAM therapies.

Although 80 percent reported that they had received substantial benefit from their use of CAM, the majority (58 percent) did not discuss the use of these therapies with their physician (Astin et al., 2000). This is of concern due to potentially harmful interactions between traditional interventions (e.g., drugs) and CAM therapies (e.g., herbs), and reflects poor communication between clients and their primary physicians (Crock et al., 1999).

Krauss et al. (1998) investigated the use of alternative therapies by adults with physical disabilities. The authors concluded that persons with physical disabilities are more likely to use alternative therapies than the general population and to see providers for alternative therapies, have their use recommended by their physicians, and be reimbursed for them by their health insurance. It is notable that a high prevalence of dysphoria (excessive pain, anguish, agitation) was found among those with disabilities. These individuals with disabilities often combined the use of alternative and conventional therapies for treatment of this disorder (Krauss et al., 1998).

Reimbursement Policies for Alternative and Complementary Therapies

Some insurance companies have conducted pilot and longitudinal surveys on the utilization of alternative and complementary therapies by their insurees. They have begun to recognize the cost savings related to lowered health care spending when holistic therapies and preventive care approaches are employed. In addition, primarily due to consumer interest and, to a lesser extent, legislative mandate and demonstrated efficacy, several prominent insurance companies and managed care organizations have begun offering coverage for CAM therapies (Pelletier, 1997; 1999). A review of the literature reveals an immense variation among insurers in terms of the types of services covered, whether or not an individual needs a physician's prescription for coverage or whether they can self-refer based on individual choice, and a marked difference in organizational policies related to both the reimburser and the health care provider.

To date, there has been little published information about the perceptions of a key link between conventional and alternative medicine—the HMOs which lie at the center of the managed-care system in the United States (Benjamin, 1997; Berman, 2000; Rossman, 1997). Results of a recent study of HMOs and alternative care showed that two-thirds of HMOs in the United States offer benefits for at least one form of alternative care (Daily, 1999). The most common offerings are chiropractic (65 percent) and acupuncture (35 percent). Of those HMOs that offer alternative care coverage, 38 percent indicated that demand among members and employers compelled them to offer CAM benefits. One objective of this study was to determine the concerns of HMOs regarding cost of this benefit. The question posed was, Will HMO coverage of CAM be a net reduction, an add-on cost, or a break-even proposition? Fifty percent of the HMOs surveyed felt that costs would be neutral or reduced as long as traditional medicine and CAM were integrated.

Chiropractors and acupuncturists are more likely to be reimbursed by insurers than naturopaths, herbalists, nutritionists, or other alternative health care practitioners (Moore,

1997). The potential for reimbursement is increased if traditional and alternative health care providers function under the same corporate umbrella, especially if the integrated care center is part of a larger health care system (Moore, 1997). In other words, managed care companies that integrate conventional with alternative therapies are more likely to cover alternative interventions when compared to nonintegrated systems of health care. Independent holistic health care providers are experiencing inconsistencies in reimbursement policies by the same insurer, for the same intervention, based on the fiscal intermediaries' "interpretation" of the insurance claim (Moore, 1996). Some alternative therapy practitioners are establishing holistic centers in response to consumer demand and managing under a reimbursement policy of "out-of-pocket" or "pay-as-you-go" by the client, who is allowed the privilege of self-referral.

A survey by Eisenberg et al. (1998) established that out-of-pocket expenditures for CAM were estimated at approximately $27 million annually for such services as chiropractic, herbs, homeopathy, massage and body work, stress management, and acupuncture. It was determined that, on average, Americans who use CAM services spend about $500 per year on out-of-pocket expenses and visit a CAM provider more than 10 times each year. Even more significant, there were 630 million visits to CAM providers in 1997 compared to 430 million visits to primary-care physicians in the same year (Eisenberg et al., 1998). Researchers concluded that this rate of utilization demanded that insurers establish reimbursement policies for coverage for CAM therapies.

A model of coverage for the practice of alternative and complementary medicine is found in the state of Washington. In 1995, Washington implemented a law that mandated all health insurance carriers to cover alternative medicine. As James Stevenson, of the State of Washington Insurance Commission, stated, this law "requires health insurance plans in the state to provide equal access to every category of health care provider to treat conditions that would be covered under the state's Basic Health Plan" (Jan. 6, 2002, personal communication). For example, treatment for chronic pain conditions is not limited to conventional medicine. The beneficiary of this state's health care plan may seek alternative approaches for the treatment of pain, such as biofeedback, chiropractic care, or nutritional approaches (to name a few).

American Western Life Insurance, managed by Prime Care Health Network, educates consumers in alternative health care practices and provides insurance coverage under the "Wellness Plan." Under this plan, beneficiaries are required to have an annual physical exam by a doctor in their network. Subscribers are encouraged to manage their own preventive care. Educational materials on healthy lifestyle and information on CAM therapies are a part of the introductory package to the insurance policy. Benefits include reimbursement for unconventional physical therapies (see Appendix 1), chiropractic care, acupuncture, nutritionists, and the like. Coverage varies by policy, and there is a set capitation for annual coverage of CAM therapies—for example, $500 per year under one of the plans.

Kaiser Permanente has a long history of integrating alternative health care practices with traditional medicine. There is no differentiation with insurance coverage. Whatever care is given is considered to be a part of treatment, health promotion, and health maintenance, whether care is provided by a conventional physician or an alternative health care practitioner. Kaiser insurance coverage specific to CAM therapies under the Kaiser plan is not an issue.

Mutual of Omaha is conducting a longitudinal study of policyholders to evaluate outcomes and determine the cost efficacy of CAM therapies (Horrigan and Ornish, 1995). At press time, it provided coverage for a selected group of alternative practices, including cardiac rehabilitation, acupuncture, naturopathy, chiropractic care, and stress management. The Preventable Medical Research Institute in collaboration with the Harvard University School of

Public Health is tracking all patients who seek alternative health care and comparing this group to a similar group that receives traditional care. Under this company's insurance, CAM therapies are covered at the same rate as conventional therapies. The information gained from this study will be invaluable in determining efficacy and cost based on outcomes of CAM therapies of every variety.

Alternative Health Benefit Services negotiates and develops alternative health plans that are underwritten by other companies, and is involved in marketing and administration of integrated health care networks in the Pacific Northwest. Under its plan, comprehensive major medical coverage is provided as well as partial reimbursement for alternative and complementary modalities. An annual maximum benefit for appropriate acupuncture and chiropractic treatments is $1,000 if there is not an established diagnosis (e.g., fracture, CVA). Massage therapy and bodywork by a certified, licensed practitioner are covered with a $25 copayment and a maximum of 25 visits annually. Homeopathic, herbal remedies, and Chinese medicine are capped at $500 annually. Mental health and substance abuse programs have a lifetime maximum benefit of $10,000 and are limited to $1,000 per year (Moore, 1997). A physician's referral is required for all alternative interventions.

A survey conducted by Oxford Health Plans found that 75 percent of its members were interested in adding alternative health services to their health plan. This company launched the first CAM program in the country (Daily, 1999). Oxford Health Plans in the Northeast provide a policy that covers alternative therapies through a credentialed network of providers. The coverage for alternative medicine is purchased as a supplement to regular coverage. The policyholder is offered a choice of traditional or alternative services based on their own personal needs and beliefs, and a primary care physician referral is not required. In order to become credentialed, a practitioner of any CAM therapies (defined by the NIH) must be licensed in the state in which he or she practices, have graduated from an accredited school, show evidence of the pursuit of continuing education, demonstrate two years of clinical experience, and maintain proper malpractice insurance. Recredentialing occurs every 2 years, and providers are subject to site inspections.

The problem most HMOs face when covering CAM is a financial one. There are no well-defined databases or sets of criteria for what insurance should and shouldn't pay for, and the utilization of guidelines for practice doesn't exist for CAM. In addressing this apparent difficulty, several legislative initiatives by federal agencies as well as professional organizations have been launched. The argument that an infinite amount of money is spent on hospitals and high-tech treatments and that CAM is high-touch, low-tech, and low-cost care, is a common theme. Many Americans believe, and in many cases have experienced, that alternative medicine may help a wide variety of health conditions. The common use of vitamins and herbs, homeopathy, acupuncture, yoga and t'ai chi, and other forms of alternative therapies makes the issue of reimbursement for CAM therapies important enough to have become a legislative issue. Without substantial research and evidence-based strategies of practice efficacy, however, the insurance companies are at a loss to establish any form of consistent reimbursement for CAM therapies.

Insurance companies appear to be increasingly willing to examine ways to reduce health care costs, and alternative and complementary therapies are being looked at seriously as a viable option. The credentialing of practitioners has been fostered as a new process toward including alternative therapies as part of health care benefits. Standardization and process management has not been addressed on a national basis and will continue to be the center of debate in years to come.

Legislative Initiatives

Although the regulation of alternative therapies in the United States occurs primarily at the state level through licensure, in recent years governmental focus upon the interests of the alternative health care community has also been evident in federal legislation. The NIH established an OAM, and the Food and Drug Administration (FDA) has initiated regulatory actions for dietary supplements. Moreover, issues concerning alternative therapies continue to take center stage with the failure of Congress to enact comprehensive health care reforms, in part because of the exclusion of alternative therapies. Recent versions of both Democratic and Republican health care proposals include alternative modalities, such as chiropractic, acupuncture, nutritional, and herbal medicine, as an integral part of the proposed reform legislation. Additionally, the Access to Medical Treatment Act (1994) reflected congressional interest in ensuring the right to administer and to receive treatments without excessive regulation by the FDA. This section of the chapter provides an overview of these developments.

The OAM was established in 1992 pursuant to a congressional directive (Federal Register, 1992). In explaining the need for the office, the Senate Appropriations Committee indicated that "the Committee was not satisfied that the conventional medical community as symbolized by the NIH had explored the potential that exists in unconventional practices" (Federal Register, 1992, p. 147). Many routine and effective medical procedures now considered commonplace were once considered unconventional and contraindicated. An example that the Committee gave was cancer radiation therapy, a procedure that is now commonplace, but once was considered to be quackery (i.e., out of the realm of responsible medical practice). In order to more adequately explore these unconventional medical practices, the Committee requested that the NIH establish within the Office of the Director an office to fully investigate and validate alternative practices. The Committee further directed that the NIH convene and establish an advisory panel to screen and select the procedures for investigation and to recommend a research program to fully test the most promising unconventional medical practices.

OAM was subsequently established under the NIH Revitalization Act. An important effect of this enactment was to predicate the existence of the office on statutory authority rather than a directive from a congressional committee, thus according the office more permanence as a governmental unit (NIH, 1993). OAM was charged with facilitating the evaluation of alternative medical treatments, including acupuncture and Chinese medicine, homeopathic medicine, and physical manipulation therapies.

Over the years there have been legislative proposals directly related to the use of CAM therapies. One example was the Access to Medical Treatment Act (1994), which sought to provide consumers with increased access to alternative treatments and to allow greater opportunity for the trial of alternative treatments by consumers that could potentially be effective. Opponents of the legislation argued that the absence of any requirement for scientific testing of treatments for safety prior to actual use could expose clients to dangerous products and undermine the bill's requirement that a client give "informed" consent before treatment. This bill, like most of those related to overhauling the nation's health care system, was not enacted.

The area of CAM that has received the most legislation from Congress is the area of herbs and supplements. In January of 1994, the FDA promulgated regulations under the Nutrition Labeling and Education Act of 1990 concerning supplements such as vitamins, minerals, herbs, and other similar substances (Nutrition Labeling and Education Act, 1990). Among other matters, the new regulations prescribe standards to govern nutritional labeling, nutrient content, and health claims made by manufacturers on the labels or in the labeling of dietary supplements.

Under the new regulations, the FDA will hold health claims made by manufacturers of dietary supplements to the same statutory standards that apply to food in conventional forms. The essence of that standard is the need for "significant scientific agreement" to support the claim. The FDA will promulgate regulations authorizing a health claim only when it determines, based on the totality of publicly available scientific evidence (including evidence from well-designed studies conducted in a manner that is consistent with generally recognized scientific procedures and principles), that there is significant scientific agreement among experts qualified by scientific training and experience to evaluate such claims and that the claim is supported by such evidence (Federal Register, 1994).

Continuing controversy concerning the FDA's dietary supplement regulations, however, prompted the enactment of the Dietary Supplement Health and Education Act of 1994. In its final form, the Dietary Supplement Health and Education Act of 1994 ultimately reflected a legislative compromise that was necessary to ensure passage of the measure in the House of Representatives and to accommodate the interests, on the one hand, of supplement manufacturers and many consumers for greater autonomy for the dietary supplement industry and, on the other hand, of proponents of continuing regulatory control by the FDA to ensure the safety of supplements for consumers.

New dietary supplements not marketed in the United States before October 15, 1994 may be marketed without prior approval by the FDA as long as there is a history of use or other evidence which establishes a reasonable expectation that the product is safe. The law establishes an independent Commission on Dietary Supplement Labels charged with studying and making recommendations concerning the regulation of labeling claims for dietary supplements, including the use of literature in connection with the sale of these products and the procedure for evaluation of manufacturers' claims. The law also creates an Office of Dietary Supplements in the NIH to explore the potential role of supplements in improving health care and to promote the scientific study of the benefits of supplements in maintaining health and preventing chronic disease and other health-related conditions (Dietary Act, 1994).

Fraud and Abuse

One very strong component of some insurance criteria for coverage of alternative and complementary therapies is the extensive credentials required, at the state level, for an alternative care practitioner to be accepted and reimbursed as a provider. The credentialing of alternative providers is an important step for any state to pursue to insure that the care received by beneficiaries is the highest quality and that the practitioner is qualified to provide that care. An example is Alternare of Washington, which contracts with several managed care insurers in the state of Washington and provides credentialing for the plan's network of alternative care practitioners. Alternare also shares its database of alternative providers with the health plans to assist with referrals and billing. Credentialing by Alternare is based on established minimum training requirements for a particular discipline. Alternare assures that practitioners hold a valid license to practice in their respective field.

The biggest concern related to CAM therapies is the number of "practitioners" who might be practicing without specific training or credentialing towards the provision of that service. Many of these practitioners are self-taught, as formal training programs do not exist. It is thus the task of the NCCAM to establish written standards of conduct and policies encouraging compliance and identifying areas of fraud and abuse. In order to accomplish this, the NCCAM proposes that within each health care organization a compliance officer and committee be established; that effective training and education programs be established and accredited; and that there be some mechanism which creates an effective process of communication to receive complaints of fraud and/or abuse. Additionally, the NCCAM, formerly OAM, has called for the establishment of well-publicized disciplinary guidelines for practice parameters with mechanisms for enforcement, monitoring and auditing (OAM Panel, 1997). Practice guidelines, established by representative organizations of each discipline, will be used to determine what is covered by insurance and what is not. Documentation will be a crucial component of the monitoring and auditing processes towards the prevention of fraud and abuse.

Documentation

As the health care delivery system becomes more costly, new demands are made on providers to justify the expenditure of both public and private dollars for their services. Both consumers and regulators want evidence of health care need and the efficacy of therapeutic interventions. All health professions, including CAM practitioners, are experiencing the requirement of more precise treatment and outcome standards; all are struggling to develop methods for meeting this demand. The system of reimbursement under Medicare, the gold standard against which other insurers measure their reimbursement policies, requires detailed and consistent documentation. The criteria for documentation applied to all traditional and now alternative services has been tightened and specifically targeted for increased scrutiny of claims in order to justify evaluation, treatment plans, goals, and expected outcomes.

The demand for better documentation is not unreasonable. Well-applied, appropriate documentation will establish the high quality of care that all health care professionals deliver collectively. The regulations are in place to provide reimbursement of proper and justified claims while insuring that inappropriate or inadequate claims are denied. A large proportion of claims are denied because of the documentation: the lack of it, the inadequacy of it, or perhaps even the imprecise entry of information in the case record or on the insurance claim form.

Complementary and alternative interventions, therapies, and outcomes of treatment have, historically, not been well documented. As the primary source of reimbursement has been out-of-pocket expenditures by the individual seeking care, CAM therapists have not been subjected to the scrutiny of third-party payer claim reviewers. With the current trend towards insurance coverage for particular CAM interventions, this lack of consistent documentation will have to change. It becomes increasingly important that specific evaluative information, treatment plans and modifications, and quantified outcomes of intervention be documented.

Systematic clinical auditing (e.g., utilization review, which is retrospective, and utilization management, which is prospective) can include the retrospective or prospective documentation of client characteristics, diagnostic and therapeutic interventions, and outcomes. Such a review is done as an objective measure, not to prove the effectiveness of a certain method, but rather to acquire reliable empirical information on what happens in actual and standard practice. As health insurance providers move towards reimbursement for complementary therapies, payment for services will most likely only include those practices which stand up to scientific quality and incorporate systematic clinical auditing (Melchart et al., 1997). This sort of management program integrates elements of structure- and process-oriented quality assurance with the development and testing of outcome-oriented evaluation and with controlled clinical trials on interventions considered relevant and promising.

The fundamental principle of documentation is quantification. The clinician must justify that the client can benefit significantly by receiving professional care, particularly since the reviewer is charged with determining whether "skilled" services were actually rendered. Under managed care, utilization review and management is now being applied by third-party payers to CAM therapies, as it has been to traditional therapies for decades, to monitor the provider's performance in comparison to standards and expectations of care. Utilization management is a response to finding variable practice patterns for the same clinical condition. This variation in practice is believed to cause unnecessary care and therefore become a cost burden to society (Foto, 1993). In other words, it is used as a "watch dog" or a means of holding practitioners accountable to necessary and quality treatment. Reviewed case by case, it ensures that each client qualifies for the level and kind of care he or she is receiving. In the current health care climate, utilization review and management serve two primary purposes: to improve the quality of care by deterring unnecessary or inappropriate treatment, and to save money by imposing cost-containment strategies.

The Health Care Financing Administration (HCFA) requires that utilization review be implemented, and other managed care companies have followed in the footsteps of government programs to ensure quality and medical necessity of treatment. The mode of review is the systematic audit of documentation of services provided relative to the evaluation, care, and outcomes specific to each patient. Documentation is often the only way reviewers can determine if the care received is appropriate. The strongest tool health care professionals have to demonstrate their unique skill, expertise, and ability to make effective interventions with clients is documentation. In other words, documentation reflects the "worth" of interventions.

A scientific evaluation of complementary medical practices commonly used in health care is urgently required. Although randomized clinical trials are the primary tool for such an evaluation, for a number of conceptual and pragmatic reasons, they cannot be the only tool for clinical research on complementary medicine. Using the concept of utilization review, systematic clinical auditing of client records can provide information on the "epidemiology" of complementary medical practices, make the processes used in the daily practice of complementary methods clearly intelligible, and give a preliminary estimation of outcomes.

Melchart et al. (1997) conducted a chart audit to determine the efficacy of Traditional Chinese Medicine (TCM) on 1,597 patients. Information on patient characteristics, diagnoses, and preventive and therapeutic interventions were collected in addition to having patients rate the intensity of their main complaints (on a scale of 1 to 10) at admission, at discharge, and at 2, 6, and 12 month intervals following discharge. Information was also harvested on the use of ICD-9 classification as a means for determining billing practices and reimbursement patterns. These researchers showed that documentation and systematic auditing of all patients admitted was feasible, and acceptable follow-up was possible. However, they also found some very substantial problems in documentation practices. First, documentation was not systematic. Consistent information was not obtained, making comparison of diagnostic groups difficult. Second, the coding of diagnoses was too imprecise. Often, only the three-figure ICD-9 classification was used, so secondary diagnoses were not coded according to ICD criteria. This makes quantitative analysis of comorbidity patterns impossible. Third, because of the poor documentation of the heterogeneity of diagnoses, defining reliable prognostic factors and characteristics was difficult. As a result of these documentation problems, reimbursement for services was often insufficient to cover the actual costs of patient care (Melchart et al., 1997). This study clearly demonstrates the importance of consistent, objective, and measurable evaluative and outcome data collection. Documentation is key for reimbursement.

Research Imperatives

The documented prevalence of alternative medicine practices in the United States warrants a critical evaluation of this field (Eskinazi, 2000). Many theories regarding the use of alternative therapies provide a framework for conceptualizing and analyzing phenomena that result from interventions using CAM therapies. However, much of what is reported is anecdotal in nature. Solid, theory-based research using randomized, controlled trials, longitudinal observations, outcomes studies, and the like are required to demonstrate effectiveness, safety, and cost effectiveness of complementary and alternative therapies (Edwards, 1997; Gatchel, 1998). Historically, practitioners of alternative therapies have not been highly trained in research methodology, and experts in research methodology have little training in or experience with alternative medical practices (Gatchel, 1998). However, as a result of NIH's involvement in establishing definitions, developing practice guidelines, and pursuing research that is appropriately conducted, many research initiatives have surfaced.

The legislative history of the NIH Revitalization Act of 1993 reflects Congress's intent that research fellowships for training should support programs and analysis as well as clinical research, particularly related to clinical outcomes. Concerning the ongoing efforts of NCCAM to develop a plan for research activities at NIH in the field of alternative medicine, Congress intends that the Center coordinate its work with that in other nations and pay particular attention to activities that emphasize cultural diversity (termed *ethnomedicine*). Further, Congress expects NCCAM to develop databases in functional support of both research and information transfer. By the end of 1994, it had awarded 42 grants for research concerning specific alternative modalities and two additional awards for exploratory centers in alternative medical research (House of Representatives, 1993).

The purpose of the database is to bring together all the existing data and literature on alternative medicine and develop organized, systematic, and up-to-date reviews of the relevant scientific data. The current database prepares and maintains a register of randomized controlled trials and other research efforts in this area, and also contains a compilation of basic and clinical research relevant to alternative and complementary medicine. This review of the literature is available to health care providers and consumers via the Internet at nih.gov/oam/database.

Summary

Until evidence-based practice and utilization of alternative interventions that have been found to be effective in specific conditions have been established, third-party reimbursement for these services will remain spotty. Without clear definition, insurers are left to establish their own perceptions of what CAM therapies are. The declining ability of healthcare providers to make independent decisions regarding client care, the declining level of reimbursement for traditional services rendered, the increased availability and use of alternative medicine, increasingly strict governmental regulations, and new questions regarding graduate medical education and clinical credentialing in CAM therapies are just a few of the changes that have confronted the health care industry in the last decade. Health care providers need to become proactive in all arenas where future health care policy will be determined. Research is the best defense for demonstrating the cost savings that could result from integrating traditional medicine with alternative medicine.

As the population that uses CAM care with greater frequency increases, both the promise and the perils of these therapies need to be further researched. Clinical and cost outcomes based on longitudinal studies need to focus on Medicare-eligible populations to determine if CAM interventions, when compared to or superimposed on traditional care, result in decreased disability, improved health status, and decreased cost. Addressing such clinical, financial, and public policy questions will have an impact on the overall health care system's provision of care in the future.

The challenges lie in building bridges between conventional, traditional medicine and alternative practices. Mainstreaming alternative practices that work is the next step. This will require acknowledging the efficacy of certain therapies in the face of irrefutable proof, and perhaps most important, putting the well-being of the client foremost as therapists determine which approach, or combination of approaches, will best achieve a state of wellness.

STUDY QUESTIONS

1. Describe one trend in CAM utilization.
2. How do legislative initiatives effect CAM?
3. Discuss why credentialing is important in combating fraud and abuse concerns related to CAM.
4. Discuss documentation concerns related to CAM.
5. Research your present or most recent health insurer. Does it cover CAM, and if it does, to what extent?

RESOURCES

Alternative Therapies in Health and Medicine
169 Saxony Road, Suite 104
Encinitas, CA 92024
(866)828–2962
www.alternative-therapies.com

National Center for Complementary and
  Alternative Medicine
nccam.nih.gov

REFERENCES

Access to Medical Treatment Act: Hearing on S. 2140 before the Senate Labor and Human Resources Committee, 103rd Congress, 2nd Session, 68–93, 1994.

Astin, J. A. (1998). Why patients use alternative medicine: Results of a national study. *Journal of the American Medical Association, 279,* 1548–1553.

Astin, J. A., A. Marie, K. R. Pelletier, E. Hansen, & W. L. Haskell. (1998). A review of the incorporation of complementary and alternative medicine by mainstream physicians. *Archives of Internal Medicine, 158*(21), 2303–2310.

Astin, J. A., K. R. Pelletier, A. Marie, & W. L. Haskell. (2000). Complementary and alternative medicine use among elderly persons: One-year analysis of a Blue Shield Medicare supplement. *Journal of Gerontology, 55A*(1), M4–M9.

Benjamin, S. (1997). Carefully embracing managed care. Point/Counterpoint. *Alternative Therapies, 3*(3), 63–68.

Berman, B. M., J. P. Swyer, S. M. Hartnoll, B. B. Singh, & B. Bausell. (2000). The public debate over alternative medicine: The importance of finding a middle ground. *Alternative Therapies, 6*(1), 98–101.

Crock R. D., D. Jarjoura, A. Polen, & G. W. Rutecki. (1999). Confronting the communication gap between conventional and alternative medicine: A survey of physician's attitudes. *Alternative Therapies, 5*(2), 61–66.

Daily, L. (1999). More HMO's covering alternative treatments and complementary care. *Physicians Financial News, 17*(9), S1–S6.

Dietary Supplement Health and Education Act of 1994, Pub. L. 103–417, 108 Stat. 4325, 1994.

Edwards, R. A. (1997). Our research approaches must meet the goal of improving patient care. *Alternative Therapies, 3*(1), 99–100.

Eisenberg, D. M., R. B. Davis, & S. L. Ettner. (1998). Trends in alternative medicine use in the United States, 1990–1997: Results of a follow-up national survey. *Journal of the American Medical Association, 280,* 1569–1575.

Eisenberg, D. M., R. C. Kessler, C. Foster, F. E. Norlock, D. R. Calkins, & T. L. DelBanco. (1993). Unconventional medicine in the United States: Prevalence costs and patterns of use. *New England Journal of Medicine, 328,* 246–252.

Ernst, E. (2000). Prevalence of use of complementary/alternative medicine: A systematic review. *Bulletin of the World Health Organization, 78*(2), 252–257.

Eskinazi, D., & D. Muehsam. (2000). Factors that shape alternative medicine: The role of the alternative medicine research community. *Alternative Therapies, 6*(1), 49–53.

Federal Register. (1992). Congressional Directive by the Senate Appropriations Committee to the National Institutes of Health for Fiscal Year 1992. No. 104, 102nd Congress, 1st Session.

Federal Register. (1994). C.F.R. § 101.14(c) (1994). Also found in: 21 U.S.C.A. § 343r (3)(B)(i) (Supp. 1994), 1994.

Federal Register. (1994). 59 Fed. Reg. 402, Jan. 4, 1994.

Foto, M., & G. Swanson. (1993). Utilization review and managed care. *Rehabilitation Management, 6*(5), 123–125.

Gatchel, R. J., & A. M. Maddrey. (1998). Clinical outcome research in complementary and alternative medicine: An overview of experimental design and analysis. *Alternative Therapies, 4*(5), 36–42.

Horrigan, B., & D. Ornish. (1995). Healing the heart, reversing the disease. *Alternative Therapies in Health and Medicine, 1*(5), 84–92.

House of Representatives. No. 100, 103rd Congress, 1st Session. Fed. Reg. 117, 1993. Reprinted in *U.S. Code Congressional & Administrative News, 299,* 1993.

Krauss, H. H., C. Godfrey, J. Kirk, & D. M. Eisenberg. (1998). Alternative health care: Its use by individuals with physical disabilities. *Archives of Physical Medicine and Rehabilitation, 79*(11), 1440–1447.

Melchart, D., K. Linde, J. Z. Liao, S. Hager, & W. Weidenhammer. (1997). Systematic clinical auditing in complementary medicine: Rationale, concept, and a pilot study. *Alternative Therapies, 3*(1), 33–39.

Moore, N. (1997). A review of reimbursement policies for alternative and complementary therapies. *Alternative Therapies in Health and Medicine, 3*(3), 26–29, 91–92.

Moore, N. G. (1996). The American holistic centers: A model in integrative care. *Alternative Therapies in Health and Medicine, 2*(5), 38–39.

National Institutes of Health Revitalization Act of 1993. Pub. L. No. 103–43, 107 Stat. 122.

Nutrition Labeling and Education Act of 1990, Pub. L. 104 Stat. 2353, 101–535, 1990.

OAM Panel on Definition and Description. (1997). CAM Research Methodology, April 1995. Defining and describing complementary and alternative medicine. *Alternative Therapies, 3*(2), 49–57.

Pelletier K. R., J. A. Astin, & W. L. Haskell. (1999). Current trends in the integration and reimbursement of complementary and alternative medicine by managed care organizations (MCOs) and insurance providers: 1998 update and cohort analysis. *American Journal of Health Promotion, 14*(2), 125–133.

Pelletier, K. R., A. Marie, M. Drasner, & W. L. Haskell. (1997). Current trends in the integration and reimbursment of complementary and alternative medicine by managed care, insurance carriers, and hospital providers. *American Journal of Health Promotion, 12,* 112–123.

Rossman, M. L. (1997). Managed care and alternative medicine: Who will manage what, and how? Point/Counterpoint. *Alternative Therapies, 3*(3), 63–68.

U.S. Senate, Committee on Labor and Human Resources, S. Rep. No. 410, 103rd Congress, 2nd Session, 14–15, 1994.

5

Researching Complementary Therapies

Judith Deutsch and Ellen Anderson

CHAPTER OBJECTIVES

♦ Understand a system for examining Complementary and Alternative Medicine (CAM) and decide whether CAM is appropriate to incorporate into a plan of care.
♦ Practice using the system.

It has been argued that the evidence supporting a complementary therapy should be as rigorous as the evidence to support "mainstream" interventions (Dossey, 1995). Important issues discussed in the CAM literature are clearly defining CAM, the challenges of designing a controlled study, and external validity of CAM research design (Gatchel & Maddrey, 1998; Dossey, 1995). Researchers within CAM are writing about the importance of well-designed and controlled studies as well (Eisenberg, 1997; Linde, 2000; Lukoff, Edwards, & Miller, 1998).

While the process of researching CAMs parallels that of researching other therapies, there are some challenges unique to CAM. Operationally defining approaches can be difficult because often there are descriptions used by the CAM practitioners that may not be clear to nonpractitioners (Federspil & Vettor, 2000). For example, in Structural Integration (SI), practitioners speak about "horizontalizing the pelvis." To the SI practitioner this has a specific meaning related to aligning the body within the gravitational field. A therapist unfamiliar with SI may require a more specific definition, such as aligning the anterior superior iliac spine in the sagittal and coronal planes. This definition in turn could be measured, while "horizontalizing the pelvis" cannot. Other challenges include the difficulty in validating CAMs approaches. This is particularly true about energy therapies that are difficult to measure. While one can observe the energy practitioner moving in a way that is consistent with sensing and modulating an energy field, it is very difficult to be certain that the energy field is in fact generated by the therapist.

In spite of these challenges, the application of a complementary therapy should follow a sound clinical decision-making process whereby the therapist systematically identifies the

This chapter is designed to provide therapists with a system for investigating complementary and alternative therapies that is integrated with the clinical decision-making process. The process is illustrated using a case study in which a therapist evaluates the appropriateness of including a CAM into the plan of care.

The process is relevant to therapists because they will encounter clients who will request information and guidance about incorporating CAM into their plan of care. Therapists will benefit from using this system to gain a perspective on the literature supporting different CAM approaches. Therapists are especially well qualified to evaluate the usefulness of CAM, contribute to the literature about CAM, and define how principles of holistic practice may enhance current theories of practice. This evaluation process will enable therapists to engage in such professional practices.

problem, generates a hypotheses, applies and measures the outcome of an intervention, and then makes decisions about efficacy. This system is consistent with using evidence to substantiate practice. This chapter describes the process of investigating and evaluating the literature to assist the therapist in the process of selecting appropriate complementary therapies.

In the following scenario, the therapist engaged in the clinical decision-making process has worked with clients with brain injuries for 5 years. The therapist has previously encountered the described clinical picture in which, despite several weeks of intervention, residual impairments persisted that interfered with the client's ability to regain complete functional independence. In a systematic way, the therapist will explore the possibility of including yoga as a complement to the existing plan of care.

A clinical decision-making process (see Figure 5–1) is proposed, which entails a sequence of steps beginning with the identification of the client's abilities and the impairments that may be interfering with independence. Embedded in this process is the crucial step of investigating the literature. The client scenario is described in Figure 5–2.

Investigating the Literature

In order to evaluate the appropriateness of yoga, the therapist needs to become familiar with the approach. Knowing that yoga is classified by the National Center on Complementary and Alternative Medicine (NCCAM) as a mind-body therapy (NCCAM, 2001), the therapist must then evaluate the evidence supporting the specific application of yoga. Several steps for investigating the literature will be presented. They include preliminary reading of textbooks, searching databases for review articles in order to survey the literature, searching databases for specific articles that relate to the clinical question, and evaluating the literature by identifying study design and purpose.

Preliminary reading can be used to identify the assumptions of the approach, the physiology, and proposed benefits. Chapter 24, "Yoga," in this text and Feuerstein and Payne's

Figure 5–1 Clinical decision making. Re-produced with permission from J. E. Deutsch and E. Z. Anderson © 1999.

Identify client and the specific impairments and abilities that need to be addressed

↓

Investigate the literature

↓

Generate a clinical hypothesis

↓

Collect relevant clinical data, being specific about measurements used and outcomes selected

↓

Intervene

↓

Evaluate the outcome of the intervention

↓

Report the results in the appropriate venue

Yoga for Dummies can serve as the preliminary reading for the scenario. Reading from the textbooks provides the background information about yoga (Feuerstein & Payne, 1999). Preliminary reading also provides a background for searching the literature. One can search the literature by using different databases. Each database has its own configuration and rules for including citations. Guidelines for searching databases and access to databases that are useful for CAM research are provided elsewhere (Allais et al., 2000; Helewa and Walker, 2000). The therapist searches three computerized databases: Index Medicus (Medline), the Cumulative Index of Nursing and Allied Health (CINAHL), and the NCCAM database.

The NCCAM Web site has a specific search engine, NCCAM on PubMed, which consists of approximately 180,000 bibliographic citations dated from 1963 to the present. The CAM citations were extracted from the National Library of Medicine's Medline database. The CAM citations were obtained using Medical Subject Headings (MeSH) controlled vocabulary terms from the *alternative medicine* tree structure, and other selected MeSH terms

A thirty-year old woman with a traumatic brain injury secondary to a motor vehicle accident. She sustained a fractured pelvis and several fractured ribs, was intubated and ventilator dependent. Her Glascow coma level was 9, and she was classified as a Rancho Los Amigos Scale III. After two months of inpatient rehabilitation the client was discharged to outpatient therapy.

INITIAL EXAMINATION
Patient report: The client reports being able to sit for 15 minutes before experiencing discomfort in both her lumbar and thoracic spine. She reports experiencing shortness of breath while speaking to an audience for greater than five minutes. At the end of the day she feels achy and has difficulty sleeping.
ROM: The client has limited ROM of the thoracic and lumbar spine with right tensor fascia latae (TFL) tightness.
Posture: sitting: thoracic kyphosis; standing: pelvic obliquity, 3/4 inch leg length discrepancy
Force generation: abdominals 3/5 and bilateral hip abductors 3/5
Function: The client is able to sit for 10 minutes, but then she experiences pain of 7/10. She complains of shortness of breath after elevations of 8 steps and is only able to stand for 5 minutes before reporting disabling pain (8/10).
Employment: The client is a reference librarian at a major university. Her job involves sitting at a computer for extended periods, walking up/down stairs, occasionally retrieving or storing books and in-service training for the faculty.
Client goals: Return to work, improve sleeping and decrease fatigue.

PLAN OF CARE
The plan of care has included strengthening of the abdominals and hips; stretching of the TFL and spine; education regarding posture, body mechanics and pursed-lip breathing; and a trial of a shoe lift. Ergonomic modifications for the work environment and a home exercise program were reviewed.

RE-EVALUATION (after six sessions, over 3 weeks)
The client is comfortable with the shoe-lift and there is a reduction in her pelvic obliquity. The client's standing and sitting endurance has increased to 20 minutes respectively with decrease in pain to 5/10. Although recommendations for sleeping postures were provided, the client reports that she is sleeping better but awakes feeling fatigued and achy.

EXPANDING PLAN OF CARE TO INCLUDE CAM
The therapist, who has been practicing yoga, now considers looking into yoga to complement the current plan of care. Specifically, the therapist identifies the following impairments that are still not completely resloved: SOB with speaking, fatigue upon waking, and pain with prolonged sitting and standing.

Figure 5–2 The case scenario.

(Allais et al., 2000). Access to Medline may not be as universal so an individual who may not be able to use Medline will find NCCAM on PubMed a useful alternative.

Using keywords such as yoga, posture, pain, and breathing, the search is limited to review articles, which will provide an overview of the literature without the researcher becoming overwhelmed by having to review all of the articles. The results of a search using several databases (conducted April 25, 2000) are summarized in Table 5–1.

Analyzing the results of the search is a useful exercise to gain an overview of the literature. The results of this search highlight the differences in number and type of references for each database. For example, there are more articles on yoga and breathing in Medline than in

Table 5–1 Search Results

Key Word	Medline	CINAHL	NCCAM
Yoga	494	102	442
Limit to review	43	4	unable
Yoga and breathing	55	12	0
Yoga and pain	15	6	7
Yoga and posture	33	1	30

CINAHL. There appears to be a history of studying yoga and breathing in the physiology literature, which is most comprehensively indexed in Medline. Using several databases allows one to learn about which disciplines are studying questions that may be of interest to you. Repeating a search over time will allow the practitioner to observe how the literature evolves. There may be additional citations and new areas of study.

Briefly surveying the literature by browsing the review articles affords the reader a broader perspective on the CAM. The reader can identify at a glance the key populations and issues that are being studied. In the case of yoga, browsing yields information about diagnostic groups that are treated with yoga: musculoskeletal, cardiac, respiratory, pain management, and cancer. Yoga is also applied in the areas of wellness, cognition, and emotional well being. The articles come from diverse literatures and are written in different languages. The disciplines identified in the search were Medicine (physical medicine and rehabilitation, cardiology, respiratory, rheumatology, gastroenterology, psychiatry), Nursing, Medical Anthropology, and Psychology. The articles are written in English, German, French, and Polish.

Additional observations were made while browsing the search. Most of the articles summarized potential applications of yoga. Only in selected articles was there a critical review of the available evidence. Those articles were in the application of yoga to cardiac, respiratory, and musculoskeletal pathology. Yoga was often grouped with relaxation or mind-body therapies, as classified by NCCAM.

After surveying the literature, the user may refine the search by using keywords and evaluating the purpose of the studies. Studies may be described in two broad categories: those that measure the outcomes of the intervention and those that aim to describe its mechanism. Searching using "yoga and pain" as keywords yielded both categories of articles. One set of articles focused on outcomes of the intervention, describing the results of applying yoga to a specific group for a specific purpose. The application of yoga for the management of musculoskeletal pain is reported in studies for patients with carpal tunnel syndrome (Garfinkel et al., 1998) and osteoarthritis of the hand (Garfinkel et al., 1994). The application of yoga for the behavioral management of pain using mindful meditation is also reported (Kabat-Zinn, 1982). The results of the search illustrate some diversity in the application of yoga as either movement-based or meditation in order to obtain specific outcomes.

In contrast, searching "yoga and posture" yielded studies that described the mechanism of the intervention. Studies that focus on mechanism aim to describe or explain the underlying physiology of an intervention. In this search the mechanism of yoga was studied in different ways. The effect of specific yoga postures as measured by blood flow responses in the kidneys and liver (Minvaleev, Kuznetsov, & Nozdrachev, 1998; 1999), changes in pulmonary function (Stanescu et al., 1981), exercise capacity (Rai & Ram, 1993), and modulation of CNS (Jain & Talukdar, 1993) are examples of studies that focused on mechanisms. The effect of breathing on equilibrium (Aust & Fischer, 1997) was also studied.

Another tool to evaluate the quality of the literature is to review the *research designs* that are used in the studies. A review of the research designs indicates that the studies clustered into three categories: descriptive, correlational, and experimental (see Table 5–2). Detailed descriptions of research designs can be found in other texts (Domholt, 2000; Portney & Watkins, 2000), and selected features are summarized here (Domholt, 2000). In descriptive studies the nature of a phenomenon is documented through systematic collection of data. The best example of a descriptive study is a case report. Correlational studies are those in which the primary purpose is to analyze relationships. An example of a correlational study would be an epidemiological study where the association between subject characteristics and the presence or absence of disease is measured (Domholt, 2000). In quasi-experimental and experimental studies, differences between groups or treatments are analyzed in a reliable way. The best example of an experimental study is a randomized clinical trial.

The interpretation of the studies goes from the lower level (describing) to an intermediate level (looking for patterns or relationships) to what is considered a higher level (attributing cause and effect). Experimental study designs are the most rigorous. Within each of the categories there are also hierarchies based on the rigor of the design. For example, in the experimental category, less rigorous studies are those in which there may be no randomization or control. Random selection is the process by which subjects are selected to insure that there is not a particular attribute that is more strongly represented in a group. This is in contrast with a sample of convenience, where subjects may be selected because they are accessible, but may not be representative of the population to which the study could be generalized. Con-

Table 5–2 Research Designs

Design	Purpose	Examples	Yoga Citations
Descriptive	Describe	Case study	Shannahoff-Khalsa and Beckett. (1996). Clinical case report: Efficacy of yogic techniques in the treatment of obsessive compulsive disorders. *International Journal of Neuroscience, 85* (1–2), 1–17.
Correlational	Analysis of relationships	Surveys, epidemiological studies	Smith, Amutio, Anderson, & Aria. (1996). Relaxation: Mapping an uncharted world. *Biofeedback & Self Regulation, 21*(1), 63–90.
Quasi-experimental and experimental	Analysis of difference	Randomized clinical trial	Garfinkel, Singhal, Katz, Allan, Reshetar, & Schumacher. (1998). Yoga-based intervention for carpal tunnel syndrome: A randomized trial. *JAMA, 280*(18), 1601–3.

trol is a mechanism to reduce experimenter bias. Control can be achieved by using a group that does not receive treatment, a control group. It can also be achieved by "blinding the experimenter." Blinding is a process by which the experimenter does not know which subject is in the intervention or the control group. More rigorous studies are those in which there are more controls, such as a double-blind randomized clinical trial.

In this yoga search, an example of a less rigorous study would be the article "An outpatient program in behavioral medicine for chronic pain patients based on the practice of mindfulness meditation: Theoretical considerations and preliminary results" (Kabat-Zinn, 1982). This study was performed on a single small group of patients and presented preliminary results. An example of the more rigorous design would be "Yoga-based intervention for carpal tunnel syndrome: A randomized trial" (Garfinkel et al., 1998).

Study design often matches the development of the area of study. Early in the development of an area, there may be more descriptive studies in which a practice is defined and applied in a limited way. This appears to be the case in the literature on yoga and pain, since the literature search identified many case studies and literature reviews, and only a couple of controlled clinical trials. Subsequent studies that look at patterns or relationships in which the important dependent variables are being identified prevail. Finally, when there are specific hypotheses and questions to test, studies move more towards the third category of looking for cause and effect. In this type of study, a hypothesis is formed in which the independent variable (that which the experimenter manipulates) is believed to affect the dependent variable (the measured or outcome variable). The designs may coexist within a specific literature, where some areas may be well defined and be tested for cause and effect, but other areas are still in the early stages, so descriptive designs are used. For example, in the literature on yoga and breathing, most of the studies are experimental, in which the effect of a variety of yoga breathing techniques have been tested on specific groups in a controlled way, although there are no large randomized clinical trials. For more information on evaluating the evidence to support an intervention see Sackett et al.'s *Evidence-Based Medicine: How to Practice and Teach EBM* (2000).

Having completed a broad overview of the literature on yoga, the therapist determines that there are resources in selected areas. Selecting and evaluating the articles that are pertinent to the client is the next step. Note that the therapist has broadly reviewed the literature to understand the context of the specific information needed for clinical decision making. To review, the therapist's goals are to identify articles that would assist with determining if the use of yoga would be appropriate to complement the intervention in order to improve the client's breathing, reduce the pain from sustained positions, and the ameliorate the fatigue and disturbed sleep. As a result of the search, the therapist found abundant literature about the use of yoga breathing techniques that have been shown to improve both physiological as well as psychological aspects of breathing. There was also some evidence for the amelioration of pain using yoga. However, neither of these literatures is applied directly to a client with a traumatic brain injury (TBI). A surprise in the search was the application of the term *posture*. The therapist expected to find articles about improving posture by using yoga; instead, the articles were about the effect of yoga postures on breathing and other body functions. Finally, the search did not reveal anything about yoga and fatigue or sleeplessness.

An additional search using selected keywords is performed. The results (indicated in parenthesis for each key term) of the search are yoga and TBI (0), yoga and fatigue (5), and yoga and sleep (12). Some of the articles from the second search are duplicates of what was found in the first search under a different category. For example, the carpal tunnel article

(Garfinkel et al., 1998) was listed under yoga and fatigue as well as under yoga and pain because both reductions in pain and fatigue were outcomes of that study. The yoga and sleep literature was not relevant to the therapist's client because it focused on comparing physiologic correlates during yoga and sleep rather than ameliorating sleep disturbances (Corby et al., 1978; Peng et al., 1999; Zhang, Zhao, & He, 1988). Specific articles are relevant to the client, in which pranayama (breathing) and Hatha (movement) yoga have been shown to reduce the perception and the sense of fatigue (Berger & Owen, 1992; Wood, 1993).

The therapist has determined that the quality of the literature is good with respect to the yoga and breathing resources. The designs are mostly experimental, there is a convergence of evidence from different labs, and the findings are consistent with the assumptions of yoga. The literature on pain and yoga has fewer studies, but there are a couple of clinical trials that are well designed and relate directly to patients with musculoskeletal pathology. And, although there are no specific citations about yoga and brain injury, the therapist decides that available literature about yoga applies to the client. The primary impairments of pain, poor posture, difficulty breathing, and fatigue that were identified as limiting this client's ability to sit, stand, speak for extended periods of time, and sleep appear to be amenable to yoga. Specifically, there are articles to support that movement-based yoga reduced pain and fatigue for patients with musculoskeletal pathology (Garfinkel et al., 1998; Garfinkel et al., 1994). There was also evidence for changes in respiratory function using a combination of movement and breathing yoga approaches (Joshi, Joshi, & Gokhale, 1992; Makwana, Khirwadkar, & Gupta, 1988; Telles & Desiraju, 1991; Vedanthan et al., 1998). Finally, there was also evidence of improved posture as a result of yoga (Savic et al., 1990).

Intervention

Having decided to use yoga as an intervention, the therapist notes that the process of investigating the literature has required a search by breaking the topic into different sections. The therapist had to search yoga and pain, yoga and sleep, and yoga and fatigue separately. However, the clinical application of yoga requires an integration of the elements of the search in order to create a holistic intervention. The therapist generates a clinical hypothesis that the impairments may be interrelated and decides to address them concurrently. The literature search implicitly supports this approach, since there were overlapping references when different search terms such as yoga and pain and yoga and sleep were used. The therapist determines that an improvement in sitting tolerance and sleeping will be the expected outcomes of the intervention. It is the amelioration of pain and improvement of posture and breathing that will be the critical elements to effect this change. The therapist will therefore examine the client using measurement tools that will capture these predicted changes, such as timed tests for sitting, sleep reports, visual analogue scores for pain, vital capacity, observation of breathing patterns, and photographs of posture. Given the lack of information on yoga and TBI, the therapist anticipates that it may be appropriate to document this experience. Books and articles about writing case studies are consulted in order to ensure collection of information in a consistent and valid manner (Lukoff, Edwards & Miller, 1998; McEwen, 1996).

Using clinical trials on patients with musculoskeletal issues as a guideline, the therapist designs the intervention (Garfinkel et al., 1998; Garfinkel et al., 1994). In both studies,

Hatha yoga, a movement-based yoga, is used as the intervention. Hatha yoga is familiar to the therapist and is relevant to this client because breathing is incorporated. Guidelines on frequency, duration, and intensity from the Garfinkel studies (1994, 1998) cannot be applied directly to the client, since the focus is on the upper extremity. The studies, however, cite as a resource a text by Iyengar (1979) titled *Light on Yoga* in which yoga postures (asanas) and breathing (pranayama) are described. While the book describes the postures comprehensively, it is difficult to link the use of the postures to specific impairments.

In an effort to select the relevant postures for the client's impairments and desired outcomes, the therapist also refers to a textbook titled *Relax and Renew*. It is written by a physical therapist who is also a yoga practitioner (Lasater, 1995). In *Relax and Renew*, the therapist finds recommendations for specific postures to alleviate problems such as back pain, insomnia, and difficulty in breathing. The therapist selects four postures: mountain-brook, elevated legs-up-the wall, seated mountain, and supported child's pose. These postures incorporate motions and positions that the therapist evaluates as empirically suitable to achieve the goals of the intervention. The positions mobilize the spine and incorporate expansion of the thoracic cavity for breath. The postures require that the client move from an elongated position of the spine in flexion to an elongated position of the spine in extension.

Importantly, general cautions and suggestions about where and when to practice yoga are offered in both texts. Suggestions such as moving slowly, being able to take a full breath in each posture (to avoid extreme ranges), and avoiding positions that produce pain are also incorporated into the plan of care. Environmental considerations such as using a flat surface, external supports as necessary, and practicing in the morning (because you are more mindful) or the evening (to reach a greater state of relaxation) are noted. The schedule of therapy is adjusted to incorporate recommendations regarding the introduction of new postures. Lasater (1995) recommends that the sessions initially be brief, as short as 5 minutes, and that new postures be added slowly. Therefore, the client is scheduled once a week for 5 more weeks.

Reporting on the Outcome

As an ongoing part of intervention, the therapist measures changes at both the impairment and ability level. The results of the intervention are mixed. Specifically, the client reports she is sleeping better, experiencing less fatigue, and able to maintain sitting for longer periods of time without pain. She no longer becomes short of breath when speaking, but continues to experience breathlessness with elevations and has pain (5/10) with standing for 30 minutes.

Excited about the outcome of the intervention, the therapist decides to write a case report about the application of yoga to a client with TBI. The therapist has determined that there is no literature on yoga and TBI, so the use of a case study is an appropriate format to begin to describe practice. This is an opportunity for the therapist to contribute to the literature supporting the use of CAM. In order to do this the therapist reads resources on the mechanics of writing the case study (Domholt, 2000; McEwen, 1996).

There are several choices for selecting a journal in to which to submit the case study. Several options would be the complementary therapy, rehabilitation medicine, or allied health literatures. Readers of these three literatures would be interested in an article on the application of yoga to a client with a TBI. Journals in these literatures have already published articles about complementary therapies, indicating an interest and willingness to publish in the area of CAM.

The process of integrating the CAM into practice and reporting on the outcome of the intervention is complete. The therapist has moved from a clinical question to investigating the literature to applying the intervention and documenting the results. The process of researching complementary therapies is integrated with clinical decision making and is accessible for therapists considering the use of CAM in their practice.

Summary

In this chapter a system for incorporating the use of literature to make decisions about including CAM into a plan of care has been described. The steps include identifying a client's relevant impairments and abilities, investigating the literature, generating a clinical hypothesis, collecting relevant clinical data (being specific about measurements used and outcomes selected), intervening, evaluating the outcome of the intervention, and reporting the results in the appropriate venue. Each of the steps is described and applied to a case scenario.

STUDY QUESTIONS

1. Perform the same search that is presented in Table 5–1 and compare your results. A word of caution: Searching the Web using a browser rather than identifying specific databases often yields resources that are not peer-reviewed and may be difficult to evaluate. However, the Web may contain relevant information about professional associations and CAM practitioners.
2. To practice the skills described in the chapter, return to the case study described in Figure 5–2. Instead of yoga, use Structural Integration or Rolfing as the intervention that the therapist is considering for the management of the client. This will also allow you to compare the literature on yoga with the literature on Structural Integration.

SUGGESTED READING

Garrard, J. (1999). *Health Sciences Literature Review Made Easy*. Gaithersburg, MD: Aspen.

Helewa, A., & J. Walker. (2000). *Critical Evaluation of Research in Physical Rehabilitation*. Philadelphia: Saunders.

Sackett, D. L., S. E. Straus, W. S. Richardson, W. Rosenberg, & R. B. Haynes. (2000). *Evidence-Based Medicine: How to Practice and Teach EBM*. (2nd ed.). London: Churchill Livingstone.

RESOURCES

Journals that Publish Complementary Therapy Exclusively

Acupuncture in Medicine

Advances in Mind-Body Medicine

Alternative Health Practitioner

Alternative Medicine Review

Alternative Therapies in Clinical Practice

Alternative Therapies in Health and Medicine

American Journal of Chinese Medicine

Biofeedback and Self-Regulation

British Homoeopathic Journal

Complementary Therapies in Medicine

Homoeopathy

Integrative Medicine

International Journal of Alternative and Complementary Medicine

Journal–American Osteopathic Association

Journal of Bodywork and Movement Therapies

Journal of Herbs, Spices and Medicinal Plants

Journal of Holistic Nursing

Journal of Manipulative and Physiological Therapeutics

Journal of Traditional Chinese Medicine

Manual Therapy

The Journal of Alternative and Complementary Medicine

Topics in Clinical Chiropractic

Journals that Have Included CAM Articles in Their Publications

American Journal of Occupational Therapy

Archives of Physical Medicine and Rehabilitation

British Medical Journal

Journal of the American Medical Association

Journal of Family Practice

Journal of Orthopedic and Sports Physical Therapy

Lancet

New England Journal of Medicine

Neurology Report

Physical and Occupational Therapy in Geriatrics

Physical Therapy Clinics of North America

Rheumatic Disease Clinics of North America

Databases that List CAM Research

AMED (portico.bl.uk/). Allied and complementary medicine database maintained by the British Library of Medicine.

CINHAL (cinahl.com/csources/csources.htm). Cumulative Index to Nursing and Allied Health. Multidisciplinary database listing articles of interest in allied health.

HERBMED (www.amfoundation.org/herbmed.htm). A free interactive database hyperlinked to articles that support the efficacy and mechanism of the herbs.

NCCAM (www.nlm.nih.gov/nccam/camonpubmed.html). Bibliographic citations from the National Library of Medicine.

TCMLARS, Traditional Chinese Medical Literature Analysis and Retrieval System. Produced by the Beijing Institute of Information and Library of the Academy of Traditional Chinese Medicine in Beijing. This resource is available in both Chinese and English. It has three databases:

    ACULARS (Acupuncture Literature Analysis and Retrieval System)
    TCM Database (Traditional Chinese Medical Literature Database)
    Chinese Material Medical Database

REFERENCES

Allais, G., D. Voghera, C. DeLorenzo, O. Mana, & C. Benedetto. (2000). Access to databases in complementary medicine. *Journal of Alternative and Complementary Medicine, 6*(3), 265–274.

Aust, G., & K. Fischer. (1997). Changes in body equilibrium response caused by breathing. A posturographic study with visual feedback. *Laryngo-Rhino-Otologie, 76*(10), 577–582.

Berger, B. G., & D. R. Owen. (1992). Mood alteration with yoga and swimming: Aerobic exercise may not be necessary. *Perceptual & Motor Skills, 75*(3), 1331–1343.

Corby, J. C., W. T. Roth, V. P. Zarcone, Jr., & B. S. Kopell. (1978). Psychophysiological correlates of the practice of tantric yoga meditation. *Archives of General Psychiatry, 35*(5), 571–577.

Domholt, E. (2000). *Physical Therapy Research: Principles and Applications.* (2nd ed.). Philadelphia: Saunders.

Dossey, L. (1995). How should alternative therapies be evaluated? *Alternative Therapies in Health and Medicine, 1*(2), 6–10, 79–85.

Eisenberg, D. (1997). Alternative medicine: Introduction and overview. Presented at Alternative Medicine. Implications for Clinical Practice; March 9–12, Boston, MA.

Federspil, G., & R. Vettor. (2000). Can scientific medicine incorporate alternative medicine? *Journal of Alternative and Complementary Medicine, 6*(3), 241–244.

Feuerstein, G., & L. Payne. (1999). *Yoga for Dummies.* Forest City, CA: IDG Books Worldwide.

Garfinkel, M. S., H. R. Schumacher, Jr., A. Husain, M. Levy, & R. A. Reshetar. (1994). Evaluation of a yoga-based regimen for treatment of osteoarthritis of the hands. *Journal of Rheumatology, 21*(12), 2341–2343.

Garfinkel, M. S., A. Singhal, W. A. Katz, D. A. Allan, R. Reshetar, & H. R. Schumacher, Jr. (1998). Yoga-based intervention for carpal tunnel syndrome: A randomized trial. *Journal of the American Medical Association, 280*(18), 1601–1603.

Gatchel, R. J., & A. M. Maddrey. (1998). Clinical outcome research in complementary and alternative medicine: An overview of experimental design and analysis. *Alternative Therapies in Health and Medicine, 4*(5), 36–42.

Helewa, A., & J. Walker. (2000). *Critical Evaluation of Research in Physical Rehabilitation.* Philadelphia: Saunders.

Iyengar, B. K. S. (1979). *Light on Yoga.* (Rev. ed.). New York: Schocken Books.

Jain, S. C., & B. Talukdar. (1993). Evaluation of yoga therapy programme for patients of bronchial asthma. *Singapore Medical Journal, 34*(4), 306–308.

Joshi L. N., V. D. Joshi, & L. V. Gokhale. (1992). Effect of short term 'Pranayama' practice on breathing rate and ventilatory functions of lung. *Indian Journal of Physiology & Pharmacology, 36*(2):105–108.

Kabat-Zinn, J. (1982). An outpatient program in behavioral medicine for chronic pain patients based on the practice of mindfulness meditation: Theoretical considerations and preliminary results. *General Hospital Psychiatry, 4*(1), 33–47.

Lasater, J. (1995). *Relax and Renew.* Berkeley, CA: Rodnell Press.

Linde, K. (2000). How to evaluate the effectiveness of complementary therapies. *Journal of Alternative and Complementary Medicine, 6*(3), 253–256.

Lukoff, D., D. Edwards, & M. Miller. (1998). The case study as a scientific method for researching alternative therapies. *Alternative Therapies in Health and Medicine, 4*(2), 44–52.

Makwana, K., N. Khirwadkar, & H. C. Gupta. (1988). Effect of short-term yoga practice on ventilatory function tests. *Indian Journal of Physiology & Pharmacology, 32*(3), 202–208.

McEwen, I. (Ed.). (1996). *Writing Case Reports: A How-To Manual for Clinicians.* Alexandria, VA: American Physical Therapy Association.

Minvaleev, R. S., A. A. Kuznetsov, & A. D. Nozdrachev. (1998). How does body posture affect the blood flow in parenchymatous organs? I. The liver. *Fiziologiia Cheloveka, 24*(4), 101–107.

Minvaleev, R. S., A. A. Kuznetsov, & A. D. Nozdrachev. (1999). How does body posture affect the blood flow in the parenchymatous organs? II. The kidneys. *Fiziologiia Cheloveka, 25*(2), 92–98.

NCCAM. (2001). [online]. Major domains of complementary and alternative therapies. NCCAM available www.nccam.nih.gov.

Peng, C. K., J. E. Mietus, Y. Liu, G. Khalsa, P. S. Douglas, H. Benson, & A. L. Goldberg. (1999). Exaggerated heart rate oscillations during two meditation techniques. *International Journal of Cardiology, 70*(2), 101–107.

Portney, L. G., & M. P. Watkins. (2000). *Foundations for Clinical Research: Applications to Practice.* (2nd ed.). Upper Saddle River, NJ: Prentice Hall Health.

Rai, L., & K. Ram. (1993). Energy expenditure and ventilatory responses during virasana-a yogic standing posture. *Indian Journal of Physiology & Pharmacology, 37*(1), 45–50.

Sackett, D. L., S. E. Straus, W. S. Richardson, W. Rosenberg, & R. B. Haynes. (2000). *Evidence-Based Medicine: How to Practice and Teach EBM.* (2nd ed.). London: Churchill Livingstone.

Savic, K., D. Pfau, S. Skoric, & J. Pfau. (1990). The effect of Hatha yoga on poor posture in children and the psychophysiologic condition in adults. *Medicinski Pregled, 43*(5–6), 268–272.

Shannahoff-Khalsa, D. S., & L. R. Beckett. (1996). Clinical case report: Efficacy of yogic techniques in the treatment of obsessive compulsive disorders. *International Journal of Neuroscience, 85*(1–2), 1–17.

Smith, J. C., A. Amutio, J. P. Anderson, & L. A. Aria. (1996). Relaxation: Mapping an uncharted world. *Biofeedback & Self Regulation, 21*(1), 63–90.

Stanescu, D. C., B. Nemery, C. Veriter, & C. Marechal. (1981). Pattern of breathing and ventilatory response to CO2 in subjects practicing hatha-yoga. *Journal of Applied Physiology: Respiratory, Environmental & Exercise Physiology, 51*(6), 1625–1629.

Telles, S., & T. Desiraju. (1991). Oxygen consumption during pranayamic type of very slow-rate breathing. *Indian Journal of Medical Research, 94,* 357–363.

Vedanthan, P. K., L. N. Kesavalu, K. C. Murthy, K. Duvall, M. J. Hall, S. Baker, & S. Nagarathna. (1998). Clinical study of yoga techniques in university students with asthma: A controlled study. *Allergy & Asthma Proceedings, 19*(1), 3–9.

Wood, C. (1993). Mood change and perceptions of vitality: A comparison of the effects of relaxation, visualization and yoga. *Journal of the Royal Society of Medicine, 86*(5), 254–258.

Zhang, J. Z., J. Zhao, & Q. N. He. (1988). EEG findings during special psychical state (Qi gong state) by means of compressed spectral array and topographic mapping. *Computers in Biology & Medicine, 18*(6), 455–463.

6

Creating an Integrative Clinic

Larry Kopelman

CHAPTER OBJECTIVES

- Identify key market issues in the creation of an integrated clinic.
- Identify options in planning programs and services for an integrated clinic.
- Understand the importance of accreditation and standards for the integrative clinic.
- Understand physical plant issues related to the integrative clinic.
- Understand some issues of funding the integrative clinic.

Integrative medicine practice emphasizes human, social, and spiritual factors in the treatment of people's problems (NIH, 1998). In clinical medicine, the principle of integration requires that the provider integrate into the care "all that is safe and effective" without subservience to one or more schools of medical thought (Ali, 1998a, p. 77). Many people see an opportunity in the development of a center that will meet the demands of the emerging health care marketplace, helping clients to take an active role in their health. As therapists who are "hands on," provide many forms of therapies, are trained in the traditional medical model, and are accepted team members in health care, physical and occupational therapists have a role in the delivery of integrated health care.

Developing a Plan

The development of an integrative practice requires a careful plan. The literature is filled with information that suggests there are demands for integrative services. To test these assumptions, a needs assessment is essential. Allen (1996) states that therapists must know their customers, know their competition, and know themselves through a comprehensive needs assessment.

Integrative health care involves more than substituting an herb for a drug; rather, it is a process that appreciates the complexity of the problems clients face daily. To create an integrative clinic, a therapist needs to develop a plan which takes into account the customer, the competition, and the therapist's own resources. Program development should naturally flow from this information.

Many factors potentially enhance the integrative clinic. Issues such as accreditation and maintenance of standards for the integrative practitioner will be important to the credibility of the practice. A cohesive treatment team can use integrative protocols (the use of a combination of therapies without subservience to one school of thought to address client needs, for example) to achieve positive outcomes. The physical plant, including auditory, visual, and aesthetic concerns, should be designed as a healing environment.

Customers

Customers include clients, other health care providers (such as referral sources), and payers (Allen, 1996). Therapists will need to know the general demographic profile of area residents, all of whom are potential clients. Socioeconomic trends and significant variances in demographics (e.g., a large community of retirees) as well as health and illness trends should be noted. This includes what services people in the community perceive themselves as needing and whether there are other services that the community needs also.

Gathering Information

Host an informal evening providing information about integrative medicine. Interacting with attendees, who should include current clients, potential future clients, and colleagues, allows you to identify trends in the community. These meetings can create potential valuable referral resources and should be held several times a year.

Informal research in the community will also help to identify needs and other service providers. Stop into the local health food store and ask what alternative and complementary services are provided in the community. Look at the bulletin boards in community areas regularly. Check out the local health newsletters and adult continuing education courses as well as health and fitness centers. Identify holistic organizations in the community and obtain membership lists. Go to local health fairs and talk to the vendors and participants. These are resources to learn not only about the competition (because they may also be advertising), but also about providers with whom you could partner to provide services. Are services you can provide provided by your competition? Are these providers your competition, or are services you can provide an addition to what is already in the community?

Therapists need to consider *other health care providers* and their needs to maintain professional relationships and generate further referrals. Respecting professional boundaries, communication, and client satisfaction may all be of concern to other health care providers (Allen, 1996).

Physicians have traditionally been an important source of referrals for therapists. Thus it is important to assess the needs of physicians and to do a physician readiness assessment to determine the degree to which physician referrals can be anticipated (Black, 1998; Freshley, 2000). Determine physicians' exposure to and knowledge about CAM strategies and the value of integrating traditional and alternative therapies (Eisenberg et al., 2000). Are clients discussing their desire to receive complementary and alternative therapies, and if so, how are physicians responding? Are they making referrals for this, and to whom? What information would be useful to the physicians to better understand the value of integrative medicine either as part of their practice or as a referral? Is there an interest in adding mid-level providers to their existing practice (if this is legally possible in the potential practice state), or would they prefer to utilize outside sources (Panel on Definition and Description, 1997)?

Another group of customers are the people who *pay* for services. Possible payers include employers, insurance companies, and in the case of self-pay services, clients. Therapists must determine what payers are willing to pay for a service and whether payers are ready to pay for holistic services. Identify opportunities for collaboration to meet the needs of employers and insurance companies by contacting them to discuss their needs. Determine what services are desired and reimbursable by insurance companies, HMOs, prospective payment organizations, and employers. Regardless of who is paying for the service, therapists need to be price-sensitive in the delivery of care.

Therapists also need to determine the future need for such services. What is the payer's perception of holistic practices? How does the insurer usually respond to the needs of its clients? Does the payer see the advantages of CAM, possibly as a market niche differentiation and in the cost-effective management of chronic disease? Some insurance companies have developed prevention models that successfully contain costs. For example, Highmark Blue Cross of Pennsylvania has recovered $9,000 per patient while paying $3,000 for added preventive services (Silberman, 2000).

Yourself

The development of any new therapy service cannot occur without careful consideration of the therapist's own resources. Therapists need to determine not only their level of professional skill and knowledge, but also their level of business and organizational skill as well as available time and money (Allen, 1996). What skills does the therapist have that can be utilized? What training is needed to develop further skills? These resources then need to be compared to the needs of the customer to determine how skills can be used to meet the needs of the community.

Program Development

Program development must flow from analysis of potential customers, the competition, and the therapist's own resources. Programs can be developed along a number of different lines, such as disease management, health categories, modalities and methods, gender, age groups, or a combination of these.

Disease management programs address health issues from either a client or caregiver perspective. Programs to manage or prevent such problems as pain, cancer, and back injuries (called *back schools*) can be developed.

Modality-specific and method-specific programs can also be developed. For example, recent literature has identified Qi Gong (Wu, 1999) and T'ai Chi (Bottomley, 2000; Chen & Snyder, 1999; Kirstens, Dietz, & Hwang, 1991) as benefiting clients in the rehabilitation setting (Chen & Snyder, 1999; Massey & Perlman, 1998; Schaller, 1996). Any modality identified as efficacious can be considered. Yoga (Taylor & Majundmar, 2000) and biofeedback (Myers, 2000; Rogers, 2001) are modalities that have applications in rehabilitation and may be incorporated into programs for stress management or altering muscle function. Pulsed magnetic fields, a relatively new modality classified as an exogenous energy therapy, can be used for treatment of stress incontinence, pain management, and wound healing (Adams 1998; Galloway, 1988; Valbona, 1997; Weintraub 1998).

Gender-specific services for groups of clients, such as those with osteoporosis, post-menopausal symptoms, or post partum issues, are an option. Age-specific services, such as fall prevention/balance and coordination programs for older adults, may be developed by combining environmental assessment with techniques such as T'ai Chi. Another approach would be to develop a healthy lifestyle program. Such services could include nutritional counseling and acupuncture for wellness (Bland, 1995) as well as more traditional services typically provided by therapists, such as addressing functional impairments or muscle strengthening. Other bodywork may add value to your program and may include, for example, massage therapy (Birk et al., 2000; Preyde, 2000; Smith et al., 1999), Feldenkrais (Stephens, 2000; Wildman, Stephens, & Aum, 2000), yoga (Taylor & Majundmar, 2000; Quigley & Dean, 2000) or rolfing (Deutsch et al., 2000).

Relaxation and stress management programs could be developed to address disease management. Mind-body services may be provided for stress management and healthy lifestyle programs, using cognitive biofeedback, guided imagery, neurolinguistic programming (Dilts, 1983; Dilts et al., 1980), hypnotherapy (Rogers, 2001; Saichek, 2000), music therapy (McCraty et al., 1998), meditation, or prayer (Luskin, 1998). Address all of the main areas (disease and health management, body, mind, and spirit work), and a complete program will emerge (Astin et al., 1999; Syrjala, 1999).

Depending on available resources, specific products and services may be provided either as additional services or as "added values"—services clients can receive at no added charge.

Program development should include consideration of possible joint ventures or partnerships with other entities. The therapist must determine whether he or she can be the sole provider of integrative services or whether an association should be developed with an entity that offers these services. Therapists, for example, may want to be the resource for aquatic therapy, cardiovascular health, orthopedics, pain management, stress management, or senior care either alone or with other health care practitioners. Partnerships can be developed between health care practitioners or between therapists and existing organizations such as local health care institutions, hospitals, community service organizations, YMCAs, community centers, or senior centers.

Accreditation

In today's competitive environment every healthcare facility must look for survival strategies for the new century. A center that is accredited and offers both high tech and high "touch" therapy may be the strongest survivor and flourish in meeting the demands of the population.

Accreditation is synonymous with quality assurance, and measures the clinical cost effectiveness and therapy product to a set standard (American Academy of Pain Management, 1999). Accreditation means compliance with peer review standards established by practitioners to represent quality treatment.

Accreditation is typically a one- to two-day process in which evaluators survey all of the aspects of the delivery of care at the integrative facility. This process is an excellent starting point in the planning and execution of survival strategies. Also, this gives a clinic the external recognition that enhances third-party reimbursement and facilitates risk management and quality assurance programs. HMOs, public funding such as Medicare, and other insurance providers see accreditation as important. Accreditation is necessary for satisfaction of licensure requirements in some states and for satisfaction for some managed care contracts.

Standards for the Integrative Practitioner

As third-party payers establish standards, issues such as educational requirements, credentialing and licensing standards, and scope of practice are becoming important for the integrative clinic. While many of the details below apply equally to the complementary and traditional therapist, they are vital to the integrative practice to prevent liability and fraud issues, which can be devastating to a practice. All of these procedures should be performed whether the provider is an employee or under a contractual arrangement.

Credentialing should be a formal procedure with the following components: all job descriptions should clearly define specific requirements for minimum education, experience, and training; and a scope of practice and competencies, if not already defined by laws governing the state, municipality or local government, should be described. Other information to be kept on file includes performance goals, medical record filing and billing practices, and other documentation requirements specific to the clinic.

Protocols for employment should be established in the application process with a signed attestation to verify completeness and correctness of the information provided, release from liability, and release of information as it pertains to the applicant. Verify current malpractice insurance is in place and covers practitioners for their occupations. Review thoroughly any history of malpractice settlements and awards, cases pending, denial of or cancellation of malpractice, and refusal to issue a license or permit. Check for discharge from other institutions and for felony conviction by any state, federal, or local municipality.

It is very important to verify educational training and practice requirements of the alternative practitioner. For example, some practitioners must practice under the supervision of another licensed practitioner. Check for board certifications. Obtain written evidence of licensure and current registrations. Review work history for 3 to 5 years.

Check professional references (three) provided by non-family members. A procedure should be in place to notify the applicant in writing that the review will proceed and to make a recommendation for approval to hire or contract, deferral pending further credentialing procedures or not accepting the applicant. Periodically review the verification of licensure, insurance, and credentialing.

Accreditation provides public confidence by demonstrating an organizational commitment to quality client care, which can increase a program's competitive edge in the marketplace. Accreditation also promotes professional improvement by recognizing and encouraging quality.

The Integrative Team

Continuous care from a single physician has become increasingly rare: Many practitioners are specialists supported by a variety of skilled personnel and medical services, often fragmented by disease categories and methods of payment (Kennedy, 1972). Each discipline tends to have its own perspective on client care and to function autonomously (Kennedy, 1972). While there is some information-sharing and cooperation, there is little care coordinated between the interdisciplinary providers. Each provider operates independently and is only responsible for a small portion of what may be called "total care" of the client. Therefore, many clients receive excellent care but still have unmet needs.

Primary caregivers currently have most of the power and act as gatekeepers for specialists. The growth of managed care in the United States has assured us of this model. It has been theorized that at least half of the money to be spent on clients will be on prevention with the emphasis on health, not disease. This shift in paradigm should cause a delegation of responsibilities of tasks from physicians to nurses, therapists, and other health professionals (Kaiser, 2000). Physicians will still be active but not necessarily the leaders of the team. A social worker or nurse may be the coordinator of care or team leader in an interdisciplinary team.

Ideally, the client, primary care practitioner, and integrative health care team members collaboratively develop a plan to address the integrative health care needs of the client. Cohesion among team members is crucial for success of this model. Overlapping roles, status perceptions, and differences in viewpoints may lead to interprofessional conflict among the team members, and should be managed to minimize problems. The team of integrative practitioners must place self-interest and egos second to the interest of the client.

Client Selection and Evaluation

The most important element of the criteria for selection is client motivation and the ability to cooperate with the program. The physiological determinants of the injury, illness, and disease are evaluated from an integrated perspective through a comprehensive team approach. Risks and cause of the symptoms, possible complications, and degree of impairment or disability are all identified. The effect of the identified problem on the client's quality of life, reduction in physical activity, changes in occupational performance, participation in sport or social function, dependence or independence in ADL, effects on psychosocial status, presence of comorbid states, financial resources, history, secondary gain provided by the injury or illness, and client commitment to time and program participation are evaluated as well.

In a comprehensive program, an appropriate team member must evaluate each of the body's systems to establish a framework for the integrative health plan. Anatomy and physiology of the nervous system, both central and peripheral, as well as cognition and interrelationships between the psycho- and neuroimmune systems must be evaluated. The structure and function of the musculoskeletal system through appropriate tests and measurements add

Table 6–1 Patient Assessment

A. Obtain Comprehensive History
  1. Observe verbal and nonverbal behaviors
  2. Identify terms used to define complaints, intensity, frequency, location, duration, character, and related factors
  3. Obtain chief complaint
  4. Review existing records, test results, and other pertinent information
  5. Evaluate medications and medication behaviors
  6. Review nutritional supplementation
  7. Obtain detailed bio-psycho-social history
      a. Role of learning in pain experience
      b. Influence of life events/experience on pain behavior or other health problem
      c. Role of home environment, job, and family dynamics associated with problems presented
      d. Economic and policy incentives/disincentives
      e. Accident-related pain or dysfunction
      f. Cultural influences on behaviors
      g. Stress assessment cycles
      h. Spiritual and religious influences on behaviors
      i. Influences of growth/development and life stages
      j. Neurolinguistics, language barriers
      k. Association between nutrition and stress, health, pain, and disease
      l. Association of habits such as alcohol, smoking, substance abuse, overeating, etc.
      m. Quality of life, relationships, sexuality, etc.
      n. Secondary gain
B. Conduct Thorough Physical Assessment/Examination
  1. General and organ-specific
  2. Psychological
  3. Cognitive, emotional, body mechanics, and posture/gait
C. Formulate Preliminary Diagnosis(es)/Impression(s)
  1. Objective vs. subjective
  2. Classify ICD-(10)
  3. DSM-IV
  4. Classify pain: acute, subacute, recurrent, chronic, nonmalignant, malignant, somatic, visceral, atypical, sympathetically mediated, neurological, muscular, vascular, odontogenic
D. Obtain Diagnostic Data as Necessary
  1. Laboratory tests
  2. Imaging and radiographic findings
  3. Electrodiagnostic tests
  4. Psychological inventories/tests, psychometric tests, and other tests such as ultrasound, thermography, microscopy
  5. Interdisciplinary consultations
  6. Reevaluate diagnosis

information for a working clinical diagnosis. Functional activities of posture, gait, and movement offer important information about the client's status. See Table 6–1 for an example of a patient assessment.

Program Management

Careful attention to organization will promote successful client care interventions. The number of team members and their professional backgrounds will vary considerably, but they must speak a common language—that of the integrative provider. It is not necessary for each member of the team to be involved with every client; however, the facility draws its strength from the collective knowledge of the multidisciplinary team. Expertise, skills, and clinical experience are necessary to achieve the desired goals of the clinic, and team communication and interaction is vital to its survival.

While the owner or operator of a small facility may wear several organizational "hats," a large facility must have a director of operations. This person should have experience in the day-to-day running of the facility and need not be a health care provider. The administrator oversees the business aspects and coordinates the efforts of the professional health care providers and the nontechnical staff. Each area must have trained support staff based on need and governmental guidelines and regulations. Requirements of state, city, and federal laws must be adhered to. The administrator is the liaison with the medical staff, owners, and operators of the facility, who may or may not be the same people in all cases.

Every staff member should be familiar with the mission statement and philosophy of the organization and be able to participate in meeting those goals and objectives. The success of the integrative clinic, large or small, depends on how closely it adheres to its mission statement and policies and procedures.

Integrative Protocols

Integrative protocols consist of care to the client utilizing all modalities that are safe and effective without subservience to one or more schools of medical thought (Ali, 1998). Integrative protocols, which can produce inspiring outcomes, may be developed and administered by one or more providers and may include a combination of therapies, such as nutritional therapies, herbals, botanical medicine, acupuncture, physical medicine, and spiritual work. The integrative team of providers may include a variety of professionals such as medical doctors, osteopaths, physician's assistants, nurses, dentists, chiropractors, massage therapists, physical and occupational therapists, and naturopaths.

A classic example of an integrative protocol would be for a client with cardiovascular disease, which is characterized by organ dysregulation and oxidative stress influenced often by lifestyle stressors, lack of physical fitness, and poor nutritional choices. The program will emphasize improvement of the client's circulatory system, and prevention of oxidative coagulopathy, including self-regulation for stress control, optimal food choices to prevent sugar overload and hyperinsulinism, appropriate supplementation of antioxidants and herbal supplements to prevent further damage to the organs, noncompetitive exercise, and chelation therapy. Special and conventional diagnostic methods will be utilized to assess the client. Dark field and phase contrast microscopy can help determine the cellular and tissue ecologic relationships (Ali and Ali, 1997). Biological terrain analysis can help the team determine metabolic shifts and tissue utilization of the oxidative processes (Yanick, 2000); Contact Regulation Thermography (CRT) or Digital Infrared Thermal Imaging (DITI) utilizing nonionizioning infrared technology can be used to assess soft tissue, vascular, and sympathetic regulation (Takahashi, Takahashi, & Moriya, 1994). Heart rate variability studies can identify the status of the sympathetic and parasympathetic nervous system and monitor the client's response to the therapeutic interventions (del Paso, 1999; Parides, 1998; Yanick, 2000).

The matrix model is a case management model of integrative service delivery. Clients will be followed by a case manager who is versed in the full spectrum of integrated services and who identifies required services. The case manager may well utilize various practitioners to intercede in the case and assist with the care and education of the client. Therapists, nurses, certified nutritional counselors, psychological counselors, or spiritual advisors all can have an important role in the outcome.

The Integrative Facility

The physical plant should be part of the healing process (Ridenour, 2000). Physical structures have an effect on consciousness and may provoke a healing response. Light, shapes, color, and soothing sounds can be very therapeutic. Natural light, textures, and inspiring art can offer an environment to transform oneself. And a therapeutic environment not only benefits clients but also staff, who should be more productive and healthier. The goal is to design space that heals.

Aesthetics are an important aspect of healing environments (Polkinghorn, 2000). Open space, light, and sound must be considered not only from the aspect of ergonomics for employees but also as factors that have a therapeutic effect. Each treatment room may have an aromatherapy diffuser to give choices for therapy for specific conditions (Buckle 1997; Schnaubelt, 1998). These can be strategically placed to provide a relaxing aroma and also to combat offensive aromas such as chlorine in the pool area or sweating from clients exercising. Live plants can be used throughout the center to enhance energy and balance as well as to add oxygen to the environment.

Auditory Aspects of the Clinic

The healing effect of music and sound is well researched and new technology has been developed that allows full spectrum three-dimensional sound (Burns et al., 2001). A sound system for the central area and each room may be provided, and tapes can be utilized for psychoacoustics therapy (see "Resources") to enhance relaxation and stress reduction—some of the most prevalent symptoms presented by clients, their families, and caregivers. Recent studies have shown a significant effect in modulation of neuroendocrine-immune parameters in healthy subjects through use of these tools (Bittman et al., 2001). The principles of resonance, rhythm, melody, harmony, pitches, timbre, and sound energy show promise as a therapeutic tool as well (Andrews, 1996; Patrick, 1999) because the concepts of modern harmonics work on the physical and spiritual levels (Khalsa & Stauth, 1999; McCraty et al.,

1998; Rosch, 1999). These modalities offer a fresh approach to working with clients by effecting energetic centers in the body through ancient methods and practices.

Every cell in the body is a sound resonator and is connected to other cells not only by direct contact but also through this resonation of sound vibrations. It is theorized that auditory stimulation produces therapeutic benefits by transferring energy to and through cells, tissues, and organs. Therapists know that through manual vibratory techniques, such as Trager, the neuromuscular system can be influenced to reorganize (Juahn, 1987). Listening to a piece of music in a specific key has effects on the chakra centers that in turn influence the body, mind, and spirit (Tiller, 1997).

At Healthworks of Staten Island, various sounds and tones are utilized with clients. Audiotapes are selected for specific quality of tone so as to have an effect on a physiological system. For example, low deep tones are used when clients report feeling stressed and the need to relax. While the client uses a modality, such as moist heat or electric stimulation, an audiotape is played to enhance the effect of the other modalities. Often, background noise or the sound of water from a stream or ocean waves crashing on the beach can be used. While there is a lack of research demonstrating the efficacy of using specific sounds with certain conditions, clients tell therapists that there is a very beneficial effect to the use of sound—that they are able to totally relax and be "in touch" with their body. The author has found this most useful with chronic pain clients. Often, after several sessions of pairing the sound with a modality, the modality can be discontinued as the use of the sound alone produces a pain-free state. Clients are then able to use these sounds, either in the clinic or at home, to reduce pain.

Visual Aspects of the Clinic

Lighting must be addressed not only for compliance with ADA and OSHA guidelines for ergonomic work practices but as a therapeutic tool (Sol & Foster, 1992; Mac Leod, 1995). Individual treatment rooms should have rheostat controls to dim the lights and enhance control of the environment.

In selected rooms, full-color spectrum should be used to enhance healing (Ott, 1985). The entire spectrum of natural sunlight is essential for optimal functioning of all living cells in plants, animals, and humans (Olzewski & Breiling, 1996). Full-spectrum fluorescent lighting is the closest approximation to natural sunlight and has been found to balance hormones and neuroendocrine functioning (Olzewski & Breiling, 1996).

Mandel discovered that red, orange, and yellow tend to stimulate or raise energy, while green, blue, and violet tend to sedate or detoxify energy (Cousins, 1996; Dinshah, 1997; Luscher, 1969). Choice of room color should follow from these effects.

Funding

Financial feasibility remains an issue to contend with, despite the fact that 58 percent of the public is paying for CAM therapies out of pocket and insurance carriers are beginning to experiment with coverage of CAM (Biedess, 2000).

How can a team of providers integrate the variety of services needed for a client with integrative protocols and make it cost effective for the client and profitable for the providers? Two of the largest centers in New York City were closed in 2000 due to multimillion dollar losses. Another integrative group, American Whole Health, closed many of its centers, with only a few in Chicago still operating and profitable (Nachman-Hunt, 2000). Only a handful of large complementary and alternative clinics have survived at press time (Biedess, 2000; Nachman-Hunt, 2000).

Most successful providers who are involved in CAM have the client self-pay (Testa, 1999). Perhaps that is still the best model, as costs escalate when the insurance industry or the government gets involved with direct client care. Client care fees, contracts, consulting fees, products, grants, and sales of nutraceuticals all can generate the income for the center.

Summary

Therapists have many options in integrative practice, ranging from practicing alone and independently to partnering with other health care professionals to developing an integrative center of health care.

Therapists must meet the demands of the population by being proactive in delivery of integrative therapies. As professionals, therapists must see that clients are treated with safe and evidence-based treatment by credentialed people, protecting both the public and their own profession. And they must teach colleagues that there are valid approaches to health care that should be integrated into traditional settings to create new environments for healing.

STUDY PROJECT

Interview 5 to 10 people, including both consumers and health care providers, about CAM, and plan an integrative clinic.

Be sure to identify the following:

- ◆ A geographic area of service
- ◆ A client population
- ◆ Health care needs, both served and underserved
- ◆ The needs of referral sources and payers
- ◆ Services that can be provided: Discuss who will provide them. What are the licensing and practice issues of these personnel? Are there scope of practice limitations to be aware of?
- ◆ Physical plant plan: What major areas of concern will need to be addressed?
- ◆ Possible sources of funding.

RESOURCES

AAIM American Association of Integrative
    Medicine
2750 East Sunshine
Springfield, Missouri 65804
(417) 881-9995
www.aaimedicine.com

American Music Therapy Association
8455 Colesville Road, Suite 1000
Silver Springs, MD 20910
(301) 589-3300
www.musictherapy.org

REFERENCES

Adams, F. (1998). Magnetic neuromedicine: An attractive promise. *American Journal of Pain, 8*(1), 17–18.

Ali, M. (1998a). Seven core principles of integrative medicine. *Journal of Integrative Medicine, 2*(2), 77–81.

Ali, M. (1998b). The principles and practice of medicine. *Journal of Integrative Medicine, 3*(7), 74–81.

Ali, M., & O. Ali. (1997). AA oxidopathy: The core pathogenitic mechanism ischemic heart disease, Part 1. *Journal of Integrative Medicine, 1,* 6–12.

Allen, D. W. (1996). Finding your place in the integrated delivery system. In J. Davis, and M. A. Freeman. *Marketing for Therapists: A Handbook for Success in Managed Care.* San Francisco, CA: Josey-Bass.

American Academy of Pain Management. Pain, Program Accreditation, 1999.

Andrews, T. (1996). *The Healers Manual: A Beginners Guide to Vibrational Therapies.* St. Paul, MN: Llewellyn.

Astin, J., J. Astin, S. L. Shapiro, R. A. Lee, & D. H. Shapiro. (1999, Mar.). The construct of control in mind-body medicine: Implications for health care. *Alternative Therapies, 5*(2), 42–47.

Biedess, P. (2000). *Operational Issues, Issues with Managed Care and Insurance Products.* Kaiser Institute for Integrative Medicine, Santa Fe, New Mexico.

Birk, T. J., A. McGrady, R. D. MacArthur, & S. Khuderet. (2000). The effects of massage therapy in combination with other complementary therapies on immune system measures and quality of life in human immunodeficiency virus. *Journal of Alternative and Complementary Medicine, 6*(5), 405–414.

Bittman, B., L. Berk, D. Felton, J. Westengard, C. Simonton, & J. Pappas. (2001, Jan.) Composite effects of group drumming music therapy on modulation of neuroendocrine-immune parameters in normal subjects. *Alternative Therapies, 7*(1), 38–47.

Black, C. (1998). Getting ahead of the competition: Strategies to market your rehab services for workers compensation referrals. *Rehab Management,* 50–55.

Bland, J. S., E. Barranger, R. G. Reedy, & K. Bland. (1995). A medical food-supplementation detoxification program in the management of chronic health problems. *Alternative Therapies in Health and Medicine, 1*(5), 62–71.

Bottomley, J. (2000). The use of Tai Chi as a movement modality in orthopedics. *Orthopaedic Physical Therapy Clinics of North America, 9*(3), 361–373.

Buckle, J. (1997). *Clinical Aromatherapy in Nursing.* Bristol, Great Britain: J.W. Arrowsmith.

Burns, S., M. Harbuz, F. Hucklebridge, & L. Bunt. (2001, Jan.). A pilot study into the therapeutic effects of music therapy at a cancer help center. *Alternative Therapies, 7*(1), 48–56.

Charnes, M. P., & L. J. Tewksbury. (1993). *Collaborative Management in Health Care.* San Francisco, CA: Jossey-Bass.

Chen, K. M., & M. Snyder. (1999, Sept.). A researched-based use of Tai Chi/movement therapy as a nursing intervention. *Journal of Holistic Nursing, 17*(3), 267–279.

Cousins, G. (1989). *Head First.* New York: Penguin Books.

del Paso, R. (1999, Mar.). A biofeedback system of barroreceptor cardiac reflex sensitivity. *Applied Psychophysiological Biofeedback, 24*(1), 67–77.

Deutsch, J., L. Derr, P. Judd, & B. Reuven. (2000, Sept.). Treatment of chronic pain through the use of structural integration (rolfing). *Orthopaedic Physical Therapy Clinics of North America, 9*(3), 411–425.

Dilts, R. (1983). *Applications of Neuro-Linguistic Programing.* Capitola, CA: Meta Publications.

Dilts, R., J. Grindler, R. Bandler, & J. DeLozier. (1980). *Neuro-Linguistic Programing Vol 1: The Study of the Structure of Subjective Experience.* Capitola, CA: Meta Publications.

Dinshah, D. (1997). *Let There Be Light.* 4th ed., Malaga, NJ: Dinshah Health Society.

Eisenberg, D., R. B. Davis, S. L. Ettner, S. Appel, S. Wilkey, M. VanRompay, & R. C. Kessles. (2000). Trends in alternative medicine use in the United States 1990–1997: Results of a follow-up national survey. In P. Fontanarosa (Ed.), *Alternative Medicine: An Objective Assessment*. Chicago, IL: American Medical Association.

Freshly, C. (2000). Developing a business plan. Kaiser Institute for Integrative Medicine.

Flynn, J. (2000). Management Technology, Administration class notes. Capital University of Integrative Medicine.

Galloway, N., R. El-Galley, R. Appell, H. Russell, & S. Carlan. (1988). Multicenter trial: Extra corporeal magnetic innervation (ExMI) for the treatment of stress incontinence. Presented at the June meeting of the International Continence Society, WHO, Monaco.

Gerber, R. (2000). *Vibrational Medicine for the 21st Century*. New York: Harper Collins.

Giandes, C., & D. I. Rosenthal. (1999, Mar.). Using hypnosis to accelerate the healing of bone fractures: A randomized controlled pilot study. *Alternative Therapies, 5*(2), 67–75.

Hartley, L. (1996). Make those blues go away: The effect of light on seasonal affective disorder and premenstrual syndrome. In J. Lieberman & B. Breiling (Eds.), *Light Years Ahead: The Illustrated Guide to Full Spectrum Light in Mind-Body Healing*. Berkley, CA: Celestial Arts.

Horowitz, S. (2000, Dec.). Update on magnet therapy: Drug-free pain relief, wound healing and immune support. *Complementary Therapies, 6*, 325–336.

Juahn, D. (1987). The Trager approach. *The Trager Journal, 2*(7), 1–3.

Kaiser, L. (2000). Changing Paradigms, 1971–1999. Kaiser Institute for Integrative Medicine.

Kaiser, L. (2000). Living on the Edge. Symposium conducted at the meeting of the Kaiser Foundation, Santa Fe, New Mexico.

Kennedy, E. M. (1972). *In Critical Condition: The Crises in America's Health Care*. New York: Praeger.

Khalsa, S., & C. Stauth. (1999). *The Pain Cure*. New York: Warner Books.

Kirstens, A. E., F. Dietz, & S. M. Hwang. (1991, June). Evaluating the safety and potential use of a weight-bearing exercise, Tai Chi Chuan, for rheumatoid arthritis patients. *American Journal of Medical Rehabilitation, 70*(3), 136–141.

Luscher, M. (1969). *The Luscher Color Test*. New York: Random House.

Luskin, F. M., K. Newell, M. Griffith, M. Holmes, S. Telles, F. F. Marvasti, K. Pelletier, & W. Haskell. (1998, May). A review of mind-body therapies in the treatment of cardiovascular disease, part 1: Implications for the elderly. *Alternative Therapies, 4*(3), 46–52.

Mac Leod, D. (1995). *The Ergonomics Edge: Improving Safety, Quality and Productivity*. New York: Van Nostrand Reinhold.

Man, D., & M. Markov. (1998). Effect of permanent magnetic field on postoperative pain and wound healing in plastic surgery. Aesthetic and Plastic Surgery and Laser Center, Mount Sinai Medical Center, NY. The Second World Congress on Electricity and Magnetism in Biology and Medicine, June 8–13, Bologna, Italy.

Markoll, R., & S. Kornhauser. (1999, June). Pulsed signal therapy: Powerful pain relief and promising potential. *American Journal of Electromedicine*, 1–6.

Massey, P., D. K. Massey, & G. M. Kislinger. (1988, Apr.). Martial arts for herniated discs and chronic pain. *Alternative and Complementary Therapies*, 128–133.

Massey, P., & A. Perlman. (1999, May). Lasting resolution of chronic thoracic neuritis using martial-arts-based physical therapy. *Alternative Therapies, 5*(3), 103–104.

Matterson, R. (2000, Apr./May). Designing our future. *Rehab Management*, 18–19.

Micozzi, M. (2000). Forward: Complementary medicine. *Orthopaedic Physical Therapy Clinics of North America, 9*(3), xi.

Myers, H. (2000). *Recent Advances in EMG Monitoring*. Montreal, Canada: Thought Technology.

McCraty, R., R. Barrios-Chaplin, M. Atkinson, & D. Tomasino. (1998, Jan.). The effects of different types of music on mood, tension and mental clarity. *Alternative Therapies, 4*(1), 75–84.

Nachman-Hunt, N. (2000, Nov./Dec.). Can complementary healthcare clinics make IT? *Natural Business Lohas Journal,* 52–54.

Nassaer, M., & B. W. Xiu. (1994). *Laser Acupuncture: Introductory Textbook for Treatment of Pain, Paralysis, Spasticity and Other Disorders.* Boston, MA: Boston Chinese Medicine.

NIH Office of Alternative Medicine Clearinghouse. (1998). Frequently Asked Questions, 1.

Olzewski, D., & B. Breiling. (1996). Getting into light: The use of phototherapy in everyday life. In J. Lieberman & B. Breiling (Eds.), *Light Years Ahead: The Illustrated Guide to Full Spectrum and Colored Light in Mind-Body Healing.* Berkeley, CA: Celestial Arts.

Ott, J. N. (1985). Color and light: Their effects on plants, animals and people. *The International Journal of Biosocial Research, 7*(1), 7–10.

Parides, Michael. (1998). A comparison of nerve express and chronos algorithms. Research Holter Laboratory, College of Physicians and Surgeons of Columbia University, 1–6.

Panel on Definition and Description. (1997). CAM Research Methodology Conference, April 1995, "Defining and Describing Complementary and Alternative Medicine." *Alternative Therapies, 3*(2), 49–57.

Patrick, G. (1999, Mar./Apr.). The effects of vibroacoustic music on symptom reduction. *IEEE Engineering in Medicine and Biology,* 97–100.

Pellitier, K. R., A. Marie, M. Krasner, & W. Haskell. (1997). Current trends in the integration and reimbursement of complementary and alternative medicine by managed care, insurance providers and hospital providers. *American Journal of Health Promotion, 12*(2), 112–123.

Polkinghorn, D. (2000). Healing design for integrative medicine. Kaiser Institute for Integrative Medicine, Edwards, Colorado.

Preyde, M. (2000, June 27). Effectiveness of massage therapy for subacute low-back pain: A randomized controlled trial. *Canadian Medical Association Journal, 162*(13), 1815–1820.

Quigley, D., & C. Dean. (2000). Yoga. In D. Novey (Ed.), *Physician's Complete Reference to Complementary and Alternative Medicine.* St. Louis: Mosby.

Ridenour, A. (2000). Designing a Healing Clinical Office Environment. In M. S. Micozzi (Ed.), *Current Review of Complementary Medicine.* Philadelphia: Current Medicine.

Rogers, D. (2001). Mind-body interventions. In M. Micozzi (Ed.), *Fundamentals of Complementary and Alternative Medicine* (2nd ed.). New York: Churchill Livingstone.

Rosch, P. (1999). Acupuncture and music. *The Newsletter of the American Institute of Stress, 4, 7.*

Saichek, K. (2000). Hypnotherapy. In D. Novey (Ed.), *Physician's Complete Reference to Complementary and Alternative Medicine.* St. Louis: Mosby.

Schaller, K. J. (1996, Oct.). Tai Chi Chih: An exercise option for older adults. *Journal of Gerontological Nursing, 22*(10), 12–17.

Schnaubelt, K. (1998). *Medical Aroma Therapy: Healing with Essential Oils.* Berkeley, CA: Frog Ltd.

Silberman, A. (2000). Symposium conducted at the Kaiser Institute, Phoenix, Arizona. Program in Integrated Medicine.

Smith, M. C., M. A. Stallings, S. Mariner, & M. Burrall. (1999, July). Benefits of massage therapy for hospitalized patients: A descriptive and qualitative evaluation. *Alternative Therapies, 4*(4), 64–71.

Sol, N., & C. Foster (Eds.). (1992). *American College of Sports Medicine's Health/Fitness Facility Standards and Guidelines.* Suppl. 10. Champaign, IL: Human Kinetics Publishers.

Stephens, J. (2000, Sept.). Feldenkrais method: Background, research, and case studies. *Orthopaedic Physical Therapy Clinics of North America, 9*(3), 375–394.

Syrjala, K. L., G. W. Donaldson, M. W. Davis, M. E. Kippes, & J. E. Carr. (1995). Relaxation and imagery and cognitive-behavioral training reduce pain during cancer treatment. *Pain, 63,* 189–198.

Takakashi, Y., K. Takahashi, & H. Moriya. (1994). Thermal deficit in lumbar radiculopathy: Correlations with pain and neurological signs and its value for assessing symptomatic severity. *Spine, 19*(21), 2443–2449.

Taylor, M., & M. Majundmar. (2000). Incorporating yoga therapeutics into orthopedic physical therapy. *Orthopaedic Physical Therapy Clinics of North America, 9*(3), 341–359.

Testa, S. (1999). The delivery of integrative health care: Examining the integrative medical model. Dissertation in partial fulfillment of the degree of master of integrative health science, Capital University of Integrative Medicine.

Tiller, W. (1997). *Science and Human Transformation: Subtle Energies, Intentionality and Consciousness.* Walnut Creek, CA: Pavior.

Valbona, C., C. Hazellwood, & G. Jurida. (1997). Response of pain to static magnetic fields in post-polio patients: A double blind pilot study. *Archives of Physical Medicine and Rehabilitation, 78,* 1198–1203.

Weeks, J. (2000, Oct.). Charting the mainstream: A review of trends in the dominant medical system. *Townsend Letter for Doctors and Patients,* 22–23.

Weintraub, M. (1998). Chronic submaximal stimulation in peripheral neuropathy: Is there a beneficial relationship? *American Journal of Pain Management, 8*(1), 1–3.

Wildman, F., J. Stephens, & L. Aum. (2000). Feldenkrais Method. In D. Novey (Ed.), *Physician's Complete Reference to Complementary and Alternative Medicine.* St. Louis: Mosby.

Wu, W., E. Bandilla, D. S. Ciccone, J. Yang, S. S. Cheng, N. Carner, Y. Wu, & R. Shen. (1999, Jan.). Effects of Qi Gong on late-stage complex regional pain syndrome. *Alternative Therapies, 5*(1), 45–54.

Yanick, P. (2000). *Quantum Medicine.* Portland, OR: Writers Service Publications.

7

Developing Therapeutic Presence

Suzanne Scurlock-Durana

CHAPTER OBJECTIVES

♦ Define therapeutic presence.
♦ Understand the concepts of being grounded and in touch with one's inner knowledge and external resources.
♦ Outline principles which can be used to develop therapeutic presence.
♦ Understand how to bring therapeutic presence into the therapeutic setting.

Therapists are trained to examine and analyze a client's physical condition as well as their motivation and attitudes in order to help them attain healthier functioning. Rarely, if ever, are therapists trained to examine and analyze their own motivation, attitudes, and role in the process. In the last decade health professionals have become aware that the outcome of any given therapeutic intervention is significantly influenced by the therapist's ability to hold a strong healing, or therapeutic, presence. This makes it necessary to include oneself in the equation of the healing process through which clients are going.

In this chapter therapeutic presence, which is the unspoken, unseen connection between therapist and client that occurs in every therapeutic intervention, will be addressed. This means knowing how to remain connected to one's resources, grounded, attuned (i.e., not feeling numb), and fully present in the face of challenging, sometimes emotional, therapy situations. It means being empathetic and feeling connected to clients without taking on their frustration, anxiety, pain, or grief. It means facilitating a healing therapy session while honoring one's own boundaries and the boundaries of the client. To accomplish this means learning how to be in touch with and nurturing of oneself, so that the therapist's therapeutic presence can catalyze and nurture the healing process for clients.

This can create a challenge, because many people have been taught that it is somehow bad to focus on their own bodies and emotions—that they should choose to ignore pains and suppress feelings. This chapter addresses the "how to" of regaining the innate sense of self

It is vital to attend to yourself as a therapist. The principles described in this chapter provide therapists with a foundation to begin to understand their own sense of inner knowledge and external resources. This should strengthen treatment interventions, optimally facilitating health in your clients and yourself, and prevent feelings of depletion and burnout that can result from not being in touch with oneself.

knowledge each person is born with. In some circles this is defined as "inner knowing." In other contexts it is called "internal and external sensory awareness" (Gendlin, 1982). Whatever it is called, the reader will learn about paying attention to the subtle cues received constantly from the body and the surrounding environment, cues the reader may have been taught to ignore, if raised in Western culture (Capra, 1983).

For those who feel they would be overwhelmed by their emotions if they were to deeply and truly feel them, this chapter will discuss how to tolerate and modulate such feelings. This allows a person to have emotions and learn from them rather than tamp them down for fear of being completely washed away by them—embarrassed or seen as unprofessional. During times of stress or personal tragedy, this is particularly important.

The chapter also addresses enhancing one's sense of external resources (see "Defining Grounded" on page 74 in this chapter) and using this sense to develop a feeling of renewal and confidence, building from experiences in the present and past.

Finally, the author will explain how to bring this inner knowing to any given therapeutic setting in order to have it inform and guide the process for a positive outcome that nurtures and promotes healing for everyone involved. This ability to hold a therapeutic presence will enhance all of the therapist's other skills, manual and verbal, and it will assist therapists in staying healthy and in not burning out with today's demands and schedules. The reader may even choose to apply these principles in other areas of life.

The Five Principles

Quantum physics has taught that on a molecular level, everyone exists in a virtual sea of energy (Capra, 1975; Gribbin, 1984; Murchie, 1967; Pert, 1997; Zukav, 1979) and that each person is an integral part of that energy field, affecting and being affected by everything around them, simply by being present. The following principles, developed by the author, provide an underlying foundation for how this unseen energy field operates in each person's life and interactions with others, especially in therapeutic relationships. It is helpful for the therapist to be able to recognize one or more of these principles when they are in action, so that knowledge of them can help to guide, rather than control, the therapist. They are all equally important in every person's life, in different ways, and they interrelate with each other all the time, so they are not hierarchical in nature. Therapists may find that in a given situation they are aware of one or more of these principles playing a major role in how they feel and act. In a sense the principles are like signs on a map. They form much of the unconscious

Being "grounded" refers to feeling connected in a steady and enduring way to inner knowledge and external resources. Being grounded is an invisible but tangible sense of connection to nurturing, nourishing energy. Metaphors for feeling grounded and methods for creating a grounded feeling vary from person to person. Some of the ways people refer to feeling grounded to an *external* resource include:

- feeling connected to a skill level.
- feeling rooted in the earth.
- feeling the energy of the sun or another aspect of nature.

   Some people refer to feeling grounded to *internal* knowledge as:

- remembering the feeling of a peak experience.
- the calm sensation of a steady, even breath.

context from which we live. And they form much of the unspoken context health professionals use in therapeutic relationships, in the treatment room or clinic.

Principle I: Connection and Separation

This principle highlights the skill of recognizing the range of internal sensations that all people have, from feeling deeply connected to what gives us joy in life, to feeling completely isolated or separate from the joy and nurturing that life offers. Recognizing whether one is feeling separate from or connected to life in any given moment provides valuable information for making life decisions, both large and small. Each person has an innate capacity to feel his or her own internal and external connection to the self and the world. If therapists know how to give and receive in a way that nurtures themselves deeply, they can often be more in touch with their internal sense of satisfaction and connection to the world that they live in. Small experiences become very important and informative; for example, a person can be renewed by taking a walk in the forest while breathing deeply, or by holding a small infant and feeling the joy of the newness of that life. Likewise, one can use "negative" experiences or information to enhance health. For example, if one is coming down with a cold and begins to feel sick and disconnected from a healthy state of being, this disconnected feeling can inform people to go take the vitamin C, a hot bath, or to rest.

When people recognize that, as human beings, they are born with this capacity for inner knowledge, then they can also note that, as they grow up in today's culture, certain experiences can cause it to slip away. In order to better recognize and reclaim one's sense of inner knowledge, it is necessary first to acknowledge the sense of separation when it crops up in one's life, private and professional. People are taught to work faster and harder, to knuckle down and push for the goal at all costs (this is true from school schedules to gift shopping). People's deeper needs, emotional and physical, are often relegated to a lesser status. People smile and say they are fine when truly they are not feeling that way at all (Pert, 1997).

The first half of this principle is recognizing how connected or disconnected one is feeling *within oneself* in any given moment, and then using that awareness (with as little judgment as possible) to begin moving back in the direction of connection to one's aliveness, the deeper sense of oneself in this world. Jon Kabat-Zinn, in his groundbreaking programs with chronic pain clients at the University of Massachusetts Medical Center, teaches the importance of internal sensation mindfulness, using different practices (following the breath, watching thoughts), in order to reach a sense of calm or quietness. When that sense of connection, or quiet, is achieved, body physiology improves (e.g., with decreased cortisol levels), pain tolerance increases and pain levels often decrease, and hopefulness, one's sense of possibilities for the future, increases (Kabat-Zinn, 1994, 1990; Pert, 1997).

The second half of this principle is to feel a sense of connection to the world and external resources from that quiet inner place. This is simple to write about, but can be more difficult to achieve. So many things in today's culture conspire to keep this from happening. The cultural context in which one is raised *can* allow people to keep their innate sense of internal and external connection that they are born with, and to deepen it as they grow (and thus to gain wisdom). However, it rarely does. Instead, people find themselves rushing through the day or planning their lives based on what they were told is the correct way to do it—without ever realizing that by learning to reconnect, internally and externally, they can tap a vast and deep reservoir of knowledge and guidance in order to live a more self-actualized life. This skill allows people to take in and understand what other people convey and sense internally, whether it rings true at that moment, and act on it accordingly.

Principle II: Acknowledging and Widening One's Perceptual Lens

This principle highlights that each person has a particular perceptual lens through which he or she experiences the world. People need to *recognize* that it is just one view of life that is unique to each person and is not necessarily reality. In order for people to be able to let in the amount and variety of information that is available, they have to *widen* their particular lens.

A person's upbringing, physiology, and all life experiences go into creating these lenses. They are invisible and unconscious in almost everyone. They can be thought of as the perceptual background context from which people live their lives. There is little that is fixed and universally true in terms of how one sees, experiences, and then interprets the events of one's life. A client was shocked several years ago to have a heart-to-heart conversation with her sister and to discover that she had an *entirely* different emotional experience of her father while growing up than her sister did. They were not that different in age, grew up in the same household, and it confounded her until she remembered this principle. Everyone interprets what they see and what happens to them, and then they create beliefs about life or themselves based on these interpretations. On a very simple level, think about how hard it is to get agreement about exactly what happened at the scene of an accident. Each witness has his or her own perception and story about what happened.

Understanding clients from a narrow viewpoint can impede therapists. When therapists judge a client's particular health care issues too narrowly, it is possible to miss what may help clients heal the fastest or what may even impair the healing process. A colleague of the author's shared an extreme example of this. Early in her career, a therapist in the same rehabilitation facility was fired for telling a young man, newly paraplegic, that his disability was God's revenge on him for something bad he had done. Needless to say, this was a crushing pronouncement to give anyone in the vulnerable state he was in at the time. Yet from her "perceptual lens," that was why he had ended up in a wheelchair.

There are many more subtle examples of judging clients. For instance, if a therapist holds the perception that no matter what he or she does for clients, it will never be enough, then this will affect how the therapist interacts with clients and interfere with his or her capacity to help clients heal. Some therapists spend too much time with each person, trying to "do enough" (to no avail) and ending each day exhausted, burnt out. Or, conversely, some therapists may not try to connect much at all, doing the minimum necessary to get by, because they are sure they won't succeed or that their efforts will not be enough—so why try? In both cases, a perceptual lens can be so much a part of the therapist's self image that he or she may not even be conscious of it.

The next key to this principle is remembering that a person's perceptual lens and belief systems will shape the nature of what people can *receive* moment by moment. It is important for a person to be open to receiving internal knowledge and external resources. If people have a particular lens that says they cannot feel vulnerable and open without disaster occurring (perhaps based on *real* past experiences of those disasters), they may also have problems receiving any internal or external sense of safety that would allow them to experience their vulnerability.

People can begin to correct this narrow viewpoint by becoming more conscious about realizing when it happens and then choosing to respond differently. For example, in the moment people realize they are perceiving a situation through a "narrower lens" than they would like, they need to make a conscious decision to perceive this experience in a new and different way. Using the example from above, they may want to imagine themselves open to the possibility that they *can* feel vulnerable *without* disaster striking so that they don't have to pull away. After people focus on the possibility of something new, they should note any changes in internal sensations and movement of energy. It may be slow and subtle initially, but important, valuable changes can take place when this principle is engaged in this way (Rossi, 1986; Erickson & Rossi, 1979).

Principle III: Reclaiming, Honoring and Reconnecting All Parts of Oneself to the Whole— Body, Mind, Spirit and Emotions

This principle recognizes that all people are unique at the core of who they are, that their spirits are one of a kind, and that they need to acknowledge their uniqueness and reconnect the parts that may feel isolated or separate. This principle also acknowledges that in order to have a clear sense of connection to oneself and to the world, it is imperative to have a good "felt sense" of one's physical body and one's spirit. Another way to describe this felt sense is knowing where one stops and the rest of the world begins. This entails having healthy boundaries: boundaries that allow the therapist to connect with what is good in the world and separate from what is not wanted. This is best done by having a nourishing sense of energy flowing through every cell of the physical body (Cohen, 1997; Eisenberg & Wright, 1987). In this principle, the author uses the metaphor of a container to symbolize the physical body and a river of energy to denote a healthy flow of life force (Erickson, 1988). This means that a person's skin and the energy field that flows through and around it is one's boundary. In the best of all possible worlds, this boundary is respected by everyone.

When a person's "container" is full and flowing with nourishing energy, the person often has a much clearer sense of himself or herself internally, as well as a sense of where his or her boundaries are. The person can choose to connect at will with the surrounding world and has a clearer choice about what to do with someone else's negative feelings. This is particularly valuable if a client is in physical or emotional pain or is expressing something that is unpleasant for him or her in the course of a treatment session. If therapists utilize the skills underlying this principle, they will be less likely to end up feeling exhausted or burnt out by the treatment process and their interactions with such clients. In other words, if therapists stay full and maintain access to whatever source of energy feeds them, they are a lot less likely to carry away a client's anxiety, pain, grief, or other emotion. It would be like trying to put more water into a glass that is full and constantly being refilled as the river flows through it.

This principle also speaks to the larger process of integration of all of the parts of a person. People have different parts of themselves that were not safe to fully experience when they were growing up, such as aspects of their sexual or creative selves. This might have to do with the culture one grew up in, with family, or religious faith or practices. However, people operate optimally when all aspects of their minds, bodies, emotions and spirit are in constant connection and dialogue. This means that whether one is making a big decision, such as what to do with life after graduation, or making a less important decision, such as choosing food from a menu in a restaurant, it is important to include all these parts of the self in the decision-making process. When therapists begin to live this integration, there is a sense of connection and an informing that occurs (some would call this intuition or knowing). People who can do this are natural guides through the maze of how to be present, what techniques to use, and what to say to a given client for the client's highest good and the therapist's own as well.

For many therapists, the hardest part of this integration is recognizing and trusting the subtle cues of the body. Most people have no problem gathering the data. They know whether the prospect of taking a given path makes them feel happy or sad, scared or anxious. But is it the best step to take at this moment, for oneself and for others?

Inner knowledge lies in the integration of all of this. The body can be thought of as a person's navigational system for inner knowledge. Its signals can give a clear indication of which direction to head in, given all the information—emotional feelings and physical sensations. Unless one knows how to feel and respond to all of the body's signals, it is difficult to use it as a navigational tool. If people live primarily in their heads, as much of today's culture does, they may make logical, reasonable decisions. But will their decisions include the wisdom of the heart? Many therapists are addicted to staying busy and having a full schedule. Often, these therapists have described being numb to their feelings and their bodily needs. They end up with severe muscular tension and exhaustion that keeps them from being able to offer 100 percent of themselves in their therapy sessions, not to mention in the rest of their lives.

Alternately, if people live dominated and overwhelmed by their emotions, they may make decisions that feel absolutely true for that moment, but are these decisions for the highest good when those closest to them, or the bigger picture of life, is considered? If people live dominated by their sexual drive, or by addiction, they may have momentary satisfaction. However, chances are those physical drives are felt to the detriment, if not obliteration, of all the deeper, more subtle, sensations of one's spirit (integrated with body-mind-emotion) that enrich and inform the totality of one's being. So, this integration, coupled with a connection to what is safe and nurturing and informing in the world (i.e., external resources), creates a powerful, deep intelligence from which to operate.

Principle IV: Continually Connecting to Your Resources

This principle builds on the last one and yet it stands alone as well. Unless people constantly remember to stay connected to their inner knowledge and external resources, they burn out. This is particularly true for those in health care. It is simply not enough to know *how* to remember the connection and establish a stronger flow of nurturing, nourishing energy. This principle emphasizes that people need to live it, to practice, to remember to *feel* this connection in each moment.

When therapists do not live in this connection to their inner knowledge and external resources, it is easy to be less focused in treatment. It might look like this: While I am in a treatment session with client A, I am thinking about client B coming next and what time I need to leave in order to make it to my dental appointment after work, as well as what I need to pick up at the store on the way home. Therapists may be vaguely aware of feeling pulled in a million directions, and their current clients are definitely not getting the therapist's best. Instead, therapists should try working with the mind, harnessing its focus and acuity to refill themselves energetically and to notice what is going on in their internal awareness as they notice what is going on in the treatment of the client.

The world, as well as one's internal environment, is incredibly complex. In order to utilize this inner navigational system that people are born with, therapists must first remember to renew their sense of energy all the time. People need to know how to listen to all of the signals, nuances, and information provided by internal knowledge and external resources. This enhances a larger sense of who they are and what they are capable of as therapists and human beings.

Principle V: Recognizing and Honoring One's Internal and External Resources

This principle notes that it is necessary to know, in the very core of one's being, that people *are* supported moment to moment by an ever-present, unconditional source of nourishing life energy. As noted earlier, people live in a sea of energy that contains a wide range of resources. Many people would agree, in concept, that this is true. In some circles this is known as faith. However, when the therapist has inadvertently lost his or her connection to this source of energy or has become depleted from stress or challenge, it is important to remember and really *feel* that support by stopping and connecting with it.

Activities to Connect to Your Resources

The experience of grounding is different for each person, because everyone accesses and then creatively expresses this life force or source in his or her own way. It could manifest as stopping and saying a prayer. Kabat-Zinn (1994) teaches people to focus inside, quiet the breath, and calm themselves. It could manifest as taking a needed nap or putting on a piece of music that helps a person calmly focus. The author teaches people imagery of connecting and filling up from the earth's field (Scurlock-Durana, 1996). Writing or drawing about something stressful can enhance inner knowledge by helping organize the experience. The reader will want to answer the following question affirmatively when identifying grounding activities: "Do I feel more of my body, or do I feel nurtured by my external resources, when I engage in this activity?"

Helpful Guidelines

Having outlined the five basic principles that provide a foundation for health care practitioners to hold a strong therapeutic presence for others and for themselves, guidelines for creating and holding that healing presence for another person are reviewed below.

1. In holding a strong, therapeutic presence for another person or situation, it is imperative that one remembers that this is a state of *being,* not a *doing* skill. Simply put, all the words, manual techniques, or protocols that therapists follow are a part of *doing* skills. What is being discussed here is the invisible, but very powerful, skill of *being* present in all that one is, in a therapeutic way for another person. When people are in this state of being, they feel connected, full, and present for other people. They can sense a flow of energy that feeds them as well as the other person. In this skill, giving and receiving essentially become one and the same (Trout, 1990).

Often, therapists have the ingrained habit of giving out all of their energy into treatment sessions (doing), and only noticing the depletion at the end of the day. By being aware of this state of *being* full as one goes through the day, therapists can continually nourish and refill themselves consciously. Take a quiet moment to take a few good deep breaths. Feel the solid support of the ground, receive what is needed from it. Say a quiet prayer or meditate on gratitude.

2. It is imperative in holding a therapeutic presence that therapists have a clear intention about it. This means that:

(a) They are aware of how *they* are doing that day, energetically. Are they feeling full and fresh, or depleted and stressed out? In any condition they may find themselves, if they can stop, check inside, and honestly admit to themselves how they are doing, rather than automatically buckling down and tightening their jaws to make it through the day, they will be much better off. When therapists find themselves depleted, it is important to simply take the time to rest back in themselves, connect more deeply to their internal knowledge and external resources, and fill up before beginning. This "conscious use of self" will be invaluable in preventing burnout.

(b) Therapists must acknowledge their skills and talents. This means trusting the quiet whispers of wisdom that are heard when connected and in a good flow of life's energy. It is important not to second-guess oneself in this area. Trust what is known and use it. Don't pull back when experiencing a knowing, intuitive force to move forward in a particular direction.

(c) Therapists must set a clear time boundary with clients, which is neither rigid and cold nor too soft and pliable. When a good strong therapeutic presence is established with someone, it is amazing how much healing can occur in a short period of time. Time is almost irrelevant. As this intention is set clearly, the life force that is being brought to bear for that client that day will show up and do all that needs to be done for that person. When therapists consistently run overtime with clients, they must ask themselves, "Is this coming out of a sense that I am not doing enough, that I need to do more to 'fix' this person?" Such an attitude leads to burn out. If therapists find themselves always looking for the right technique in course after course, the one that makes them feel like they know enough, then the right technique may not be an active *doing* skill, it may be learning how to hold a strong therapeutic presence, how to *be* with clients in a new and more relaxed way.

(d) Therapists need to know and acknowledge the space in which they are working. This means understanding its limitations, but also letting themselves be surprised by how much can happen under any circumstances. The author has seen good therapists working in situations where there is little privacy or time, and the clients know it, yet manage to heal and release all kinds of things in ways appropriate to the space and time. Obviously, this is not optimal. But, the therapeutic presence held for clients, under any external circumstances, can become the dominant force in that healing situation—not the external details.

3. Therapists must remember to constantly access their internal knowledge and external resources for nourishing energy. This must continue throughout the session, although they will find that they don't need to be "intending" it constantly once this habit is well established. When people know how to fill themselves and continually access their resources for energy, then they are not depleted as they hold a therapeutic presence for other people. In fact, they will often be in a much more expanded, delightful state of awareness due to this constant filling process. As mentioned earlier, therapists will also find that if clients are in pain or discharging something that is unpleasant, therapists will not absorb that other energy as it is discharged. Remember the image of trying to put more water into a glass that is already full. When people stay full and maintain access to the resources that feed them, then they are less likely to walk away with other people's anxiety, fear, pain, or grief.

A corollary to that guideline is to remember that each therapist is not the only source or resource for that client. This understanding should prevent therapists from becoming overly responsible for any other person's healing process. The signal that indicates a therapist is accepting too much responsibility for the healing of clients is the thought, "I'm not doing enough." Or, the therapist may feel that he or she has not done enough until a client's entire healing process takes place or comes to completion. This is not to suggest that therapists ever leave anyone in the middle of a crisis. However, if they are holding a therapeutic presence for someone with a long-term illness or a very serious injury, they may have to hold that therapeutic presence on many different occasions to have the *whole* healing come to completion. And it is important to understand that the therapist cannot be the judge of that unfolding, its pace, or time frame. If therapists try to hold it all in one space in time, they may find themselves exhausted and depleted. Everyone has other resources and unseen support. When therapists insist on doing it all themselves, it is as though they don't trust that support.

4. Remember that the therapist will be holding a space of unconditional positive regard for the client—an acceptance of whatever that person must do, at whatever pace, in order to bring that healing moment forward for himself or herself. In holding this unconditional space for another person, therapists may even find themselves able to be a therapeutic presence for the dying process in a way that creates healing even into death.

The corollary to this guideline is that the easiest way to hold unconditional positive regard for another is to hold it for oneself as well. This needs to be noted, because sometimes in this process, therapists hold such an empathic space that they forget to keep filling themselves and holding their own "container" of being. This may feel like slipping forward energetically into the other person because of the strong empathy for what that person is going through. The key, again, is to continually remember to remain connected to one's own sense of internal knowledge and external resources.

5. Remember that one's body is like an incredible navigation system. People hear and sense their inner knowledge best when they are focused on the present. When people's focus moves from the present, they begin to miss the signals and lose contact with their own inner

knowledge and external resources. Or, they become so connected with someone's pain that they miss the cue that reminds them to sit further back in their body and ground, connecting to their resources, so that the client can feel a foundation for what he or she is working on.

Summary

The five principles and guidelines discussed help create a strong therapeutic presence. When a therapist begins working with clients it is important, in order to achieve the greatest results, to maintain this presence. By continually connecting to one's inner knowledge and external resources not only will therapists be able to hold a strong unconditional therapeutic presence for clients, but they will also likely end the session full of energy, despite the intensity of what transpires.

STUDY QUESTIONS

1. What is therapeutic presence?
2. What is the significance of therapeutic presence?
3. Briefly discuss the five principles described in this chapter.
4. Describe two activities (one internal and one external) that help you feel grounded, and reflect on how this feeling can be used in your work as a therapist.

RESOURCES

Healing From the Core: A Journey Home to Ourselves (audio series)
Suzanne Scurlock-Durana
11417 Tanbark Drive
Reston, VA 20191
www.healingfromthecore.com

REFERENCES

Capra, F. (1975). *The Tao of Physics*. Berkeley, CA: Shambhala Publications.

Capra, F. (1983). *The Turning Point: Science, Society and Rising Culture*. New York: Simon & Schuster.

Cohen, K. (1997). *The Way of Qigong*. New York: Ballantine.

Eisenberg, D., & T. Wright. (1987). *Encounters with Qi: Exploring Chinese Medicine*. New York: Penguin Books.

Erickson, H. (1988). Modeling and role-modeling: Ericksonian techniques applied to physiological problems. In J. K. Zeig & S. Lankton (Eds.), *Developing Ericksonian Therapy: State of the Art*. New York: Brunner/Mazel.

Erickson, M., & E. Rossi. (1979). *Hypnotherapy: An Exploratory Casebook*. New York: Irvington Press.

Gendlin, E. (1982). *Focusing* (Rev. ed.). New York: Bantam Books.

Gribbin, J. (1984). *In Search of Schrodinger's Cat: Quantum Physics and Reality*. New York: Bantam Books.

Kabat-Zinn, J. (1990). *Full Catastrophe Living: Using the Wisdom of Your Body and Mind to Face Stress, Pain, and Illness*. New York: Hyperion.

Kabat-Zinn, J. (1994). *Wherever You Go There You Are*. New York: Hyperion.

Murchie, G. (1967). *Music of the Spheres—Volume II. The Microcosm: Matter, Atoms, Waves, Radiation, and Relativity*. New York: Dover Publications.

Pert, C. (1997). *Molecules of Emotion: Why You Feel the Way You Feel*. New York: Simon & Schuster.

Rossi, E. (1986). *Mind-Body Communication in Hypnosis: The Seminars, Workshops, and Lectures of Milton H. Erickson, Volume III*. New York: McGraw-Hill.

Scurlock-Durana, S. (1996). *Healing From the Core: A Journey Home to Ourselves* (Cassette recording ISBN No. 1-893996-00-X). Reston, VA: Lion Recording.

Trout, S. (1990). *To See Differently*. Washington, D.C.: Three Roses Press.

Zukav, G. (1979). *The Dancing Wu Li Masters: An Overview of the New Physics*. New York: William Morrow & Company.

8

Introduction to Asian Medical Systems

Maureen McKenna

CHAPTER OBJECTIVES

◆ Understand the basic principles of Traditional Chinese Medicine.
◆ Understand the basic principles of Ayurveda.

Asian medicine and therapies encompass many different philosophies from different countries. All have ancient origins. During the past 40 or 50 years, there has been a proliferation in the dissemination of knowledge and an increase in practice of these disciplines in the Western world. One of the best known of these is Traditional Chinese Medicine (TCM), which dates back several thousand years (Ziyin & Zelin, 1994).

Traditional Chinese Medicine

The first academic written account of TCM theories and clinical experiences was documented in 18 volumes of the Nei Jing, or Nei Ching. The material from which they were compiled over several subsequent dynasties was thought to have originated approximately 3,000 to 4,000 years ago (Ziyin & Zelin, 1994). Mann (1973) names the Hungdi Neiging Suwen, written in 200 BC, as the original title that was translated in contemporary times by Professor Ilza Veith. There are various alternate titles of these volumes: *The Yellow Emperor's Classic of Internal Disease* (Mann, 1973) and the *The Yellow Emperor's Canon of Internal Medicine*, which was recorded in the form of a dialogue of questions and answers between the Yellow Emperor and his physician (DuBrin & Keenan, 1974). In addition, Ziyin and Zelin refer to bone and turtle shell inscriptions depicting various medical interventions and surgical techniques (1994), and Mann states that the oldest records of acupuncture were found in 1600 BC on bone etchings as well (1973).

The four basic concepts of the Nei Ching are as follows: the opposing forces of yin and yang; the Tao, which is the way or method of attaining harmony between earth and heaven with the human beings between those two dimensions; the theory of the five elements; and the combination of all of these in the application to medicine (Omura, 1982). In order to attain and maintain a healthy state of being, the fundamentals of TCM require a balance between the forces of yin and yang, and between the five basic elements and the qi, or chi (Ziyin & Zelin, 1994).

Perhaps the most important and distinctive theories of TCM are the concepts of yin and yang, the five elements, and Qi, because they are so important for health. In recent years, these terms have been widely used in the Western world, although perhaps not as widely understood. There are discrepancies in the origin of written references to these balancing forces. Maciocia (1989) indicates that the first references to yin and yang date back to 1000 BC, whereas DuBrin and Keenan (1974) state that the yin and yang doctrine was first mentioned in the I Ching in 800 BC.

Yin and Yang

In contrast to the Cartesian dualism of the Western model and the inherent dichotomy of the mind and matter, Chinese metaphysics divides the world into yin and yang (Diebschlag, 1997). DuBrin and Keenan (1974) quote one passage from *The Yellow Emperor's Canon of Internal Medicine*, which introduces this dichotomy:

> *The principle of Yin and Yang is the basic principle of everything in creation. It is the principle of the entire universe. It is the parent of every change; it is the root and source of life and death; it is also found within the temples of the gods. Heaven was created by an accumulation of Yang, the light element, while earth was created by an accumulation of Yin, the dark element. Through their interactions and their functions, Yin and Yang, the negative and the positive principles in nature, are the causes of diseases which befall those who are in rebellion against the laws of nature, or those who do not conform to them. (p. 96)*

In TCM health is partly based on the dynamic balance and harmony between the fundamental principles of yin and yang. The symbol of this balance is a circle divided into two equal portions by a serpentine line. One half is black with a white "eye," and the other half is the opposite combination. The white area is known as the yang and represents a positive, bright, warm, expanding force. Conversely, the black area is known as the Yin and represents the negative, the dark, the cool, and the diminishing or shrinking force. The human body is described as having positive and negative physical aspects, which correspond to yin and yang. For example, the exterior (yang) is active, light, and positive, and the interior (yin) is passive, dark, and negative. They are interdependent forces because one dimension cannot exist without its complementary counter balance (Leong, 1974; DuBrin & Keenan, 1974). The yang dimension (the functional activities of the human body) is supported by the yin (the body fluids). The yin in turn supports the yang by the production of nutrients to enable the physical bodily activities of yang to occur.

Each portion of the human body is assigned a yin or yang character depending on its function. The yang is contained in those parts that are on the exterior (skin and muscle), that are superior in location (the head and above the waist), that are posterior (the back), and that are lateral (outer aspects of limbs). The yin parts are the opposite of these: the front of the chest, the abdomen, some of the interior organs, parts below the waist, and the inner or medial surface of limbs. The meridians mark the flow of qi along those same general pathways. The yang channels are along the back and serve to protect the body from exterior pathogenic factors. By contrast, yin's channels are interior and function to nourish the body. The yang channels begin and end at the head. They also include some of the internal organs but only those that excrete and have a connection with the exterior, such as the bladder, intestines, and stomach. The yin organs store nutrients, blood, and body fluids (Maciocia, 1989).

Diseases are believed to be caused by an imbalance between yang and yin. For example, if there should be a disruption in the internal organs (yang), then the yin is affected and the function of digesting nutrients is impaired. In another illustration, in a client who develops an infection, who has a high fever and flushed face, rapid pulse and dry lips, the symptoms are those attributed to yang, while someone who develops septic shock would exhibit the yin symptoms of pallor, sweating, chills, and a weak pulse. As conditions improve with the application of the appropriate intervention, the balance of yang and yin changes to restore and maintain the healthy equilibrium of the functions of the body (Ziyin & Zelin, 1994)

Meridians

Acupoints are specific areas on the body where there is an accumulation of qi, or energy, and they are categorized into three different types. There are the channel points, which are located along specific paths or channels, called meridians, in a predictable pattern and serve to regulate or stimulate an organ or vessel to which they are linked. There are 361 of these points located along the meridian channels. In the second category are 200 extraordinary points, which do not relate to any of the meridians. The third category has unspecified points that elicit pain or discomfort on palpation (Ziyin & Zelin, 1994). There are 12 main pairs of meridians in the human body, plus two that are not paired. They are named for the organs and vessels that they influence: the lungs, large intestine, stomach, spleen, heart, small intestine, bladder, kidney, pericardium, gall bladder, liver, and the "triple warmer" or "triple energizer" located on the posterior aspect of the arm traversing from the ring finger across the posterior shoulder to the temporal area.

The 12 paired meridians are also balanced between six yin organs—the more solid ones—and six yang organs—the hollow ones (DuBrin & Keenan, 1974; Eagle, 1980). These meridians are used extensively in differential diagnosis in TCM, which then guides the practitioner to the appropriate treatment.

Qi or Chi

The qi (pronounced *chee*) or chi, has no literal translation from the Chinese. It has been called the vital energy, life force, matter, and ether, and is said to circulate around the body in the meridian channels. Qi is energy that manifests on both the physical and spiritual levels simultaneously, and its form is in a constant state of flux between rarefied and dense according to its locality and function. It is said that in the healthy individual, qi remains moving and flowing, and the stagnation of qi, or its altered flow, creates disease. For example, poor circulation of qi, which becomes pathologically dense, can create lumps, masses, and tumors (Maciocia, 1994).

The flow of qi is determined by taking the pulses at the wrist, not in the same way that in Western medicine the radial artery pulse is monitored at the wrist, but in a more subtle palpation of the meridian pulses. Six of these invisible meridians pass through the wrist of the right hand and six through the left. The experienced TCM practitioner can detect up to twenty-eight different pulse qualities that indicate the quality and quantity of the vital energy flow through different organs (Eagle, 1980). Qi deficiencies manifest as clusters of symptoms and pulse types. For example, qi deficiencies in the lung and spleen can manifest in the following signs: fatigue, empty pulse, breathlessness and a weak speaking voice, poor appetite, and loose stools. Qi stagnation, however, can produce feelings of abdominal distention, depression and altered mood states, and a "wiry" or "tight" pulse (Maciocia, 1994).

The Five Elements

The ancient Chinese divided everything in the world into five categories—the elements of earth, fire, metal, water, and wood. Until recent times, four of these (excluding wood) were commonly used in Western medicine. The names of the elements do not denote a literal element but rather a symbolic association with the idea (Mann, 1973).

The concept of the five elements may have originated from the ancient Chinese people's observations of nature. For example, they observed that trees grow upon the earth, depleting it by taking nutrients from it, that plants can crack rocks and break up soil, and thus concluded that "wood acts on earth" (Maciocia, 1989; Mann, 1973; Ziyin & Zelin, 1994). A diagrammatic representation of the creative theory can be depicted in a pentagonal shape with each of the five elements in a systematic and logical position of creative influence at the apex of each of the five angles. For example, wood (liver and gall bladder) will burn to form a fire (heart and small intestine), the ashes of which form the earth (spleen and stomach). Metals (lungs and large intestines) and minerals can be obtained from the earth and when they are heated become molten like water. Water (kidneys and bladder) is essential for the growth of plants and wood. This completes the cycle of creativity. By contrast, and to insure balance, there is a cycle of destructive influence. The elements are again depicted in the same five-pointed star arrangement but with the influence translating across the circle rather than around the perimeter of the pentagonal shape, creating a five-pointed star within it.

The water element corresponds to winter, which is the darkest and coldest time of the year. It represents the will to trust and survive, as well as procreation, self-actualization, and willpower. Water includes the function of the kidneys, bladder, bones, and endocrine system. The out-of-balance dimension manifests as fear, struggling for survival, reduced sexuality, fatigue, and lack of trust. Problems with the urinary tract, infertility, hypertension, and endocrine disorders are additional medical symptoms.

The fire element corresponds to summer and is characterized by warmth and light, the period of greatest activity and growth. In the individual person, fire represents the capacity to establish warm, intimate, loving relationships, passion and playfulness, relaxation, and enthusiasm. Fire organs are the heart, the small intestine, and the functions of the autonomic nervous system. Physical symptoms may involve insomnia, tinnitus, cardiac disease, and digestive problems. When the fire element is out of balance, the person exhibits a lack of warmth, inability to create or maintain relationships, doubt, depression, and a lack of joy.

Wood corresponds to the spring season with new growth, longer days, and increasing activity. In the individual, this is represented by having the ability to organize, to have a vision of the future, and to appropriately express emotion. When out of balance, there is difficulty in making decisions, controlling anger, and relaxing, and the person experiences a low tolerance for frustration. This element includes the function of the liver, biliary, musculoskeletal, and ocular systems. Imbalances may present with the symptoms of fibromyalgia, chronic muscular and vision problems, and headaches.

The metal element corresponds to the autumn season with the decreasing daylight, colder temperatures, and shorter days. This manifests in the person as a sense of self-worth, vitality, endurance, the ability to release grudges and emotionally charged issues. The function of the lungs, the skin, and the colon are in this category. When out of balance, metal corresponds to sadness, depression, poor self-esteem, inability to recover from loss, and rigidity. The physical symptoms may include asthma, eczema, and lower bowel disorders.

The earth element corresponds to the season of late summer, harvest, as well as the capacity for nourishment, security, stability, empathy, and caring. The organs of digestion, the stomach, spleen, and pancreas are included in this category. When there is an imbalance in this element, the person may exhibit obsessive characteristics manifesting in physical symptoms such as eating disorders, gynecological problems, sinusitis, and both upper and lower gastrointestinal diseases.

Using the Concepts for Healing Diseases

In the 12th and 13th centuries physicians began exploring different aspects of TCM, such as the need to balance the body's diseases with an opposite force or condition. One belief held that the weather and the external environment affected health, therefore a "hot" disease was treated with a "cold" medicine. Another belief held that there was a need to balance the masculine (yang) and feminine (yin) forces and to rid the body of evils by the use of purgatives, and yet another sought to optimize the function of the stomach and spleen to speed recovery from illness.

One of the main differences between TCM and Western medicine is that TCM diagnoses focus on external observation (i.e., physical symptoms, personality characteristics, and observation of the tongue), palpation of pulses, and the treatment and prevention of chronic conditions, while Western medicine's focus is on treating acute trauma through surgery and the use of post mortems (Ziyin & Zelin, 1994). Therefore, TCM is reduced to the basic theory of yin and yang and the effect they have on the physiology, pathology, diagnosis, and treatment of diseases.

In attempting to balance the cause of disease or disequilibrium in the body by using the principles of TCM, these principles need to be understood and taken into consideration when planning related treatment approaches and interventions.

The healing arts of acupuncture, acupressure (Shiatsu), the use of Chinese herbs, and Qi Gong involve the restoration of the body's harmony. It is the purpose of each of these interventions to ensure that qi energy remains moving and flowing. T'ai Chi is a system of moving meditation and physical exercise, which is also based on the belief that flowing qi results in good health. During the practice of T'ai Chi, the relaxing, flowing movements of the form and the attention to the breath are focused on the Hara center (or the lower Dan Tien), an area located just below and posterior to the navel. This is believed to be the reservoir of the qi, which is circulated by breathing in an imaginary loop from the navel, up the back, over the head, and down the front of the body to the original starting point. Each cycle purifies the breath and builds the qi (Lee, 1976).

According to Liao (1990), the search for a constructive and harmonious way to realize the full potential of the human spirit and the body's natural homeostasis began a few hundred years ago with the development of the T'ai Chi exercise system. The basic premise of T'ai Chi practice is to integrate and balance the mind with the body. T'ai Chi utilizes the concepts of yin and yang, moving the body forward and upward in the exhalation phase of the breath (yang), and down and back in the inhalation phase (yin) (Kessenich, 1998). It is a discipline of gentle repetitive exercises involving continuous movements of the body accompanied by deep diaphragmatic breathing (Cerrato, 1999). This concentrated attention and general awareness of rhythm and form leads the practitioner into a state of peaceful mindfulness.

Ayurveda

One of the ancient healing systems in India is the 5,000-year-old practice of Ayurveda, also known as Maharashi Ayurveda in more contemporary times. It is a holistic healing science, the name of which is derived from two Sanskrit words, *ayu* (meaning life) and *veda* (meaning science). Therefore, Ayurveda is the science of life. The goals are to maintain good health for those people who are well and to alleviate illness in those who are sick. It is similar to TCM in its emphasis on achieving balance and perfect health in all the functions of life, such as eating, drinking, playing, working, and exercising (Chopra, 1991).

Chopra (1991) describes the purpose of Ayurveda:

> *. . . to tell us how our lives can be influenced, shaped, extended, and ultimately controlled without interference from sickness or old age. The guiding principle of Ayurveda is that the mind exerts the deepest influence on the body, and that freedom from sickness depends upon contacting our own awareness, bringing it into balance, and then extending that balance to the body. (p.6)*

Doshas

According to the Ayurvedic tradition, there are three body types, Kapha, Pitta, and Vata, also known as *doshas,* which are the fundamental metabolic principles governing the functioning of the human body. Most people are a combination of more than one primary type. By determining a person's predominant dosha, optimal choices can be made in the areas of exercise, eating, and relaxation. Again, as in the other traditions, the goal is to identify the imbalance and to find the complementing factors.

Chopra (1991) has an assessment quiz that determines an individual's primary body type or the combination of types. People can be classified as a single-dosha type, a two-dosha type, or a three-dosha type. Most people find that they fall into the two-dosha type. The person's primary trait will be reflected by the higher score on this section of the quiz, but attention is paid to the influences of both types when considering ways to reestablish the body's natural balance, according to these principles. These three primary doshas also relate to the principle of the five elements described in the TCM section in which there are both abstract and material concepts. Vata is the dry energy and is composed of air and space, Pitta is hot and is composed of fire and water, and Kapha is heavy and is composed of water and earth (Chopra, 1991).

Kapha refers primarily to a body structure generally described as being of a solid and powerful build, tending towards obesity, and possessing a slow, steady energy. The "pure" Kapha body type describes these people as having a tendency to gain weight faster and to lose it more slowly; they require at least eight hours of sleep at night; they do not do well with cool and damp weather; and they possess a calm disposition and a steady energy level. This heaviness of the Kapha type, due to excess water, will make these people prone to chest congestion and blocked sinuses. The combination of the viscous mucus watery component and the heaviness of the earth quality makes these people typically "down to earth" (Chopra, 1991).

People with Pitta characteristics often exhibit the opposite qualities. They tend to be warm, have a faster metabolism, are of medium build and strength, and are frequently irritable and prone to anger. Additionally, they are noted to have a sharp intellect and an articulate form of speech and to be orderly and precise in their activities. They also like the extreme cold temperature of ice-cold drinks and ice cream. Although this type of person is generally physically warm, energetic, and aggressive due to the fire element, the water element will make them prone to excess sweating (Chopra, 1991).

Vata refers to all movement in the body; therefore, people with this prominent profile have a thin physique, are very active mentally and physically, and as a consequence, do not fall asleep readily or remain soundly asleep. They are quick learners but also forget information quickly. Vata energy is also referred to as the "wind," and too much air in this form creates too much Vata. A Vata person will complain of intestinal gas, for example (Chopra, 1991).

Each main dosha category has five sub-doshas that relate to specific body parts, functions, and locations. This examination of the sub-doshas is important to the Ayurvedic physician practitioner in order to arrive at the origin of a disease and to make an accurate diagnosis before prescribing treatment. The sub-doshas address the actual areas of the body involved, such as the circulatory system, the stomach and intestinal organs, and the throat, lungs, head, and brain.

Ayurveda and Yoga

Ayurveda, which has been practiced for over 5,000 years in India (Chopra, 1991), includes various aspects of yoga. Yoga, classified as a mind-body intervention by the NCCAM, is a pivotal concept in the Indian culture, the word having derived from a Sanskrit root verb that means to bind, join, unite, and control. It is the art of creative and harmonious living between the self and the source of spiritual power, of the individual with the universal reality, the mortal with the eternal (Chaudhuri, 1965).

Although yoga is an internally focused discipline with spiritual connections, it is not a religion, nor are there fixed, rigid rules, dogmas or scriptural injunctions to which practitioners should conform. Yoga offers ways by which inner consciousness can grow, leading each person ultimately to a greater understanding of the nature of reality, to replace doubt with critical self-inquiry and faith into an actual lived experience. Yoga can be interpreted as a technique by which to fulfill the ultimate destiny of life. All the different forms of yoga seek union with a higher power, and they guide practitioners in ways to rise above differences between people and factors in the outside world that cause separation from others and from the divine. Thus, people of all faiths can participate in this universal "religion" without abandoning their own affiliations (Chaudhuri, 1965).

Ayurveda notes that each person has a different psychological type with variations on the spectrum of introvert/extrovert, emotional/analytic, and contemplative/active. Different forms of yoga have been developed to address these personality types, using different pathways to attain the ultimate goal of self-discipline, union, and control. In each of these practices, breathing and an internal focus of attention are common components (Chaudhuri, 1965). In order to achieve a measure of balance, each person should practice the principles of yoga that best develop the qualities needed to attain balance in the personality and "the full-flowering of the individual as a unique creative center of the cosmic whole" (Chaudhuri, 1965, p. 22).

It is important for the individual to recognize the imbalance and use a corresponding type of yoga. Some of the yoga forms include strenuous postures and exercises, all of which are designed to activate certain functions of the body or the mind (Law, 1974). These types of yoga, for example, might best be used with people who overuse the brain at the expense of the body or who develop muscles instead of the brain.

In the Western world, the medical benefits of yoga are only just being established. While therapists can direct the use of yoga for therapeutic outcomes, it must be remembered that each person derives something different and personal from yoga practice and that the ultimate aim of yoga is to attain the "realization of life," not necessarily to cure mental or physical ailments.

Summary

Modern Western society typically rewards and emphasizes the speed of task accomplishment and the attainment of some form of instant gratification. In contrast to this, interventions based on TCM and Ayurveda provide the practitioner the opposite rewards of quiet contemplation and freedom from the stresses of everyday life, from chronic pain and illness, fatigue, anxiety, depression, confusion, and physical instability (Jin, 1989, 1992). As society continues its interest in these interventions, therapists are professionally encouraged to become educated in the basic concepts behind these interventions and to be able to communicate a full understanding of each approach to their clients and colleagues.

STUDY QUESTIONS

1. What are yin and yang, and how do they affect illness in TCM?
2. How does TCM view the relationship between chi, health, and illness?

3. Describe three methods of diagnosis in TCM.
4. What is the relationship between the five elements and health and illness?
5. How does Ayurveda view health and illness?

REFERENCES

Cerrato, P. (1999). Tai chi: A martial art turns therapeutic. *RN, 62*(2), 59.

Chaudhuri, H. (1965). *Integral Yoga*. Wheaton, IL: Theosophical Publishing House.

Chopra, D. (1991). *Perfect Health*. New York: Harmony.

Diebschlag, F. (1997). *Psychospiritual aspects of Traditional Chinese Medicine*. Notes from a talk at East West seminar at Bore Farm, July 1997.

DuBrin, S., & J. Keenan. (1974). *Acupuncture and Your Health*. Chatsworth, CA: Books for Better Living.

Eagle, R. (1980). *A Guide to Alternative Medicine*. London: BBC.

Jin, P. (1989). Changes in heart rate, noradrenaline, cortisol and mood during Tai Chi. *Journal of Psychosomatic Research, 33*(2), 197–206.

Jin, P. (1992). Efficacy of Tai Chi, brisk walking, meditation, and reading in reducing mental and emotional stress. *Journal of Psychosomatic Research, 36*(4), 361–70.

Kessenich, C. (1998). Tai Chi as a method of fall prevention in the elderly. *Orthopedic Nursing, 17*(4), 27.

Law, D. (1974). *A Guide to Alternative Medicine*. New York: Doubleday.

Lee, D. (1976). *Tai Chi Chuan: The Philosophy of Yin and Yang and Its Application*. Burbank, CA: O'Hara.

Leong, L. (1974). *Acupuncture: A Layman's View*. New York: Signet.

Liao, W. (1990). *T'ai Chi Classics*. Boston: Shambala.

Maciocia, G. (1989). *The Foundations of Chinese Medicine*. New York: Churchill Livingstone.

Mann, F. (1973). *Acupuncture: The Ancient Chinese Art of Healing and How It Works Scientifically*. New York: Vintage.

Omura, Y. (1982). *Acupuncture Medicine: Its Historical and Clinical Background*. Tokyo: Japan Publications, Inc.

Ziyin, S., & Zelin, C. (1994). *The Basis of Traditional Chinese Medicine*. Boston: Shambhala.

9

Introduction to Energy Therapies

Ellen Zambo Anderson

CHAPTER OBJECTIVES

◆ Understand the division of energy therapies into biofields and electromagnetic fields.
◆ Understand the concepts of qi and universal polarity.
◆ Understand the concepts of prana and chakras.
◆ Understand basic concepts of electrical stimulation.
◆ Understand concepts central to sound and music therapy.

Energy therapy or energy medicine can focus on either biofields, defined as energy fields originating within the body, or on electromagnetic fields that originate from sources other than the body (NCCAM, 2000). For health care providers who practice traditional Chinese, Ayurvedic, or other Eastern medical systems, the notion of energy and its role in health have been acknowledged for thousands of years. For Western health care providers, the idea that subtle and electromagnetic energy principles are relevant to health management is relatively new. Chopra (1990), Dossey (1999), Gerber (1988, 2000), Pelletier (2000), Weil (1983), and others have suggested that a shift in the Western paradigm of healing toward a more holistic approach will be one that considers principles of energy systems in its quest for health and well being.

Biofields with Internal Sources

Vital Life Forces

Eastern medicine assumes human beings to be multidimensional organisms made up of dynamic and interactive energy systems. This energetic network is nurtured by a vital life force or energy known as *qi* or *chi* in Chinese, *prana* in Sanskrit, and *ki* in Japanese. It is through the flow of energy that the body and mind are thought to be inextricably connected and that a healthy state is achieved when all systems are in balance and the energy of life can flow freely. When energy flow is restricted or unbalanced, a person is at risk for being ill or impaired.

Traditional Chinese Medicine (TCM) is an ancient system of medicine that continues to be used in various forms by approximately one quarter of the world's population (Pelletier, 2000). According to TCM, qi travels through the human body and its organs via a complex network of channels and meridians. The 12 major meridians are thought to be related to a specific organ-energy system that regulates that system's vital functions (Reid, 1994). These major meridians and their particularly sensitive energy points, called *hsueh,* are the basis for acupuncture and acupressure techniques that seek to manipulate the flow and balance of vital energy flow (Reid, 1994).

Universal Polarity

Another tenet of TMC is the concept of universal polarity. TCM assumes that energy moves and is transformed by virtue of the tension between electromagnetic fields with opposite poles. The negative pole, known as the yin, is associated with the feminine, passive, dark, and inner qualities. The positive pole, known as the yang, is associated with masculine, active, light, and outer qualities. In ancient Chinese philosophy every form, object, and event in the universe consists of both yin and yang, with the relationship between the two defining things as they are (Veith, 1970). For living creatures, yin and yang must be in balance for health to exist.

Prana and Chakras

Ayurvedic medicine is considered to be the oldest system of natural medicine and has been practiced for approximately 5,500 years. This ancient healing system was first described around 3500 BC in the ancient Hindu texts known as the *Vedas,* which means "science of life" (Pelletier, 2000). Similar to TCM, Ayurveda assumes that all life is based on an underlying energy or vital force. This vital life force, or prana, is thought to be part of an energy system that includes energy centers known as *chakras* (Karagulla & Kunz, 1989). These chakras, which means "wheels" in Sanskrit, are said to resemble whirling vortices of subtle energy and are located at seven points along a vertical line ascending from the base of the spine to the head (Kunz, 1991). Each chakra is associated with a particular nerve plexus and endocrine

---

Therapy Focus

Therapists need to be interested in the underlying assumptions of interventions that are promoted to help individuals improve their health and well-being. By understanding the theories or assumptions of energy therapies as well as evidence that exists for their use and application, a therapist may be better able to assist his or her client in making decisions regarding the utilization of such therapies.

gland and is thought to function as a type of energy transformer (Gerber, 1988). The chakras in turn are connected to each other and to physical-cellular structures within the body via subtle-energy channels known as *nadis*. Although nadis are viewed to be different from meridians, they are thought to form a network of energy pathways that are interwoven with the physical nervous system (Gerber, 2000). Assuming that the mind, body, and spirit are connected by the chakras and nadis, Ayurveda suggests that all aspects of life, including emotional issues and relationships, play a role in health. In energetic terms, Ayurvedic medicine suggests that emotional stress can produce imbalances at the chakras that in turn may lead to illness due to an altered flow of prana to vital organs (Chopra,1990).

Polarity Therapy

Asian medical systems and their assumptions have provided the basis for many complementary and alternative therapies currently being offered by Western practitioners. Polarity therapy, for example, was developed in the mid-1900s by Dr. Randolf Stone, a chiropractor, osteopathic physician, and naturopath. Through his study of Asian medical systems, herbal remedies, and spiritualism, Stone suggested that a dynamic relationship between positive and negative charges exists at every level of organization within the universe and that the pulsation of energy between two oppositely charged poles is the basis for a life force or energy (Sills, 1990). Consistent with Asian medical systems, Stone further suggested that disease or illness is due to a disruption of this energy flow. Stone proposed that polarity therapy could release blocked energy and manipulate energy flow between negative and positive charges (Sharp, 1997). Unfortunately, despite an extensive body of writings left behind by Dr. Stone, there is a paucity of experimental studies in the area of polarity therapy. In 1999, Benford and colleagues investigated the fluctuation of electromagnetic fields during polarity therapy and found a reduction in gamma radiation at four different treatment sites, but an explanation and implications for such a reduction have not be identified.

Reiki

Reiki is an energetic healing practice with origins consistent with ancient Tibetan Buddhist teachings. As with other healing approaches based on Asian medical systems, an underlying assumption of Reiki is that imbalance of one's energy field can result in physical or emotional dysfunction or illness (Horan, 1992). During a Reiki session, the practitioner intends to channel vital energy from the universe into the client's energy field to facilitate balance and healing (Barnett & Chambers, 1996). Further discussion of this intervention can be found in a subsequent chapter in this book.

Therapeutic Touch

Therapeutic touch (TT) is a contemporary interpretation of the ancient health practice of laying on of hands. Developed by Dolores Krieger, PhD, RN, professor emeritus at New York University and Dora Kunz, and a mystic and healer, TT is based on the Hindu concepts of prana and chakras and the assumption that disease or impairment reflects an imbalance in the flow of vital life energy. The intention for all TT sessions is to restore balance in the client's energy field and flow, thereby promoting an environment for self-healing (Krieger, 1997). A more detailed description of TT can be found in a subsequent chapter in this book.

External Sources of Biofields

In addition to life energies, the terms *energy medicine* and *energy therapy* also include interventions that utilize electromagnetic energy in the form of electricity, magnetism, light, and sound waves to facilitate health and healing. In *The Body Electric* (1985), physician-researcher Robert Becker describes his early work on salamander regeneration and how this work led to the discovery of the existence of bioelectrical currents throughout the body and nervous system. Since then, much research in the area of electrical stimulation and tissue healing has been conducted, and for many health care providers, electrical stimulation is considered to be fairly mainstream. Abeed, Naseer, and Abel (1998) and Zamora-Navas and colleagues (1995) have demonstrated the benefits of using capacitively coupled electrical stimulation (CCEST) in nonunion fractures of long bone. Goodwin and colleagues (1999), Mooney (1990), and Kane (1988) have reported successful use of electrical stimulation for lumbar spinal fusions. Other research has supported the use of electrical stimulation for chronic wound healing (Baker et al., 1997; Gardner, Frantz, & Schmidt, 1999; Kloth & McCulloch, 1996).

Transcutaneous electrical nerve stimulation (TENS) is another form of electrical stimulation that is often recommended by mainstream health care providers as a way to interrupt the transmission of pain messages to the brain, thereby decreasing the client's pain (Melzack, 1983; Yurtkuran & Kocagil, 1999). Electrical stimulation is delivered to specific nerve and/or muscle points via topical electrodes that are connected to a stimulator that can be worn like a pager. Other studies by Ghoname and colleagues (1999a, 1999b) not only demonstrated that TENS is effective in reducing low back pain and sciatica, but also determined that a different form of stimulation, known as percutaneous electrical nerve stimulation (PENS) is even more effective. Unlike TENS, which is noninvasive, PENS involves the electrical stimulation of acupuncture-like needles that are placed into soft tissue and/or muscle. PENS has been effective in reducing diabetic neuropathic pain (Hamza et al., 2000) and headache (Ahmed et al., 2000).

Magnets

Interventions that utilize other energy forms, such as magnetism and sound waves, are not as supported in the scientific literature. The suggestion that magnets can be used to promote health and healing has been offered since the late 18th century when Franz Anton Mesmer (1734–1815), an Austrian physician, proposed that humans possess a form of energy called *animal magnetism* and that he could manipulate animal magnetism using magnets. Early treatments consisted of moving real magnets over a client's body to regulate fluid in the tissues, but Mesmer eventually abandoned the magnets all together, believing his hands possessed electrical properties that could produce improvement in unhealthy conditions (Gerber, 1988).

In this century, companies that distribute therapeutic magnets have suggested the use of magnets to relieve pain. Despite millions of dollars being spent on magnets, only a handful of studies have investigated the efficacy of magnets in the management of pain, and the results have been conflicting. In one randomized, double-blind study Vallbona, Hazlewood, and

Jurida (1997) reported that persons with postpolio syndrome who used a 300–500 Gauss magnetic device experienced a significant reduction of trigger point pain as compared to subjects in the placebo group. In a later study, however, Collacott and colleagues (2000) reported that the use of bipolar magnet therapy had no therapeutic benefits for persons with chronic low back pain when compared to a sham treatment.

Sound

Sound therapy, which incorporates sound healing and music therapy, is an intervention that uses auditory and vibrational input to facilitate changes in physiology, emotions, and behavior. Sound healing, which has its roots in ancient and Native American healing traditions, may involve many different methods, such as chimes, chanting, or drumming. Practitioners of sound healing suggest that specific sound frequencies delivered at certain intervals can promote health and healing through a wide range of mechanisms. When searching for scientific evidence for sound healing, however, only one article was identified. Bittman and colleagues (2001) investigated the role of group drumming in the alteration of stress-related hormones, cell-mediated immunity, and anxiety. Although the researchers identified some neuroendocrine and immunologic alterations in drumming subjects as compared to controls, they acknowledge the need to address such issues as timing and duration of the intervention. The magnitude of effect should also be considered, given the finding that no pre- or post-differences existed in drumming subjects compared to controls in depression or anxiety.

Music

Music and music therapy, on the other hand, has received quite of bit of attention in the literature. People have written that listening to certain types of music can lower blood pressure and heart rate (Barnason, Zimmerman, Nieveen, 1995; White, 1999), reduce pain and anxiety (Barnason, Zimmerman, Nieveen, 1995; LeScouarnec et al., 2001; Schorr, 1993), and alter mood (McCraty et al., 1998). Recent studies on the effects of music and music therapy have not only investigated stress and behavioral alterations, but have also measured direct changes in neuroendocrine and neuroimmune values (Burns et al., 2001; Kumar et al., 1999). While there have been a few studies in which the researchers did not find music to significantly benefit a pre- and postoperative patient population, the literature generally supports music therapy as a useful therapeutic intervention for different client populations (Broscious, 1999; Gaberson, 1995; Good et al., 1999). Investigators have identified the need to advance research in music and music therapy by conducting studies with more rigorous designs, greater number of subjects and consistent psychological and physiological markers (Kneafsey, 1997; LeScouarnec, et al., 2001).

Summary

Energy medicine or therapies are approaches that utilize either internal or external sources of energy for client health and healing. Medical systems that acknowledge internal sources of energy are Traditional Chinese Medicine and Ayurveda. Approaches that utilize internal sources of energy include Reiki and therapeutic touch. Approaches that use external sources of energy include electrical stimulation, magnets, music, and sound. Evidence to support each approach varies.

STUDY QUESTIONS

1. How are energy approaches classified?
2. Define qi and universal polarity.
3. Describe the concepts of prana and chakras.
4. Discuss basic concepts of electrical stimulation.
5. Discuss basic concepts central to sound and music therapy.

RESOURCES

American Polarity Therapy Association
PO Box 19858
Boulder, CO 80308
(303) 545-2080
hq@polaritytherapy.org
www.polaritytherapy.org

American Music Therapy Association, Inc.
8455 Colesville Road, Suite 1000
Silver Spring, MD 20910

(301) 589-3300
info@musictherapy.org
www.musictherapy.org

British Institute of Magnet Therapy
Lower Race, Pontypool, Torfaen,
   NP4 5UH
01-495 752122
bimt@mag-lab.com; bimt@cogreslab.co.uk
www.maglab.co.uk/bimtnews.htm

REFERENCES

Abeed, R. I., M. Naseer, & E. W. Abel. (1998). Capacitively coupled electrical stimulation treatment: Results from patients with failed long bone fracture unions. *Journal of Orthopedic Trauma, 12*(7), 510–513.

Ahmed, H. E., P. F. White, W. F. Craig, M. A. Hamza, E. S. Ghoname, & N. M. Gajraj. (2000). Use of percutaneous electrical nerve stimulation (PENS) in the short-term management of headache. *Headache, 40*(4), 311–315.

Baker, L. L., R. Chamber, S. K. DeMuth, & F. Villar. (1997). Effects of electrical stimulation on wound healing in patients with diabetic ulcers. *Diabetes Care, 20*(3), 405–412.

Barnason, S., L. Zimmerman, & J. Nieveen. (1995). The effects of music interventions on anxiety in the patient after coronary artery bypass grafting. *Heart Lung, 14*(2), 124–133.

Barnett, L., & M. Chambers. (1996). *Reiki Energy Medicine: Bringing Healing Touch into Home, Hospital, and Hospice.* Rochester, VT: Healing Arts Press.

Becker, R. O., & G. Selden. (1985). *The Body Electric.* New York: William Morrow.

Benford, M. S., J. Talnagi, D. B. Doss, S. Boosey, & L. E. Arnold. (1999). Gamma radiation fluctuations during alternative healing therapy. *Alternative Therapies in Health and Medicine, 5*(4), 51–56.

Bittman, B. B., L. S. Berk, D. L. Felten, J. Westengard, O. C. Simonton, J. Pappas, & M. Ninehouser. (2001). Composite effects of group drumming music therapy on modulation of neuroendocrine-immune parameters in normal subjects. *Alternative Therapies in Health and Medicine, 7*(1), 38–47.

Broscious, S. K. (1999). Music: An intervention for pain during chest tube removal after open heart surgery. *American Journal of Critical Care, 8*(6), 410–415.

Burns, S. J., M. S. Harbuz, F. Hucklebridge, & L. Bunt. (2001). A pilot study into the therapeutic effects of music therapy at a cancer help center. *Alternative Therapies in Health and Medicine, 7*(1), 48–56.

Chopra, D. (1990). *Perfect Health—The Complete Mind/Body Guide*. New York: Crown Publishers.

Collacott, E. A., J. T. Zimmerman, D. W. White, & J. P. Rindone. (2000). Bipolar permanent magnets for the treatment of chronic low back pain: A pilot study. *Journal of the American Medical Association, 283*(10), 1322–1325.

Dossey, L. (1999). *Reinventing Medicine: Beyond Mind-Body to a New Era of Healing*. New York: HarperCollins.

Gaberson, K. B. (1995). The effect of humorous and musical distraction on preoperative anxiety. *AORN Journal, 62*(5), 784–788.

Gardiner, S. E., R. A. Frantz, & F. L. Schmidt. (1999). Effect of electrical stimulation on chronic wound healing: A meta-analysis. *Wound Repair Rejuvenation, 7*(6), 495–503.

Gerber, R. (1988). *Vibrational Medicine: New Choices for Healing Ourselves*. (Rev. ed.). Santa Fe, NM: Bear & Company.

Gerber, R. (2000). *Vibrational Medicine for the 21st Century*. New York: HarperCollins.

Ghoname, E. A., P. E. White, H. E. Ahmed, M. A. Hamza, W. F. Craig, & C. E. Noe. (1999a). Percutaneous electrical nerve stimulation: An alternative to TENS in the management of sciatica. *Pain, 83*(2), 193–199.

Ghoname, E. A., W. F. Craig, H. E. Ahmed, M. A. Hamza, B. N. Henderson, N. M. Gajraj, P. J. Huber, & R. J. Gatchel. (1999b). Percutaneous electrical nerve stimulation for low back pain: A randomized crossover study. *Journal of the American Medical Association. 281*(9), 818–823.

Good, M., M. Stanton-Hicks, J. A. Grass, G. Cranston-Anderson, C. Choi, L. J. Schoolmeester, & A. Salman. (1999). Relief of postoperative pain with jaw relaxation, music and their combination. *Pain, 81*(1–2), 163–172.

Goodwin, C. B., C. T. Brighton, R. D. Guyer, J. R. Johnson, K. I. Light, & H. A. Yuan. (1999). A double-blind study of capacitively coupled electrical stimulation as an adjunct to lumbar spinal fusions. *Spine, 24*(13), 1349–1356.

Hamza, M. A., P. F. White, W. F. Craig, E. S. Ghoname, H. E. Ahmed, T. J. Proctor, C. E. Noe, A. S. Vakharia, & N. Gajraj. (2000). Percutaneous electrical nerve stimulation: A novel analgesic therapy for diabetic neuropathic pain. *Diabetes Care, 23*(3), 365–370.

Horan, P. (1992). *Empowerment Through Reiki*. (2nd ed.). Wilmot, WI: Lotus Light.

Kane, W. J. (1988). Direct current electrical bone growth stimulation for spinal fusion. *Spine, 13*(3), 363–365.

Karagulla, S., & D. Kunz. (1989). *The Chakras and the Human Energy Field*. Wheaton, IL: Theosophical Publishing House.

Kitts, B. (1988). Polarity therapy. In F. M. Tappen (Ed.), *Healing Massage Techniques: Holistic, Classic and Emerging Methods*. Englewood Cliffs, NJ: Prentice-Hall.

Kloth, L. E., and J. M. McCulloch. (1996). Promotion of wound healing with electrical stimulation. *Advances in Wound Care, 95*(5), 42–45.

Kneafsey, R. (1997). The therapeutic use of music in a care of the elderly setting: A literature review. *Journal of Clinical Nursing, 6*(5), 341–346.

Krieger, D. (1997). *Therapeutic Touch Inner Workbook: Ventures in Transpersonal Healing*. Santa Fe, NM: Bear & Company.

Kumar, A. M., F. Tims, D. G. Cruess, M. J. Mintzer, G. Ironson, D. Loewenstein, R. Cattan, J. B. Fernandez, C. Eisdorfer, & M. Kumar. (1999). Music therapy increases serum melatonin levels in patients with Alzheimer's disease. *Alternative Therapies in Health and Medicine, 5*(6), 49–57.

Kunz, D. (1991). *The Personal Aura*. Wheaton, IL: Theosophical Publishing House.

LeScouarnec, R., R. Poirier, J. E. Owens, J. Gauthier, A. G. Taylor, & P. A. Foresman. (2001). Use of biaural beat tapes for treatment of anxiety: A pilot study of tape preference and outcomes. *Alternative Therapies in Health and Medicine, 7*(1), 58–63.

McCraty, R., B. Barrios-Choplin, M. Atkinson, & D. Tomasino. (1998). The effects of different types of music on mood, tension, and mental clarity. *Alternative Therapies in Health and Medicine, 4*(1), 75–84.

Melzack, R., P. Vetere, & L. Finch. (1983). Transcutaneous electrical nervous stimulation for low back pain: A combination of TENS and massage for pain and range of motion. *Physical Therapy, 63*(4), 489–493.

Mooney, V. (1990). A randomized double blind prospective study of the efficacy of pulsed electromagnetic fields for interbody lumbar fusions. *Spine, 15*(7), 708–712.

National Institutes of Health, National Center for Complementary and Alternative Medicine. (2000). [Online]. Available: *http://altmed.od.nuh.gov/nccam/what-is-cam/classify.shtml*.

Pelletier, K. R. (2000). *The Best Alternative Medicine*. New York: Simon & Schuster.

Reid, D. (1994). *The Complete Book of Chinese Health and Healing*. Boston: Shambhala.

Schorr, A. (1993). Music and pattern change in chronic pain. *Advances in Nursing Science, 15*(4), 27–36.

Sharp, M. B. (1997). Polarity, reflexology and touch for health. In C. M. Davis (Ed.), *Complementary Therapies in Rehabilitation*. Thorofare, NJ: Slack.

Sills, F. (1990). *The Polarity Process: Energy as a Healing Art*. Dorset, UK: Element Books.

Vallbona, C., C. F. Hazlewood, & G. Jurida. (1997). Response of pain to static magnetic fields in postpolio patients: A double–blind pilot study. *Archives of Physical Medicine and Rehabilitation, 78*(11), 1200–1203.

Veith, I. (1970). *The Yellow Emperor's Classic of Internal Medicine*. (I. Veith, Trans.). Los Angeles, CA: University of California Press.

Weil, A. (1983). *Health & Healing—Understanding Conventional & Alternative Medicine*. Boston: Houghton Mifflin.

White, J. M. (1999). Effects of relaxing music on cardiac autonomic balance and anxiety after acute myocardial infarction. *American Journal of Critical Care, 8*, 220–230.

Yurtkuran, M., & T. Kocagil. (1999). TENS, electroacupuncture and ice massage: Comparison of treatment for osteoarthritis of the knee. *American Journal of Acupuncture, 27*(3–4), 133–140.

Zamora-Navis, F., V. A. Borras, L. R. Antelo, A. J. Saras, & R. M. Pena. (1995). Electrical stimulation of bone malunion with the presence of a gap. *Acta Orthopedica of Belgium, 61*(3), 169–176.

10

Introduction to Manual and Body-Based Approaches

Judith Deutsch

CHAPTER OBJECTIVES

- Understand the basic purpose of chiropractic and osteopathic medicine.
- Understand and differentiate between the general components of manual and movement therapies.
- Understand the general scope of current research knowledge of different body-based systems.

Manual and body-based therapies are considered a distinct complementary and alternative medicine (CAM) domain in the National Center for Complementary and Alternative Medicine classification (NCCAM, 2001). Manual therapies are defined as those therapies in which the methods are based on manipulation and/or movement of the body. This domain is divided into three categories: osteopathy, chiropractic, and massage and bodywork. Therapies in the bodywork category, which are included in this book, are craniosacral therapy (CST), Feldenkrais, myofascial release, and Structural Integration (Rolfing). Other therapies, such as the Alexander technique and Pilates, not presented in this book, are also classified as bodywork. While not included in NCCAM's listing as manual body-based therapies, reflexology, yoga, and T'ai Chi could potentially be included in this category. Reflexology has some similarities with the manual tissue-based therapies, while T'ai Chi and forms of yoga have elements that are similar to the movement therapies. Typically, yoga and T'ai Chi are classified as mind-body approaches.

Osteopathic Medicine and Chiropractic

Osteopathic medicine and chiropractic practices, in their original conceptualization, were designed to treat abnormalities of structure and function (Greenman, 1996). Generally practi-

100

tioners of both approaches examine body muscle tension and restricted movement, applying manual techniques such as thrusts (chiropractors) and muscle energy (osteopaths) in order to restore alignment and movement. Thrusts are direct manipulations of the spine, while muscle energy techniques use the tension that can be developed by a muscle's contraction to restore joint alignment (Nyberg, 1993). Recently, both osteopathy and chiropractic have developed a broader scope of practice, but practitioners still use bodywork techniques when clients have musculoskeletal pathology.

Contributions from osteopathy and chiropractic can be found in the manual therapies. For example, the craniosacral approach is a derivative of osteopathy. The evidence to support osteopathic and chiropractic medicine has been reviewed elsewhere (Vickers & Zollman, 1999a). For more detailed reading on osteopathic and chiropractic approaches, refer to Greenman (1996), Kaptchuk & Eisenberg (1998), and Thomas and colleagues (2002).

Massage and Bodywork

Massage and bodywork comprise the third category of body-based therapies. Many forms of massage are influenced by the system of medicine on which they are based. For example, most practitioners of Shiatsu masssage (i.e., accupressure) follow many of the principles of Traditional Chinese Medicine, such as use of meridians and the flow of chi (Sasaki, 1988).

Massage has been used to promote relaxation, treat painful muscular conditions, and reduce anxiety. Reportedly, it is used to improve sleep disorders and pain, conditions known to be exacerbated by anxiety, as well as improve self-image in conditions such as physical disabilities and terminal illnesses (Vickers, 1999b). Systematic reviews of massage executed by the Cochrane Collaboration found support for the use of massage with low-birthweight infants by increasing their weight and decreasing their length of hospital stay (Vickers et al., 1998), but not for improving developmental outcomes in infants (Vickers et al., 2001) or as a stand alone intervention for low back pain (Furlan et al., 2001). In random clinical trials it has also been shown that massage reduces anxiety in young psychiatric patients (Field, 1992) and has psychophysiologic benefits for postcardiac patients (Stevensen, 1995). The use of reflexology was shown to decrease premenstrual syndromes when compared to a sham reflexology condition (Oleson & Flocco, 1993). Interestingly, massage is often used as a control condition for testing other complementary therapies. For example, massage was compared with acupuncture for the treatment of chronic neck pain and found to be less effective (Irnich et al., 2001).

Bodywork

The bodywork therapies that are presented in the following chapters can be divided into movement awareness (such as Feldenkrais, T'ai Chi, and yoga), tissue-based approaches (such as Rolfing, myofascial release, and reflexology), and energy-based approaches (craniosacral therapy [CST]). Some approaches are named for their originator (e.g., the Feldenkrais Method and Rolfing), while others are derivatives of specific techniques (e.g., craniosacral therapy from osteopathy) or describe their actions (e.g., myofascial release). With the exception of yoga and T'ai Chi, all of the approaches were developed in the 20th century. This suggests that their practice is rather new and perhaps the levels of evidence to support them are just being developed.

Tissue-based approaches are similar to the osteopathic and chiropractic approaches in the sense that the relationship between structure and function is central and the intervention is aimed at restoring function by modifying the structure of the individual. Structure is modified by direct and indirect manual techniques. The fascial system, which connects all the structures in the body, is central to these approaches. However, there are some important differences. Myofascial release is recommended as a component of a comprehensive intervention. Structural Integration is a complete approach which includes elements of tissue work and movement reeducation. In craniosacral therapy the examination and intervention balances energy fields and therefore affects not only the musculoskeletal but the also the immune and nervous systems. Barnes (2003) has suggested a hypothesis about the mechanisms that may underlie the tissue-based therapies in Chapter 16, "Myofascial Release." Refer to the chapters on energy therapies and therapeutic touch in this book for more information on mechanisms of energy therapies.

The movement therapy approaches, as their name suggests, are indicated for teaching efficient movement. T'ai Chi, yoga, and Feldenkrais have in common an emphasis on ease, efficiency, and awareness of movement. In yoga the emphasis is on focusing the mind to allow the body to enhance health, while in Feldenkrais the sensory system is heightened to increase awareness about the effects of movement. T'ai Chi, Feldenkrais, and some forms of yoga can be considered movement reeducation tools and are indicated for clients who need or wish to relearn movement, either due to illness or disability or to enhance wellness.

Indications and Evidence-Based Therapy

The movement therapies appear to be indicated for a wide range of client populations, which include people with cardiovascular disease as well as neurologic and musculoskeletal conditions. There is some evidence to support most of these suggested applications. The tissue-based approaches appear to be indicated primarily for musculoskeletal conditions, but both Structural Integration and craniosacral therapy are recommended for neurologic conditions as well. Evidence, although preliminary, to support these indications can be found for Structural Integration (Cottingham & Maitland, 2000; Deutsch, Judd, & DeMasi, 1997; Perry, Jones, & Thomas, 1981), Shiatsu, and reflexology. See individual chapters for references.

The evidence to support the efficacy and efficiency of the bodywork approaches spans a broad range. There are no cited efficacy studies in the myofascial release and craniosacral therapy literatures, while there are several clinical trials and a large number on articles that deal with the mechanisms of yoga and T'ai Chi. Between these two extremes of evidence are approaches such as Structural Integration and awareness through movement (ATM), an aspect of the Feldenkrais Method (see Chapter 15, "The Feldenkrais Method," for references as well as Lake, 1985; Gutman, Herbert, & Brown, 1977; Bearman & Shafarman, 1999; and Stephens et al., 2001)—approaches in which some clinical efficacy study exists. With the exception of Johnson and colleagues' investigation (1999), none have been large-scale trials. Yet in their modest literatures, Shiatsu, Structural Integration, reflexology, and ATM have supported some of their assumptions.

Criteria to become a practitioner vary greatly. Structural Integration, reflexology, the Feldenkrais Method, and craniosacral therapy organizations provide certification after intensive training. Craniosacral therapy organizations provide intermediate levels of training, and one can begin to learn ATM principles in four-day courses. There are no short courses on Structural Integration. T'ai Chi, myofascial release, and yoga instruction is provided in a continuing education model. While practitioners of each approach will improve skills with practice and training, extensive personal development of one's practice in yoga and T'ai Chi is highly recommended for teachers. Such differences in training requirements may account for the frequency with which therapists practice these approaches.

Summary

When taken as a group, the manual and body-based therapies are relevant to the therapist's practice. Concepts of alignment, muscle balance, ease of movement, and performance of static and dynamic exercises are part of the foundation of our training. Elements of many of these approaches are taught in entry-level training and do complement therapy practice. As the evidence to support these approaches increases, so will therapists' confidence in choosing them as part of therapy interventions. It is important to note, however, that for some of these approaches, Structural Integration and FM for example, there is extensive training in order to be certified, and therefore therapists may need to collaborate with trained practitioners or seek training themselves.

STUDY QUESTIONS

1. Provide general definitions for chiropractic and osteopathic medicine.
2. Describe relevant information about the following approaches. Include general information about each approach's definition, NCCAM classification, research support, and training.
   craniosacral therapy
   Feldenkrais Method
   myofascial release
   reflexology
   Shiatsu
   Structural Integration
   T'ai Chi
   yoga

REFERENCES

Barnes, J. F. (2003). Myofascial release. In J. Carlson (Ed.), *Complementary Therapies and Wellness: Practice Essentials for Holistic Health Care*. Upper Saddle River, NJ: Prentice Hall.

Bearman, D. & S. Shafarman. (1999). Alternative medicine. The Feldenkrais Method in the treatment of chronic pain: A study of efficacy and cost effectiveness. *American Journal of Pain Management, 9*(1), 22–7.

Cottingham, J. T., & J. Maitland. (2000). Case reports. Integrating manual and movement therapy with philosophical counseling for treatment of a patient with amyotrophic lateral sclerosis: A case study that explores the principles of holistic intervention. *Alternative Therapies in Health & Medicine, 6*(2), 128, 120–127.

Deutsch, J. E., P. Judd, & I. DeMassi. (1997). Structural Integration applied to patients with a primary neurologic diagnosis: Two case studies. *Neurology Report, 21*(5), 161–162.

Field, T., C. Morrow, C. Valdeon, S. Larson, C. Kuhn, & S. Schanberg. (1992). Massage reduces anxiety in child and adolescent psychiatric patients. *Journal of the American Academy of Child and Adolescent Psychiatry, 31,* 125–31.

Furlan, A. D., L. Brosseau, V. Welch, & J. Wong. (2001). Massage for low back pain. [Systematic Review] Cochrane Back Group. *Cochrane Database of Systematic Reviews,* Issue 2.

Greenman, P. E. (1996). Manipulative medicine. In P. E. Greenman (Ed.), *Principles of Manual Medicine* (2nd ed.). Baltimore: Williams and Wilkins.

Gutman G. M., C. P. Herbert, & S. R. Brown. (1977). Feldenkrais versus conventional exercises for the elderly. *Journal of Gerontology, 32*(5), 562–72.

Johnson S. K., J. Frederick, M. Kaufman, & B. Mountjoy. (1999). A controlled investigation of bodywork in multiple sclerosis. *Journal of Alternative & Complementary Medicine, 5*(3), 237–43.

Irnich, D., N. Behrens, H. Molzen, A. Konig, J. Gleditsch, M. Krauss, M. Natalis, E. Senn, A. Beyer, & P. Schops. Randomised trial of acupuncture compared with conventional massage and "sham" laser acupuncture for treatment of chronic neck pain. *British Medical Journal, 322*(7302), 1574–8.

Kaptchuk, T. J., & D. M. Eisenberg. (1988). Chiropractic: Origins, controversies and contributions. *Archives of Internal Medicine, 158,* 2215–2224.

Lake, B. (1985). Acute back pain: Treatment by the application of Feldenkrais principles. *Australian Family Physician, 14,* 1175–1178.

NCCAM. (2001). Major domains of complementary and alternative therapies, NCCAM. [Online] Available: www.nccam.nih.gov.

Nyberg, R. (1993). Manipulation: Definitions, types and application. In J. V. Basmajian & R. Nyberg (Eds.), *Rational Manual Therapies.* Baltimore: Williams and Wilkins.

Oleson, T., & W. Flocco. (1993). Randomized controlled study of premenstrual symptoms treated with ear, hand, and foot reflexology. *Obstetrics & Gynecology, 82*(6), 906–11.

Perry J., M. H. Jones, & L. Thomas. (1981). Functional evaluation of Rolfing in cerebral palsy. *Developmental Medicine & Child Neurology, 23*(6), 717–29.

Sasaki, P. (1988). Shiatsu: An overview. In F. M. Tappan (Ed.), *Healing Massage Techniques: Holistic, Classic, and Emerging Methods* (2nd ed.). Norwalk: Appleton & Lange.

Stephens, J., D. DuShuttle, C. Hatcher, J. Schmunes, & C. Slaninka. (2001). Improvements in balance and confidence resulting from the use of Awareness Through Movement, a structured, group motor learning process: A randomized, controlled study in people with Multiple Sclerosis. *Neurology Report, 25,* 39–54.

Stevensen, C. (1994). The psychophysiological effects of aromatherapy massage following cardiac surgery. *Complementary Therapies in Medicine, 2,* 27–35.

Thomas, F., D. C. Bergman, H. David, D. C. Peterson, J. Dana, & D. C. Lawrence. (2002). *Chiropractic Techniques* (2nd ed.). Philadelphia: Churchill Livingstone.

Vickers, A., A. Ohlsson, J. B. Lacy, & A. Horsley. (1998). Massage therapy for premature and/or low birth-weight infants to improve weight gain and/or to decrease hospital length of stay. In Cochrane Collaboration, *The Cochrane Library.* Issue 3. Oxford: Update Software.

Vickers, A., A. Ohlsson, J. B. Lacy, & A. Horsley. (2001). Massage for promoting growth and development of preterm and/or low birth-weight infants. [Systematic Review] Cochrane Neonatal Group. *Cochrane Database of Systematic Reviews.* Issue 2.

Vickers, A., & C. Zollman. (1999a). Clinical Review: ABC of complementary therapies: Osteopathy and Chiropractic. *British Medical Journal, 319,* 1176–1179.

Vickers, A., & C. Zollman. (1999b). Clinical Review: ABC of complementary therapies: Massage therapies. *British Medical Journal, 319,* 1254–1257.

11

Introduction to Mind-Body Interventions

Jodi L. Carlson

CHAPTER OBJECTIVES

- Define psychoneuroimmunology and understand related concepts.
- Describe different concepts of placebo.
- Discuss the importance of mind-body concepts in Eastern medicine.
- Discuss self regulation and mind-body therapies.
- Describe the importance of information theory and state-dependent learning on mind-body therapies.

Mind-body interventions are defined by NCCAM as interventions that ". . . employ a variety of techniques designed to facilitate the mind's capacity to affect bodily function and symptoms" (NCCAM, 2001, p. 3). This generally refers to interventions that can be taught to clients to affect themselves, as opposed to interventions directed by the intention of another person, such as in energy therapies. Some mind-body interventions overlap with other domains of alternative therapies. For example, T'ai Chi is classified by NCCAM as both a mind-body and body-based method. Other interventions, such as Qi Gong, incorporate multiple domains of approach, such as imagery and internal focus (mind-body approaches) as well as an external focus, which is an energy therapy.

The body of knowledge supporting and explaining the workings of mind-body interventions is diverse. Many facets of mind-body interventions have been demonstrated through research, but much is still theoretical. The purpose of this chapter is to introduce the reader to the research and theory relevant to mind-body interventions.

Many professionals refer to seeing *with* or *in* the mind's eye when discussing mind-body approaches such as imagery, meditation, and visualization. The notion of seeing or "directing" the mind's eye (Samuels, 1975) for healing alludes to the effect the psyche can have on the physical body. Approaches to treatment that utilize the effect of the psyche on the body in nontraditional ways are called mind-body interventions. The mechanisms behind mind-body work are increasingly being studied and understood. To enhance the use of mind-body approaches, therapists need to understand the research and related theories.

Psychoneuroimmunology

The field of psychoneuroimmunology (PNI) and its sister disciplines—neuroimmodulation, psychoneuroendocrinology, and behavioral medicine (Pert, Dreher, & Ruff, 1998)—contribute the strongest scientific support for the notion that the mind affects bodily function and symptoms. PNI is defined as ". . . the study of interactions among behavior, neural and endocrine function, and immune system processes" (Ader, Felten, & Cohen, 2001, p. xxi). The "psyche" aspect of these fields addresses more than behavior. It also includes aspects of human experience, such as psychological and sociological traits.

In 1975, Ader and Cohen showed that animals can be taught to alter behavior and immune function via classical conditioning. The researchers inadvertently taught rats to vomit *and* depress their immune systems when given sweetened water by initially pairing sweetened water with cyclophosphamide, a chemotherapy agent that induces vomiting and depresses immune function. Since then, Ader and Cohen (2001) note that while selected studies have not demonstrated a conditioning effect (e.g., Booth, Petrie, & Brook, 1995), animal research and some research on humans does support conditioning responses overall. Further research is needed to determine why conditioning occurs in some populations and under certain conditions but not others.

In general, many PNI studies have shown relationships and some causation between the psyche and disease, disease and immunity, and the psyche and immunity. Delahanty, Dougall, and Baum (2001) found that the current body of research supports endocrine and immune changes after both natural disasters and traumatic stress, and that human-caused disasters are associated with increased persistency in immune changes. Turner-Cobb, Septon, and Spiegel (2001) note that "the role of social support provides the strongest evidence of psychosocial impact on illness . . ." (p. 572), and the public has been aware for years of the negative effects of personality traits such as hostility and the Type A personality, which increase risk for chronic cardiac disease. Such bodies of knowledge in PNI stem from correlation studies, which measure relationships, as opposed to stemming from causation studies, which seek to measure origination of effects.

An example of the state and limits of knowledge in PNI at press time is in the area of acute exercise. Hoffman-Goetz and Pedersen (2001) reviewed the effects of acute exercise on immune response. A significant amount of research shows that acute exercise stress produces nonspecific immune response such as prolonged neutrophil action, increased monocytes and macrophages, and natural killer cell action; and some evidence suggests that certain immune responses decrease after exercise. Research also demonstrates the immune-related affects of acute exercise on many physiological systems (e.g., exercise increases the heart rate, which increases blood flow to skeletal muscles), but only theorizes how increased blood flow can enhance immune function. Causative interactions, and their clinical significance, remain to be shown (Ader & Cohen, 2001; Hoffman-Goetz & Pedersen, 2001).

Reviewing psychosocial effects on immune function and disease progression in human cancers, Turner-Cobb, Septon, and Spiegel (2001) note that "any psychosocial factor that can upregulate immune mechanisms that defend against cancer may also have the potential to retard the progression of disease with some varieties of tumors. However, much research is needed to determine the combinations of psychosocial factors and types of tumors in which such mechanisms may operate" (p. 568). Theoretically, "cancer" and "tumors" can be replaced with a more generic "illness," since the principle is the same—any factor that enhances immune function might potentially be used to prevent the progression of illness.

Another set of overlapping but not exclusive effects are those of stress reduction paradigms in altering infectious and inflammatory illness (Sternberg, 2000). Noting that different cultures have utilized mind-body interventions for centuries, Sternberg (2000) comments:

> . . . meditation, psychotherapy, prayer and exercise all share components which could change an individual's perception of stressful stimuli, thus changing the degree to which stress-responsive neuroendocrine systems are brought into play in response to such stimuli. If psychological and neurohormonal responses can be altered by relaxation techniques, such approaches could also ultimately modulate immune responses after stress exposure, through modulating the many neurohormonal and neurotransmitter pathways through which the nervous and immune systems communicate. (p. 40)

The relevance of PNI and related disciplines for therapists lies in support for structuring interventions and the environment for maximal health and healing, as well as preventive efforts, such as harnessing the power of stress reduction paradigms or other behavioral factors, to reduce risk and morbidity associated with illness. The next frontier of PNI research will involve connecting the areas of psyche, disease, and immunity to demonstrate causation, and determining the clinical significance of these interactions to enhance evidence based practice.

The Psychosomatic Network

> The bodymind can no longer be wholly characterized as a hierarchical system of hard-wired connections that descend down from a putative ruling station (the brain), but rather as an expansive network of free-flowing information transmitted by molecules that enter at any nodal point and move rapidly to any other point. (Pert, Dreher, & Ruff, 1998, p. 32)

Typically, many scientists and health professionals have thought of the body and mind as two separate but interconnected entities. The *psychosomatic network* is a term used to illustrate a new vision of the body and mind. As described by Pert and colleagues (1998), the old conceptualization of body and mind is being set aside for a vision of ". . . inseparable components of a dynamic mind-body system" (p. 30). Literally, the psychosomatic network describes how each part of the body, down to cells and DNA, has access to neural messages. This conceptualization is increasingly supported by research. Pert and colleagues reviewed related research that supports, among other notions, this infusion of the body with neural components, ". . . bidirectional communication between neuropeptides and the immune system" (p. 32), and how "biochemical substrates of *emotion* play crucial roles in *directing the movement of immune cells throughout the body*" (p. 33) (emphasis added).

The notion of a psychosomatic network is relevant to mind-body interventions not only because of the strong research support in PNI that backs it up, but also because it transforms conceptualization of the body and mind.

Placebo

The placebo response has generated a great deal of research and theory related to CAM and PNI. Placebos are "treatments" that appear similar to active treatments but that are not intended to affect specific illnesses or conditions (Hrobjartsson & Gotzsche, 2001). Beecher (1955) initially suggested that placebos are effective treatments for a variety of symptoms and illnesses, but his methodology has been criticized by Kaptchuk for intentionally hiding weak treatment effects (Horrigan, 2001). Nevertheless, studies have shown that placebos do produce clinically significant changes in people.

Other authors relate the placebo response to people's holistic being. Kaptchuk (Horrigan, 2001) defines the placebo effect as

> . . . an inherent capacity within a person to evoke renewed senses of well-being, intactness, and authenticity. This endowment is especially elicited by the symbolic and behavioral activities of the patient-healer encounter. The mediums through which such placebo effects seem to work include the power of belief, expectation, hope, imagination, will, intention, preference, and commitment, as well as the ability human beings have to change their relationship to disease and its meaning. (p. 102)

The placebo response works because something other than "active" treatments effect changes in people. The assumption has been that placebo effects can occur because the mind believes it is receiving an active treatment and directs the body to heal, implying the immense power the mind has in healing. If the mind has the power to heal the body when it believes active treatment is present, it is possible that there are other conditions under which the mind can direct the body to heal without active treatments. The relevance of placebo for therapists lies in support of the power of the mind in healing during the patient–healer encounter.

Eastern Medicine

It is significant that the notion that mind and body systems influence each other, as supported by PNI, is similar to how Traditional Chinese Medicine (TCM) and Ayurveda describe the body and the mind—as inseparably connected.

Kaptchuk notes ". . . mind and will are seen in the context of what the Chinese call spirit. For the Chinese, spirit is the dimension of human life that is not restricted to ordinary time and space. Mind is that aspect of spirit that describes the consciousness of possibilities" (Horrigan, 2001, p. 107). Furthermore, he notes that "one of the things I learned as a practitioner of Chinese medicine was that there is always room for transformation. . . . In any situation, there's always a possibility for people to have a different relationship with themselves" (p. 106). Eastern medicine systems promote the conscious use of mind-body interventions (although they call them by other names) such as meditation and the use of breath, as well as other factors such as exercise/activity, nutrition, and physical manipulation to enhance balance, prevent and/or treat illness. As a result of this conceptualization, interventions based in TCM or Ayurveda (such as T'ai Chi and yoga, respectively) often simultaneously address body and mind.

Self-Regulation

Most mind-body approaches can be understood to enhance health and healing by increasing self-regulation. Biofeedback uses visual and auditory cues to teach skills such as muscle reeducation, changed perception of pain, and autonomic control. Yoga uses breath work (Sovik, 2000) and, as with T'ai Chi, mindful participation in movement to enhance control of the body and mind. Imagery uses linguistic and sensory cues to increase control over physical and mental performance as well as emotional responses. And meditation and breath use mindful focusing to enhance health.

While topics discussed previously, such as PNI and the placebo effect, all have bearing on mind-body work in explaining the brain-body connections, they do not answer questions about optimum conditions to develop this connection for healing. E. L. Rossi's *The Psychobiology of Mind-Body Healing: New Concepts of Therapeutic Hypnosis* (1993) is notable for its compilation of information related to mind-body approaches and optimum conditions. Rossi (1993) notes: "Virtually all modern approaches to mind-body communication attempt to facilitate the process of converting words, images, sensations, ideas, beliefs, and expectations into the healing, physiological processes in the body" (p. 26). In discussing optimum conditions for mind-body interventions, then, words, images, beliefs, and the like seem to be harnessed for healing. For example, in the placebo response, its activity seems to be triggered, or optimally conditioned, by belief and expectation of healing.

One optimal condition for responses to mind-body approaches seems to be certain altered states of consciousness (Rossi, 1993). An altered state of consciousness (ASC) is defined as "a shift in a person's subjective experience from a usual state of awareness; may be induced by daydreams, dreams, deep relaxation, meditative practice, pharmacologic agents, including anesthesia, sudden psychophysiologic shift (blood loss, anoxia, dehydration, etc.)" (Dossey, 1988b, p. 24). ASC, as described above, includes healthy states as well as pathological states (Dossey, 1988b). ASC with the mastery of deep states of relaxation is referred to as optimal states of consciousness (OSC).

OSC, a state described as calm, quiet (Dossey, 1988b) and/or still, can be induced by psychophysiologic self-regulation (PPSR). PPSR balances brain hemisphere function and induces a relaxation response (Dossey, 1988b). The three components of PPSR are "body and inner self awareness, relaxation and visualization, and making effective choices" (Dossey, 1988b, p. 34). Many activities (e.g., jogging, writing) and mind-body approaches utilize methods that deliberately induce OSC.

Information Processing and State-Dependent Learning

OSC and PPSR seem to allow the mind to receive information, although the mechanisms behind this are not well understood. Theories of information processing and state-dependent learning describe possible mechanisms to understand how altered states of consciousness may be important in enhancing the mind's receptivity to enhance the therapeutic effect of mind-body therapies (Rossi, 1993).

Rossi's definition of PNI alludes to the mechanisms behind his theories: that the mind and body are *information transducers*. He provides an example of biofeedback, which he sees as ". . . biological energy of tension transduced into visible information of a measuring device" (p. 23) and goes on to say: "Mind and body are both aspects of one information system. Life is an information system. Biology is a process of information transduction. Mind and body are two facts or two ways of conceptualizing this single information system" (1993, p. 67). The notion that the mind and body are both aspects of one information system is supported by research such as Pert's findings about neuropeptides, which are vital communicators of the mind and body.

State-dependent learning is defined by Rossi: "What is learned and remembered is dependent on one's psychophysiological state at the time of the experience" (1993, p. 47). State-dependent learning is important because it may explain how stressful experiences are imprinted on a person's psyche, and possibly even on the physical body so that they perpetuate themselves (Cheek, 1981), and how altered states of consciousness may act to "release" a person from learned ways of being and provoke or induce a healing response. State-dependent learning may do this by enhancing the ability to focus on or access optimum health. In yoga, for example, researchers have shown that yogic breathing practices enhance the ability to consciously alter one's brainwaves and active control of body functions such as blood flow and heart rate (Green, Green, & Walters, 1979).

Summary

Mind-body interventions hold enormous promise for health professionals and their clients in expanding treatment options and optimizing both traditional and complementary approaches. While there is a need for further research, given the relatively small occurrence of unwanted side effects, enough evidence exists to support health professionals in integrating mind-body interventions into treatment.

STUDY QUESTIONS

1. Define psychoneuroimmunology.
2. Provide two definitions for placebo.
3. Describe how mind-body therapies enhance self-regulation.
4. Discuss how information theory and state-dependent learning can explain mechanisms of mind-body therapies.

REFERENCES

Ader, R., & N. Cohen. (1975). Behaviorally conditioned immunosuppression. *Psychosomatic Medicine, 37,* 333–340.

Ader, R., & N. Cohen. (2001). Conditioning and immunity. In R. Ader, D. Felton, & N. Cohen (Eds.), *Psychoneuroimmunology.* San Diego: Academic Press.

Ader, R., D. Felton, & N. Cohen. (2001). Preface. In R. Ader, D. Felton, & N. Cohen (Eds.), *Psychoneuroimmunology.* San Diego: Academic Press.

Beecher, H. K. (1955). The powerful placebo. *Journal of the American Medical Association, 159,* 1602–1605.

Booth, R. J., K. J. Petrie, & R. J. Brook. (1995). Conditioning allergic skin responses in humans: A controlled study. *Psychosomatic Medicine, 57,* 492–495.

Cheek, D. (1981). Awareness of meaningful sounds under general anesthesia: Considerations and a review of the literature, 1959–1979. *Theoretical and Clinical Aspects of Hypnosis.* Symposium Specialists, Miami, FL.

Delahanty, D. L., A. L. Dougall, & A. Baum. (2001). Neuroendocrine and immune alterations following natural disasters and traumatic stress. In R. Ader, D. Felton, & N. Cohen. (Eds.), *Psychoneuroimmunology.* San Diego: Academic Press.

Dossey, B. M. (1988b). The transpersonal self and states of consciousness. In B. M. Dossey, L. Keegan, C. E. Guzzetta, & L. G. Kolkmeier (Eds.), *Holistic Nursing: A Handbook for Practice,* Rockville, MD: Aspen.

Green, E. E., A. M. Green, & E. D. Walters. (1979). Biofeedback for mind/body self-regulation: Healing and creativity. In E. Peper, S. Ancoli, and M. Quinn (Eds.), *Mind-Body Integration.* New York: Plenum Press.

Hoffman-Goetz, L., & B. K. Pedersen. (2001). Immune responses to acute exercise: Hemodynamic, hormonal, and cytokine influences. In R. Ader, D. Felton, & N. Cohen (Eds.), *Psychoneuroimmunology.* San Diego: Academic Press.

Horrigan, B. (2001). Ted Kaptchuk, OMD: Subjectivity and the placebo effect in medicine. *Alternative Therapies in Health and Medicine, 7*(5), 100–108.

Hrobjartsson, A., & P. C. Gotzsche. (2001). Is the placebo powerless? An analysis of clinical trials comparing placebo with no treatment. *New England Journal of Medicine, 344*(21), 1594–1602.

NCCAM. (2001). Major domains of complementary and alternative medicine. [Online] Available: www.nccam.nih.gov.

Page, S. J. (2000). Imagery improves upper extremity motor function in chronic stroke patients: A pilot study. *Occupational Therapy Journal of Research, 20*(3), 200–212.

Parker, J. A. (2000). *Complementary Care: Alternative Paths to Wellness.* White Plains, NY: Oxford Medicare Advantage.

Pert, C. B., H. E. Dreher, & M. R. Ruff. (1998). The psychosomatic network: Foundations of mind-body medicine. *Alternative Therapies in Health and Medicine, 4*(4), 30–41.

Rossi, E. L. (1993). *The Psychobiology of Mind-Body Healing: New Concepts of Therapeutic Hypnosis.* New York: W. W. Norton.

Samuels, M. (1975). *Seeing with the Mind's Eye: The History, Techniques, and Uses of Visualization.* New York: Random House.

Sovik, R. (2000). The science of breathing—The yogic view. In E. A. Mayer & C. B. Saper (Eds.), *Progress in Brain Research, 122,* 491–505.

Sternberg, E. M. (2000). Interactions between the immune and endocrine systems. In E. A. Mayer & C. B. Saper (Eds.), *Progress in Brain Research, 122,* 35–42.

Turner-Cobb, J. M., S. E. Septon, & D. Spiegel. (2001). Psychosocial effects on immune function and disease progression in cancer: Human studies. In R. Ader, D. Felton, & N. Cohen (Eds.), *Psychoneuroimmunology.* San Diego: Academic Press.

12

Introduction to Health Promotion

Elicia Dunn Cruz

CHAPTER OBJECTIVES

- Describe current trends in public health.
- Define terms relevant to health promotion.
- Describe health promotion theories that focus on individual, interpersonal, and community levels of intervention.

Traditional medicine deals with discrete illnesses and their treatment. A person enters the traditional medical model after a diagnosis has been given regarding their health. Health promotion is concerned not just with a person's diagnosis and treatment but also with the person's behavior and its implications in regards to present as well as future illness or disease. This chapter introduces concepts that are central to health promotion and presents a sampling of theoretical models that guide health promotion programs.

Concepts Central to Health Promotion

The general aim of health promotion is to enable people "to increase control over, and to improve, their health" (World Health Organization, 1986, p. 1). This definition was articulated in the Ottawa Charter, which was developed during the World Health Organization's First International Conference on Health Promotion in 1986. The Charter defined health broadly as "a resource for everyday life . . . a positive concept emphasizing social and personal resources as well as physical capabilities" (p. 1) and further stated that "the fundamental conditions and resources for health are peace, shelter, education, food, income, a stable ecosystem, sustainable resources, social justice and equity" (p. 1).

The scope of practice for therapists has always included prevention and health promotion; however, therapists have often been restricted to engaging in these activities within the confines of the medical model and its reimbursement system—leaving them to work mainly with people who are already ill or disabled. Today, however, changes in society's needs and in the public health arena's focus and methods have handed therapists an opportunity to extend beyond these restrictions. Health is perceived as a "resource for living" rather than merely as the absence of disease; further, the issue of *quality* of life is now more important than merely *sustaining* life.

Contemporary public health aims to improve people's capacity for living via prevention and health promotion. The knowledge and experience that therapists bring to public health are valuable. Therapists have a unique focus on functional performance during day-to-day life. Public health professionals have well-developed theories about people's behavior, why they choose their behavior, and how we can help them choose and actualize healthy choices. Combing the knowledge base of these two fields can improve the efficiency of treatment and enhance people's health and wellness, whether through traditional or complementary approaches.

During the last century, health professionals have implemented various activities aimed at enabling people to maintain and enhance their health (Glanz, Lewis, and Rimer, 1997). As a result, health promotion has evolved from simple disease prevention and health education to a comprehensive dynamic approach that not only prevents disease, but also promotes health and wellness. This section defines concepts of health promotion and discusses the evolution of contemporary health promotion.

Terminology

Prevention focuses on identifying risk factors that correlate with the onset, greater severity, and longer duration of health problems, as well as on the protective factors that serve to improve people's resistance to risk factors and to subsequent health problems (Coie et al., 1993). Risk factors are characteristics such as genetic makeup, behavior, and sociocultural and physical environmental factors that increase the probability that the individual exposed to the risk will develop a specific disease or disability (Green & Kreuter, 1999). Prevention of such factors occurs at three levels. *Primary prevention* occurs prior to the onset of disease or overt symptoms of disease and focuses on identifying and reducing factors that place people or society at risk for the development of illness. *Secondary prevention* focuses on early detection of health problems and efforts to stop or slow the progression of the problem (Kniepmann, 1997). *Tertiary prevention* occurs when a health problem has occurred and has left residual damage; it aims to maximize remaining function (Sultz & Young, 1999).

Wellness refers to social, emotional, and spiritual aspects of health that extend beyond the absence of disease and disability. Wellness includes movement toward a greater awareness of and satisfaction from all aspects of life, including fitness, good nutrition, positive relation-

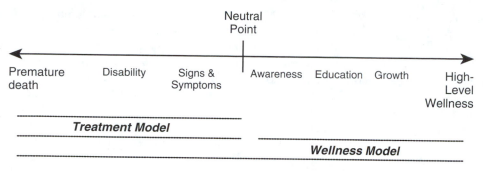

Figure 12–1 The illness–wellness continuum. *Adapted from Edelman and Fain (1998).*

ships, stress management, a life purpose, a consistent belief system, commitment to self-care, and environmental sensitivity and comfort (Murray & Zentner, 1993).

The term *health education* is sometimes used synonymously with health promotion. According to Green and Kreuter (1999), health education is only one approach to health promotion and is defined as "any combination of learning experiences designed to facilitate voluntary actions conducive to health" (p. 27). Health educators use teaching-learning strategies to facilitate the development of health-related knowledge, attitudes, and skills designed to facilitate voluntary adoption of healthy behaviors (Hooper, 1998).

Health promotion has a broader scope than health education (Breckon, Harvey, & Lancaster, 1998). It is "any planned combination of educational, political, regulatory, and organizational supports for actions and conditions of living conducive to the health of individuals, groups, or communities" (Green & Kreuter, 1999, p. 506). Health promotion is not simply the provision of information about risk factors; it is also the facilitation of and support for proactive decision making in all aspects of health. Unlike health education, health promotion encompasses both passive and active strategies to facilitate health through education and support (Edelman & Fain, 1998).

The full breadth of health promotion is better understood when it is viewed in relation to the illness–wellness continuum. This continuum, illustrated in Figure 12–1, places the absence of illness at a neutral point in the center of the continuum. Movement from the center of the continuum to the left indicates a worsening state of health, typically hallmarked by signs, symptoms, disability, or death. Movement to the right reflects increasing levels of health. This end of the continuum may be termed health, wellness, or high-level wellness. Health promotion activities can legitimately address any point along the illness–wellness continuum (Green and Kreuter, 1999), and a single health promotion activity may have outcomes at more than one point on the continuum (Breslow, 1999).

Evolution of Contemporary Health Promotion

Preventive health approaches were formally initiated during the 19th century. The first era of public health attended to the illness end of the illness–wellness continuum because it focused solely on establishing programs to help people avoid communicable diseases such as polio and tuberculosis (Green & Kreuter, 1991). In the early 20th century, as communicable diseases became less of a public health problem, chronic diseases, such as cardiovascular disease and diabetes became the prevalent health problems. Concurrently, epidemiologists began to note that certain habits of eating, physical activity, and tobacco and alcohol use closely correlated with the development of many chronic diseases (Breslow, 1999). These trends led to the next major era of public health. Health professionals broadened their focus to changing individuals' health-related behaviors through education.

The second era of public health was moderately successful. Mortality rates from chronic noncommunicable diseases decreased, particularly from cardiovascular disease and some cancers. Nevertheless, professionals noted that even with widespread health education and promotion programs, chronic illness continued to be prevalent. They questioned the lukewarm success rates and began to look to sources other than the individual as facilitating change. They endorsed a more multidisciplinary approach to health promotion, one that contributed to a broader understanding of personal, social, organizational, and environmental determinants of health (Breslow, 1999).

With the eradication of communicable diseases and the prevention of some chronic diseases came increased longevity and a larger population of older adults. This change in the population and its health led to the advent of the goal of compressing morbidity (Fries, Green & Levine, 1989), which attempts to limit the time in which one has an acute or chronic illness or disability, thereby increasing the years of life that are morbidity free. Today, morbidity is more of a problem than is mortality because chronic diseases, which typically occur later in life, have significant consequences on quality of life. Contemporary public health concerns tend to center on the quality, not the quantity, of life (Breslow, 1999; Fries, Green, & Levine, 1989).

Further influencing the shift in the focus of health promotion has been an evolving conceptualization of health. No longer is health defined as the absence of disease; instead, health is *a capacity for living*. People want more than to live disease free; they also want life "to include being able to move about freely, enjoying food and sex, feeling good, remembering things, and having family and friends" (Breslow, 1999, p. 1032).

In the United States health care system, therapists have largely practiced within medical systems, focusing on the illness end of the illness–wellness continuum. Changes in reimbursement systems have caused an increased demand for health professions to focus on the wellness end of the continuum by working to prevent morbidity in the first place and to improve the quality of life of people with chronic disabilities who are not served by the traditional medical system. Therapists' unique focus on functional performance during day-to-day life has much to offer public health efforts that aim to improve people's capacity for living.

The national agenda for improving health in the United States is articulated in *Healthy People 2010*. This agenda updates *Healthy People 2000*, which introduced and quantified health goals based on the 1979 report *Healthy People: The Surgeon General's Report on Health Promotion and Disease Prevention*. This document sets health priorities for the nation and has three overarching goals: (1) increase years of healthy life, (2) reduce disparities in health among different population groups, and (3) ensure that all citizens have access to preventive health services. Specific objectives identify the most preventable threats to health and provide a "roadmap" to improved health for all individuals in the nation (U.S. Department of Health and Human Services, 2000).

Another program that not only reflects the broad understanding of health and how to promote it, but also illustrates the exciting opportunities that rehabilitation professionals have to promote health, is Healthy Communities/Healthy Cities. This initiative of the World Health Organization uses a community development approach toward promoting the health of individuals and the communities in which they live. Community development is an ecological approach that aims to promote equity in order to promote health (Mittelmark, 1999).

Both the *Guide to Physical Therapy Practice* (American Physical Therapy Association, 2001) and the *Guide to Occupational Therapy Practice* (Moyer, 1999) articulate a role for therapists in prevention and promotion of health and wellness. Examples of prevention and health promotion activities that therapists may be involved in include screening activities, such as screening children for idiopathic scoliosis, identifying elders who are at risk for falls or depression and conducting health promotion programs to improve fitness and promote quality of life. Such goals can be addressed through both traditional and complementary approaches.

Strategies for Health Promotion

When designing intervention strategies, it is useful to use theoretical models that have previously been studied and critiqued in basic and applied research. Different situations call for different theoretical frameworks. Effective health promotion requires the application of the theoretical framework that best targets the unit of interest (Glanz, Lewis, & Rimer, 1997). Health promotion frameworks typically fall into one of three levels of change: individual, interpersonal, or community or aggregate levels (Glanz, Lewis, Rimer, 1997).

Individual Level

Health Belief Model

The health belief model (HBM) is one of the most widely studied and applied conceptual frameworks in health promotion (Strecher & Rosenstock, 1997). This model is based on attitudes and beliefs, and is used to predict and explain what motivates people to change. In general, according to this model, people who do not believe that their behavior will affect their health are not likely to change (Rippe, O'Brien, & Taylor, 1999).

The HBM is rooted in two psychological theories: (1) the stimulus response theory, which posits that behavior is shaped by its consequences, or reinforcements; and (2) the cognitive theory, a value-expectancy theory, which posits that reinforcements actually influence expectations about a situation rather than influencing behavior directly. When applied to a health context, the values and expectancies influence the desire to avoid or recover from illness and the belief that actions will be effective (Strecher & Rosenstock, 1997).

CORE CONSTRUCTS

According to the HBM, a person's perceptions about health and its related behavior are critical to his or her decision about whether or not to engage in health-related behavior. Perceived threats, which are a combination of perceived susceptibility and severity; perceived benefits; and perceived barriers influence the likelihood of one's engaging in health behaviors. Other factors that influence one's likelihood of action are personal characteristics, such as age, personality, and knowledge; cues to action; and self-efficacy (Rosenstock, 1990).

- *Perceived susceptibility* refers to the extent to which a person believes he or she is vulnerable to a given health problem.
- *Perceived severity* describes perceptions about the relative severity of the problem (Simons-Morton, Greene, & Gottlieb, 1995).
- *Perceived benefits* are beliefs about the effectiveness of various available actions in reducing the disease threat.
- *Perceived barriers* are people's opinions about the tangible and psychological costs of the advised action (Strecher & Rosenstock, 1997).

Several other potentially motivating factors have been added to the model over time. *Cues to action* mobilize people to become conscious of and to act on relevant beliefs related to health behavior. Cues may be incidental or planned. Another factor that influences a person's likelihood for action is *self-efficacy,* which describes a person's conviction that he or she can successfully execute the behavior required. Self-efficacy encompasses both a person's belief in his or her ability to change behavior and his or her belief in the potential for success of that outcome.

Transtheoretical Model

The transtheoretical model (TTM), sometimes called stages of change, was designed primarily to enhance self-control. Much of the original and ongoing research of this model has focused on initiation and cessation of addictive behaviors, such as smoking and substance abuse (DiClemente & Prochaska, 1998). The TTM is based on the assumption that people are at various motivational points in a systematic process of change. This change process is made up of five stages. The first two stages are experienced internally, as affect or thoughts, and the last are more action-oriented. This theory assumes that behavior change unfolds over time and that most people are not ready for action immediately; rather, they need to progress through the model's first two stages before they can successfully move through the latter action-oriented stages. The model offers specific processes, or principles of change, that can be applied at specific stages to facilitate movement to the next stage (Prochaska, Redding, & Evers, 1997; Valesquez, Carbonari, & DiClemente, 1999).

CORE CONSTRUCTS

There are two main organizing constructs to the TTM: stages of change and processes of change.[1] Stages of change offer a way to segment the process of change into meaningful steps in which specific tasks are completed in order to successfully achieve and sustain behavior change (DiClemente & Prochaska, 1998). The five sequential stages are described below.

- *Precontemplation* is the stage in which people are not ready to make change and have no intention of doing so.

---

[1]A third organizing construct, levels of change, has been added to this model. This construct has been the least researched construct of the TTM and will not be presented here. See DiClemente & Prochaska (1998) for a description of this construct of the model.

- *Contemplation* is the stage in which people are thinking seriously about changing. Like people in the precontemplation stage, those in the contemplation stage are not ready for action-oriented programs.
- *Preparation* is the stage in which the person is getting ready to make a change, typically within the next month. Often, these individuals have attempted to make changes in the last year and have taken some steps toward action (Prochaska, Redding, & Evers, 1997).
- *Action* is the stage in which people are ready to make change and have made an overt modification to their lifestyles in the last six months.
- *Maintenance* is the stage in which people are working to support the behavior change and to integrate and firmly establish the change into their lifestyles in order to prevent a relapse of the problem behavior (Valesquez, 2000).

The processes of change are the cognitive and behavioral mechanisms that move people through the stages of change. According to the TTM, applying certain processes at particular stages facilitates movement through the change stages. There are 10 processes that have been broken down into the two main categories of experiential and behavioral processes. Studies have shown that experiential processes are the most important during the early stages, and behavioral processes are more prominent later. Refer to Valesquez (2000) and Prochaska and colleagues (1997) for a detailed description of the ten processes of change.

APPLICATION OF THE MODEL

The TTM offers "a simple, convenient, and effective way of categorizing a target population—segmenting a market, so to speak—for programmatic attention and for creating intervention components" (Simons-Morton, Greene, & Gottlieb, 1995, p. 277). The TTM may be used to move a target population from one stage to another stage. Because each stage calls for unique skills, beliefs, and attitudes, practitioners can develop intervention guidelines for each stage in order to facilitate success within and between each of the stages. In 1994, the developers of the TTM published a self-help style guide to apply the TTM toward behavioral change (Prochaska, Norcross, & DiClemente, 1994).

Interpersonal Level

Social Cognitive Theory

Social cognitive theory (SCT) is based on a rich history of research about how people learn and maintain behavioral patterns and about the identification of intervention strategies that are effective in increasing the likelihood of behavioral change. SCT evolved from social learning theory. Social learning theory posited that reinforcements and rewards shape future behavior. The name was later changed from social learning theory to social cognitive theory because it was believed that simple learning theories did not adequately explain behavior change. The cognitive concept of self-efficacy was incorporated into the revised SCT. Current SCT holds that behavior is learned and maintained through expectancies and incentives that are shaped by a dynamic relationship between behavior, personal factors, and environmental influences. Application of this theory involves using techniques designed to influence underlying cognitive variables (such as expectancies and incentives) in order to facilitate behavioral change (Baranowski, Perry, & Parcel, 1997; Hooper, 1998).

CORE CONSTRUCTS

SCT proposes that behavior can be explained and predicted by a number of constructs that describe factors within the individual, his or her behavior, and the environment. SCT's central constructs include such concepts as expectations within the person, reinforcements for behavior, and environmental factors external to the person. An additional construct, reciprocal determinism, provides an organizing framework for the constructs. Reciprocal determinism is the constant dynamic interaction of the person, the behavior, and the environment within which the behavior is enacted (Baranowski, 1996). An implication of reciprocal determinism is that if there are any changes within any of the constructs, then the situation as a whole changes. All health promotion programs need to be multifaceted so that they consider changes in the individual and in the environment (Baranowski, Perry, & Parcel, 1997), and therefore work within the reciprocal determinism dynamic.

APPLICATION OF THE MODEL

A health promotion program called Gimme 5 is an excellent example of the application of SCT. This program was developed based on the results of an ongoing line of SCT-based research about school-aged children's consumption of fruits and vegetables (e.g., Domel et al., 1996; Kirby et al., 1995). This research found that children's personal preferences and their access to and the availability of fruits and vegetables (F&V) are key factors in predicting adequate F&V consumption. The goals of the intervention program were to enhance students' ability to ask for and prepare F&V, to increase the availability of F&V in home and school environments, and to change the students' expectancies (or affect) related to F&V. Although program results did not indicate that Gimme 5 significantly increased F&V consumption overall, it did increase fruit consumption and F&V knowledge, and it broadened student preferences for F&V by helping students realize that they liked more fruits and vegetables than they previously realized.

Community Level

Health promotion programs that work to improve health by improving the community as a whole have been applied and researched since the early 1900s (McKenzie & Pinger, 1997). It is only recently, however, that rehabilitation professionals have turned their attention to this level of health promotion. In the last century, community health promotion (CHP) has, by and large, been conducted by public health professionals from disciplines such as sociology, psychology, political science, and anthropology.

The nature of practice with communities is quite different than that of working with individuals. CHP occurs at a systems or public policy level rather than at an individual level. In this practice, community members often lead the project by working with professionals to negotiate power relations and to name problems. CHP practitioners work at the *macro-level* to organize and support community groups in their identification of important concerns and their implementation of strategies to resolve them. The focus is on the health of the entire community rather than on the health of one or more individuals. In CHP healthy individuals are the *consequence* of a healthy community; they are not the indicators of its health.

Various theoretical approaches guide health promotion at the community or aggregate level. These include community building, organizing, development, empowerment, and participation (Labonte, 1997; Minkler, 1997). According to Rothman (1979), these approaches fall into three general categories: locality development, social planning, and social action. In locality development, professionals rely on community residents' participation in identifying and solving a problem. Social planning may be conducted by outsiders to the community who study an issue and plan and problem-solve its resolution. The social action approach is usually applied to situations rooted in conflict; it involves facilitating shifts in power, usually in favor of disadvantaged groups.

CORE CONCEPTS OF CHP

Communities are groups of people who have much in common. They share social relationships and political agendas (Brownson, 1998; Grady, 1995) as well as location, environment, and fate (McKenzie & Pinger, 1997). Alexis de Tocqueville, impressed by communities in his visit to America in 1835 (1945), described them as associations of citizens who exerted their power to identify problems and to resolve them. In 1997, McKnight contended that communities hold the power for addressing health concerns.

For a community to be healthy, it must make both private and public efforts to promote, protect, and preserve the health of its members (Green & Anderson, 1986). A healthy community requires strong public policy and associations working interdependently for the common good. Its policies and associations support community members' desire for health and allow citizens to act powerfully in those associations (Minkler, 1997).

Community empowerment is often the central feature of CHP projects (Minkler, 1997). It means giving power to all group members (McKenzie & Pinger, 1997) and enabling them to make decisions that shape and determine outcomes (Alinsky, 1972). Community empowerment is characterized by: 1) enhanced participation of community members, 2) enhanced sense of community among community members, 3) increased opportunities for and satisfaction with collective action, and 4) increased sense of control over life and community experiences (Bracht, Kingsbury, & Rissel, 1999).

CHP uses a *process* that is different from typical intervention models that rehabilitation professionals use. Rehabilitation professionals typically employ a process that includes a needs assessment; specific interventions, chosen by the rehabilitation professional, aimed at changing knowledge, behaviors, and health outcomes; and program evaluation. CHP projects, on the other hand, often modify the process by presenting the needs assessment to the community and allowing the community members and social and political leaders to choose and pursue interventions based on this information.

Summary

Through health promotion models, seemingly diverse health problems are actually linked by the potential to prevent further problems and to improve people's sense of wellness—with or without their having a medical diagnosis. The conceptual and theoretical approaches presented in this chapter provide promising options for improving the lives of people and the communities in which they live.

STUDY QUESTIONS

1. Compare and contrast health education, health promotion, and community health promotion.
2. Describe the illness–wellness continuum.
3. Think about your own lifestyle. Identify one aspect of your sense of wellness that you would like to change.
   - What behaviors are associated with this aspect of your life?
   - How does your social and physical environment influence this aspect of your life?
   - How does the nature of your community influence this aspect of your life?
4. For the situation described in question 3, choose the level of intervention that would best assist you with changing this aspect of your life (individual, interpersonal, community). Describe why this level of intervention is a good fit.
5. Choose a theoretical approach that best fits the change you wish to make. Apply this theoretical model to your situation by thinking about how each of the core constructs of that model are relevant to your situation. Then apply the model of change by making a plan for yourself based on that theoretical model.
6. Discuss ways in which the theoretical models described here can be incorporated into traditional and complementary rehabilitation practice.

REFERENCES

Alinsky, S. D. (1972). *Rules for Radicals.* New York: Random House.

American Physical Therapy Association. (2001). Guide to physical therapy practice (2nd ed.). *Physical Therapy, 81*(1), 9–746.

Baranowski, T. (1996). Psychological and sociocultural factors that influence nutritional behaviors and interventions: Cardiovascular disease. In C. Garza, J. P. Haas, & J. Habicht (Eds.), *Beyond Nutritional Recommendations: Implementing Science for Healthier Populations.* New York: Cornell University Press.

Baranowski, T., G. S. Perry, & C. L. Parcel. (1997). How individuals, environments, and health behavior interact: Social cognitive theory. In K. Glanz, F. M. Lewis, & B. K. Rimer (Eds.), *Health Behavior and Health Education: Theory, Research, and Practice* (2nd ed.). San Francisco: Jossey-Bass.

Bracht, N., L. Kingsbury, & C. Rissel. (1999). A five-stage community organization model for health promotion: Empowerment and partnership strategies. In N. Bracht (Ed.), *Health Promotion at the Community Level* (2nd ed.). Thousand Oaks, CA: Sage.

Breckon, D. J., J. R. Harvey, & R. B. Lancaster. (1998). *Community Health Education: Settings, Roles, and Skills for the 21st Century* (4th ed.). Maryland: Aspen Publishers.

Breslow, L. (1999). From disease prevention to health promotion. *Journal of the American Medical Association, 281*(11), 1030–1033.

Brownson, C. A. (1998). Funding community practice: Stage 1. *American Journal of Occupational Therapy, 52,* 60–64.

Coie, J. D., N. F. Watt, S. G. West, J. D. Hawkins, J. R. Asarnow, H. J. Markman, S. L. Ramey, M. B. Shure, & B. Long. (1993). The science of prevention: A conceptual framework and some directions for a national research program. *American Psychologist, 48*(10), 1013–1022.

DiClemente, C., & J. Prochaska. (1998). Toward a comprehensive, transtheoretical model of change. In W. Miller & N. Heather (Eds.), *Treating Addictive Behaviors* (2nd ed.). New York: Plenum Press.

Domel, S. B., W. O. Thompson, H. C. Davis, T. Baranowski, S. B. Leonard, & J. Baranowski. (1996). Psychosocial predictors of fruit and vegetable consumption among elementary school children. *Health Education Research, 11*(3), 299–308.

Edelman, C. L., & J. A. Fain. (1998). Health defined: Objectives for promotion & prevention. In C. L. Edelman & C. L. Mandle (Eds.), *Health Promotion Throughout the Lifespan* (4th ed.). St. Louis: Mosby.

Fries, J. F., L. W. Green, & S. Levine. (1989). Health promotion and the compression of morbidity. *The Lancet, 1*, 481–483.

Glanz, K., F. M. Lewis, & B. K. Rimer. (1997). The scope of health promotion and health education. In K. Glanz, F. M. Lewis, & B. K. Rimer (Eds.), *Health Behavior and Health Education: Theory, Research, and Practice* (2nd ed.). San Francisco: Jossey-Bass.

Grady, A. (1995). Building inclusive community: A challenge for occupational therapy. *American Journal of Occupational Therapy, 49*, 300–310.

Green, L. W., & C. L. Anderson. (1986). *Community Health.* St. Louis: Times Mirror/Mosby.

Green, L. W., & M. W. Kreuter. (1991). *Health Promotion Planning: An Educational and Environmental Approach* (2nd ed.). Mountain View, CA: Mayfield Publishing.

Green, L. W., & M. W. Kreuter. (1999). *Health Promotion Planning: An Educational and Environmental Approach* (3rd ed.). Mountain View, CA: Mayfield Publishing.

Hooper, J. I. (1998). Health education. In C. L. Edelman & C. L. Mandle (Eds.), *Health Promotion Throughout the Lifespan* (4th ed.). St. Louis: Mosby.

Kirby, S. D., T. Baranowski, K. D. Reynolds, G. Taylor, & D. Binkley. (1995). Children's fruit and vegetable intake: Socioeconomic, adult-child, regional, and urban-rural influence. *Journal of Nutritional Education, 27*(5), 261–271.

Kniepmann, K. (1997). Prevention of disability and maintenance of health. In C. Christiansen & C. Baum (Eds.), *Occupational Therapy: Enabling Function and Well-Being* (2nd ed.). Thorofare, NJ: Slack.

Labonte, R. (1997). Community, community development, and the forming of authentic partnerships: Some critical reflections. In M. Minkler (Ed.), *Community Organizing and Community Building for Health.* New Brunswick, NJ: Rutgers University Press.

McKenzie, J. F., & R. R. Pinger. (1997). *An Introduction to Community Health.* Sadbury, MS: Jones & Barlett Publishers.

McKnight, J. L. (1997). Two tools for well-being: Health systems and communities. In M. Minkler (Ed.), *Community Organizing and Community Building for Health.* New Brunswick, NJ: Rutgers University Press.

Minkler, M. (1997). Introduction and overview. In M. Minkler (Ed.), *Community Organizing and Community Building for Health.* New Brunswick, NJ: Rutgers University Press.

Mittelmark, M. B. (1999). Health promotion at the communitywide level: Lessons from diverse perspectives. In N. Bracht (Ed.), *Health Promotion at the Community Level* (2nd ed.). Thousand Oaks, CA: Sage.

Moyer, P. (1999). The guide to occupational therapy practice. *American Journal of Occupational Therapy, 53*, 247–322.

Murray, R. B., & Zentner, J. P. (1993). *Nursing Assessment and Health Promotion: Strategies Through the Lifespan* (5th ed.). Norwalk, CT: Appleton & Lange.

Prochaska, J. O., J. C. Norcross, & C. C. DiClemente. (1994). *Changing for Good.* New York: Avon Books.

Prochaska, J. O., C. A. Redding, & K. E. Evers. (1997). In K. Glanz, F. M. Lewis, & B. K. Rimer (Eds.), *Health Behavior and Health Education: Theory, Research, and Practice* (2nd ed.). San Francisco: Jossey-Bass.

Rippe, J. M., D. O'Brien, & K. Taylor. (1999). Lifestyle strategies for risk factor reduction and treatment of coronary artery disease: An overview. In J. M. Rippe (Ed.), *Lifestyle Medicine.* Boston, MA: Blackwell Science.

Rosenstock, I. M. (1990). The health belief model: Explaining health behavior through expectancies. In K. Glanz, F. M. Lewis, B. K. Rimer (Eds.), *Health Behavior and Health Education: Theory, Research, and Practice*. San Francisco: Jossey-Bass.

Rothman, J. (1979). The interweaving of community intervention approaches. In M. Weil (Ed.), *Community Practice: Conceptual Models*. New York: Hawthorne.

Simons-Morton, B. G., W. H. Greene, & N. H. Gottlieb. (1995). *Introduction to Health Education and Health Promotion* (2nd ed.). Prospect Heights, IL: Waveland Press.

Strecher, V. J., & I. M. Rosenstock. (1997). The health belief model. In K. Glanz, F. M. Lewis, & B. K. Rimer (Eds.), *Health Behavior and Health Education: Theory, Research, and Practice* (2nd ed.). San Francisco: Jossey-Bass.

Sultz, H. A., & K. M. Young. (1999). *Healthcare USA: Understanding Its Organization and Delivery* (2nd ed.). Gaithersberg, MD: Aspen Publishers.

Tocqueville, A de. [1835] (1945). *Democracy in America*. New York: Harper and Row.

U.S. Department of Health and Human Services. *Healthy People 2000: National Health Promotion and Disease Prevention Objectives*. Washington, DC: US Dept of Health and Human Services publication No. PHS 91-50212.

U.S. Department of Health and Human Services. *Healthy People 2010*. 2nd ed. Understanding and Improving Health and Objectives for Improving Health. 2 vols. Washington, DC: U.S. Government Printing Office, November 2000.

Valesquez, M. M., J. P. Carbonari, & C. C. DiClemente. (1999). Psychiatric severity and behavior change in alcoholism: The relation of the transtheoretical model variables to psychiatric distress in dually diagnosed patients. *Addictive Behaviors, 24*(4), 481–496.

Velasquez, M. M. (2000). Developing interventions using the transtheoretical model. Paper presented at the University of Texas School of Public Health, Houston, Texas.

World Health Organization. (1986). Ottawa charter for health promotion. *Health Promotion International, 1*, iii–iv.

13

Biofeedback

Larry Kopelman

- Define biofeedback and understand its history.
- Describe basic types of biofeedback.
- Understand how biofeedback can be used in therapy settings.

Each and every day people are involved in biofeedback processes. Just getting on the bathroom scale in the morning is a form of biofeedback. People gather information about body mass and consciously or unconsciously make critical decisions about the data. Yes, dessert can be eaten, or no, starve another day.

Unlike weight, many internal events usually occur without an individual taking notice. For example, there are changes in muscle contraction, heart rate, gastrointestinal activity and brain function that are constantly changing but not perceived by an individual. In some cases psychophysiology is brought to one's attention under stressful conditions as a perception of the environment causes a change such as a rapid heart rate or rapid breathing. With the aid of biofeedback instrumentation and behavior interventions, these subtle changes may be identified and used to re-regulate physiological processes.

Biofeedback, classified by NCCAM as a mind-body method, is one of the most widely accepted modalities of the complementary family of interventions. It is a nonpharmacological and noninvasive approach to assist clients in altering physiological responses. It is not painful and has few adverse reactions. With a nearly 70 percent or better success rate of clinical improvement, biofeedback may be considered effective in the amelioration or reduction of symptoms such as headache, irritable bowel disease, and hypertension with measurable outcomes (Sabo & Giorgi, 2000). This cost-effective modality is the treatment of choice in many instances where the client is partnered with the health care provider in the health restoration process.

Biofeedback can be used in conjunction with other behavioral and stress management techniques, such as visualization, cognitive restructuring, and autogenic training. It is a learn-

125

Individual experience can be thought of as events that elicit physical, emotional, and mental responses that are stored in the body-mind. Biofeedback is the process of receiving and using feedback about responses to events to correct problems. It is used to help clients access their own healing potential with self-regulatory skill acquisition. Many different biological processes can be harnessed to provide feedback for learning. These include temperature, heart rate, and electrical muscle activity.

Biofeedback is one of the most widely used and accepted alternative therapies. It can be used to treat a variety of problems, including headaches and other pain conditions, muscle tone irregularities, and anxiety.

ing technique that allows the client to become as responsible for his or her health as the therapist, empowering the client to participate equally with the therapist in the planning and implementation of a therapeutic program.

Background

Biofeedback uses instrumentation in order to produce a desired behavioral response by collecting data and presenting it as a reinforcement. For example, by using a blood pressure monitor, a client is made aware of changes in blood pressure, and with the aid of visual and auditory signals, which change as the blood pressure changes, he or she is trained to consciously control the blood pressure.

O. Hobart Mowrer pioneered instrumented biofeedback in 1938, when he used an alarm system triggered by urine to stop bedwetting in children (Goldberg, 1995). Biofeedback as we know it was popularized in the late 1960s when Barbara Brown, Ph.D., at the Veterans Hospital in Sepulveda, California, and Elmer and Alyce Green in Topeka, Kansas, used EEG to study altered states of consciousness induced by yogis (Green & Green, 1977).

The Greens went to India in the 1970s and studied the electroencephalogram, heart rate, respiration, and other physiological functions of yogis. They compiled a great deal of information about self-regulation skills and practices, detailing them in their book *Beyond Biofeedback* (Green & Green, 1977). The pioneering work of the Greens provided scientific legitimacy to recognizing the basic connection of the mind and the body. Medical practitioners in many disciplines were introduced to the idea that biofeedback was a valid treatment modality that could help their clients without the use of drugs. Table 13–1 lists conditions treated with biofeedback.

Methods of Biofeedback

The methods of biofeedback, including electromyography, thermal, galvanic (electrodermal), pulse monitoring, EEG, virtual reality, and newer noncognitive biofeedback, are too numerous to detail within the scope of this chapter. Refer to Basmajian (1989), Basmajian and

Table 13–1 Conditions Treated with Biofeedback

- Anger states
- Anxiety
- Asthma
- Backache/neck pain
- Balance disorders
- Cardiac arrhythmias
- Carpal tunnel syndrome
- Chronic fatigue syndrome
- Depression
- Dysmennorrhea
- Essential hypertension
- Fecal/urinary incontinence
- Frigidity
- Headache/migraine
- Hyperventilation
- Impotence
- Insomnia
- Irritable bowel syndrome
- Muscle reeducation: hypotonic/hypertonic/spastic tone
- Menstrual dysfunction
- Neurodermatitis/eczema
- Postural dysfunction
- Reynaud's syndrome
- Scoliosis
- Sinus tachycardia
- Temporomandibular joint dysfunction

De Luca (1985), and Tiller (1997) for a complete description of these methods. The section below describes some of the main biofeedback methods.

Heart Rate Variability

The sympathetic nerves to the heart cause its beat to accelerate while the parasympathetic nerves cause it to decelerate. The interaction between these two systems produces a time periodic variable called the heart rate variability (HRV). HRV, with the electrocardiogram (ECG), are closely correlated measures of the regulation of the autonomic nervous system (Tiller, 1997). Normally, individuals exhibit a balance between the sympathetic and parasympathetic nervous systems (Nolan, 2000). HRV can be utilized as an index of stress on the human body.

It has been confirmed in the laboratory that input from the cardiovascular system is the only known non-nerve input to the brain that will inhibit the activity of the brain's cortex (Tiller, 1997). Through practice, one can be taught to balance electrophysiological energies into a harmonic state of coherence related to self-management of mental and emotional states. HRV may also be used as a noncognitive reading of the body to measure responses to other physiological interventions, because an immediate shift in the HRV analysis is an objective measurement of the body's response to such interventions.

Electromyography

Overcontraction of muscles, either by force or duration, may lead to problems from overload, strain, or fatigue (Sella, 1995). Undercontracting muscles can be problematic as well, because other muscles overcompensate for undercontracting muscles. While the muscle contraction itself is not accessible, the electrical activity of the contraction is studied through an electromyogram.

When clients present with problems due to muscle contraction, surface electromyography (s-emg) may be utilized to identify which muscles are involved. The process is simple: By placing sensors on the skin over the muscles, electrical activity within the muscle may be identified and recorded. Qualitative and quantitative data can be obtained, and those muscles at risk of overload or fatigue can be treated through the use of feedback.

The muscles should be evaluated while in different postures. The therapist can obtain information about both the effort of a normal myoelectric picture (i.e., muscle contractions that produce no symptoms) and problematic, maladaptive muscle contractions. An example is the identification of problematic muscle contraction during keyboarding to prevent carpal tunnel syndrome (Peper et al., 1994).

S-emg and Muscle Sequencing

S-emg can also answer diagnostic questions about whether flexors and extensors are working in or out of sequence. Often, there is the appearance that if a person can perform a movement that appears correct, he or she is using proper muscles efficiently and recruiting muscles in a proper sequence (Headley, 1994). Headley has observed, however, that a person will change his or her motor strategy if there is the presence of a painful condition. This change in motor planning may remain as a new muscular pattern. The new pattern may become a source of pain and discomfort due to altered biomechanical forces, which can lead to distinct pathology. S-emg is used in such cases to identify dysfunctional movement patterns and imbalances between flexors and extensors of different body areas, such as the cervical spine, wrist, or hand.

Other Methods of Biofeedback

Other popular modalities used in biofeedback are temperature training and galvanic skin response. Most people are not conscious of the temperature of the hands unless their attention is focused on the hands or there is a significant sensory problem, such as Reynaud's syndrome or diabetic neuropathy. Skin temperature is regulated by blood flow through the peripheral arterioles in the skin. Both visual and auditory feedback can be used from a machine that can detect subtle temperature changes. Temperature biofeedback has been found to be very useful in the treatment of a variety of conditions, including hypertension, headache, anxiety, and

Reynaud's syndrome (Green & Green, 1989). Temperature biofeedback works by feeding back information on vasoconstriction and vasodilation.

Galvanic skin response, or electrodermal response (EDR), is also mediated by the sympathetic nervous system and is simple to measure. Electrodes are placed on two sites on the skin, and the electrical conductance between them is measured. A decrease in EDR is associated with arousal states and is a direct result of the impedance change between the two electrodes. (The reaction of the sweat glands in the skin is responsible for the change in impedance.) Hyperhydrosis and some anxiety states may be treated successfully using EDR.

Virtual Reality

The ultimate biofeedback technique is virtual reality. Often, clients feel frustrated at the long time it takes for the rehabilitation process, exhibiting a lack of interest and motivation. They may feel isolated and prefer not to interact with others. By setting up a virtual environment, clients can feel liberated. They may be able to function at a higher level in the virtual world, offering them hope and freedom from their bodies. Improved performance in a virtual world may motivate them to perform better in the real world. Clients can focus and take chances in a protected environment (Wilson, Foreman, & Stanton, 1998). Gupta and colleagues (2000) note that this technology has significant potential for use in neurological pain and in pediatric clients.

Biofeedback with Specific Conditions

Biofeedback and Headache

Biofeedback is one of the most effective treatments for frequent migraine and tension type headaches (Mauskop, 1991), and almost every headache clinic offers biofeedback as a therapy. Biofeedback in headache control teaches clients to control certain functions of the autonomic nervous system, including heart rate, skin temperature, blood pressure, muscle tension, and brainwave activity. These, in turn, decrease the frequency, duration, and severity of headaches. The goal is headache cessation.

Sarafino and Goehring (2000) studied the effectiveness of biofeedback in headache patients at different ages. Results showed that both children and adults had substantial improvements in headache activity, with children showing significantly greater improvement than adults.

Biofeedback and Pain

Biofeedback is not only clinically effective with headaches, but also with a wide variety of pain conditions, including reflex sympathetic dystrophy (RSD), now known as regional complex syndrome I or II, and trigger points (Gellman & Nichols, 1997; Roy, De Luca, & Casavant, 1989). Gellman and Nichols (1997) suggest that newer therapies, such as electroacupuncture and biofeedback, can be used most effectively when a diagnosis is made early. Recent studies with TMJ patients at the University of Texas Southwestern Medical Center at Dallas have shown biofeedback to be more effective compared to a no-treatment group and biofeedback with cognitive behavioral skills treatment group (Mishra, Gatchel, & Gardea, 2000). A meta-analysis of biofeedback treatment for TMJ concluded that s-emg biofeedback is an effective method of treating TMJ dysfunction (Crider & Glaros, 1999).

Myofascial pain is another area in which biofeedback has been used with great success. When comparing biofeedback with other modalities in the treatment of chronic musculoskeletal pain, the biofeedback group showed the most substantial change. In a study by Flor and Birbaumer (1993), at 6- and 24-month follow-ups, only the biofeedback group maintained significant reductions in pain severity, decreased affective distress, and a decrease in pain-related use of the health care system.

PAIN AND EMOTIONAL RESPONSES

A client's psychophysiological state of mind will influence the experience of pain. The pain experience is related to past experience, fear and anxiety, and the significance of the pain (Bartol & Courts, 1997). For example, pain from cancer may be perceived as more intense than from another type of disease. Personal beliefs, values, and goals influence the perception of pain. Loss of hope and aspirations, and fear of the unknown, stimulate the hypothalamus and the sympathetic nervous system. The adrenals will be activated, which secrete epinephrine and norepinephrine, recognized by the body as a stress signal.

Biofeedback can assist the client with down regulation of the sympathetic nervous system by helping the client learn to recognize the physiological events associated with increased sympathetic tone, including damp cold hands and feet, rapid heart rate, increased muscle tension, and/or rapid breathing. Observing physiological change with instrumentation allows the client to recognize subtle changes that ordinarily would not be detected.

Biofeedback and Ergonomics

The high incidence of cumulative trauma disorders has been attributed to three factors: excessive force, repetition, and faulty posture while force is being applied (Parker & Imbus, 1992). Forceful static or repetitive contractions of muscles cause the corresponding tendons to stretch and affect surrounding microstructures, leading to decreased circulation, tearing, and inflammation of tissues. The magnitude of force exerted may be related to the development of musculoskeletal injury. Fixed and limited or deviated postures can overload the muscles and load the joints in an asymmetrical and/or uneven manner. Different levels of strength in any posture through a dynamic range of motion have different physiological demands. It is therefore useful to utilize myoelectric feedback mechanisms to have clients alter their stress response not only on a cognitive level but also on a purely physiological level.

Assessment

When a client is seen in the office, a clinical interview using a stress inventory is performed. The interview seeks to identify areas of stress and the precipitating factors or areas that exacerbate the problematic condition. The intake interviewer utilizes questions that identify if there are physical, cognitive, and/or emotional stressors.

A certified biofeedback clinician should have passed a rigorous examination and had supervised experience by trained biofeedback therapists. The Biofeedback Certification Institute of America (BCIA) is a single certifying group for biofeedback credentialing. Many schools and organizations offer certifications for their programs, but the BCIA certification examination is currently the only peer-recognized certification.

The American Association of Psychotherapy and Biofeedback (AAPB) is a membership organization open to licensed professionals using biofeedback in their practices. It is a multidisciplinary organization, offering training and workshops around the country. It has many state and local chapters, which hold meetings for members to discuss applications and interventions using biofeedback.

Multiple baseline physiological measurements are then taken. Thermal (skin temperature), EMG (electromyographic), GSR (galvanic skin response), and EDR (electrodermal response) measurements are simultaneously monitored. The most poorly regulated parameters are then identified and targeted for treatment. Prioritization is developed from interview scores and the physiological response at baseline measurements.

Typical Practice

After assessment determines baseline measures and priorities, treatment commences. A threshold setting is used for the client to reach a specific goal in each session. The client is hooked up to the biofeedback instrument of choice, and the therapist manipulates the sensitivity of the controls so that behavior is shaped. The client is challenged to reach more difficult goals by setting the auditory and visual feedback to specific levels. Once the threshold is reached, a change in feedback signals the client that the goal was reached.

The client is encouraged to experience and feel the subjective internal events happening, and with practice is able to reproduce the internal subjective feelings without the aid of instrumentation. With practice, most clients in a very short time are able to control and meet the targeted behaviors as long as the neuromuscular system is intact.

Case Studies

Severe Whiplash

A 26-year-old female who sustained a severe whiplash in a motor vehicle accident was seen for eight visits for standard physical therapy treatment. Therapeutic exercises for posture correction and reduction of the forward-head posture were administered. Her chief complaint was of stiffness of the cervical spine, difficulty sleeping, frequent headaches lasting 6 to 8 hours, and parasthesia of the upper extremities in a C5–C6 myotome distribution pattern. Physical modalities and manual techniques were used in treatment. She was given a home program and was very compliant. She was seen three times a week for several weeks, with minimal reduction in her subjective complaints and minimal change in actual range of motion.

During the next therapy visit, surface electromyographic biofeedback with visual and auditory augmented feedback display from the frontalis area and hand temperature-warming techniques were used. Imagery phrases, breathing, and relaxation training protocols were also used to produce reduction of muscle activity from the frontalis muscle and to increase hand warming over the course of the session. After 30 minutes of feedback, this client's EMG values were lowered and hand temperature rose. Sessions were 45 minutes in a darkened room.

At the end of the initial intake and training session, the client was given a home-practice heat-sensitive card that changes colors in relationship to the change in finger temperature. The client was instructed to use the card one to two times daily for 5 to 10 minutes until she was able to change the color of the card. These colors are associated and correlated with the feedback during the training sessions so that as the client felt the sensation of relaxation, she related that sense of well-being with the objective data presented in numerical form.

The headaches reduced in frequency and intensity over the next 3 days, and since the second session, the client has been headache free. The client received a total of three sessions of biofeedback and was discharged and sent back to the referring neurologist. She remains pain-free, has full range of motion of the cervical spine, and has no muscle spasms of the neck or periscapular musculature.

Muscle Ligament Tears

A 45-year-old male truck driver sustained acute severe muscle ligament tears to his back while unloading his truck. He presented with a severe functional scoliosis of the lumbar and thoracic paravertebral muscles as well as spasms of the quadratus-lumborum and psoas-major, unilaterally. He participated in traditional physical therapy, including deep heat massage and a stretching exercise program to restore strength and power to the thoracic and lumbar spine. He had good strength but still experienced symptoms of muscle spasms of the back and hip when he attempted to return to work. A work-hardening program was instituted, and as part of the training, a lumbar motion monitor was utilized to help him identify poor body mechanics. A mercury-switch biofeedback device was clipped onto the back of his shirt collar. The device gave a loud auditory signal—a buzzing sound—if it exceeded 50° of an angle from the vertical. Training in lifting boxes and packages was done while wearing the motion monitor, and in three sessions, the client had improved his body mechanics and no longer reported having back pain.

The use of a simple device to give feedback during a dynamic activity is an inexpensive and highly motivating therapeutic intervention. These devices can be worn during work, and involvement from other workers is experienced as a supportive part of an injury prevention program.

Head Posture Control in Cerebral Palsy Client

A 7-year old child with cerebral palsy (CP) was seen for biofeedback to help with head posture control. Born with CP, as she grew she developed habits that caused her to cock her head to one side and shift her shoulders to the opposite side, causing a torsion and lateral bend while sitting in the wheelchair. Her posture was disturbing to her parents and impaired her classroom performance, as eye contact between student and teacher was difficult. Her cognitive status was appropriate for her age. She was able to understand the concepts needed to connect the external stimuli and how it related to her attempts at movement. S-emg biofeedback training was provided, attaching sensors to the sternocleidomastoid on the side with increased muscle tone. The therapy was effective, as she was able to conceive of the movement that was observable through feedback.

This client was seen three times a week for three weeks and then reduced to two times a week for three weeks. A portable trainer was provided for home use. The parents were instructed in the settings and application of the sensor electrodes. With treatment, the child was able to sit with her head in an erect posture for durations of 20 minutes or more. Improved body spatial orientation was accomplished. She had few spasms of the sternocleidomastoid, and when she did have a spasm, she was able to correct it so her posture was maintained. Her teachers stated her progress was carried over to the classroom, making learning and concentration more effective.

Summary

There is great potential in the use of biofeedback for therapists. Biofeedback fits into the medical model, while empowering clients to help themselves. It is not only one of the better-studied complementary therapies, but it is also one of the more widely used. Research has shown that biofeedback is effective in treating headache and other types of pain and imbalances in muscle contraction. Clinicians experienced in biofeedback also report that many other conditions are amendable to the use of biofeedback, including anxiety and depression.

STUDY QUESTIONS

1. Define biofeedback.
2. Describe how heart rate variability is an objective measure of stress, and discuss its clinical applications in biofeedback.
3. Discuss the clinical applications and rationale of using s-emg as biofeedback.
4. Describe the clinical applications and rationale of using temperature training and galvanic skin response or electrodermal response as biofeedback.

5. Choose a clinical problem for which there is research to support the use of biofeedback, and discuss what type of feedback would be used and why.
6. What are the requirements to be a certified biofeedback practitioner?

SUGGESTED READING

Andreassi, J. H (1989). *Psychophysiology: Human Behavior and Physiological Response* (2nd ed.). Mahwah, NJ: Erlbaum.

Basmajian, J., & C. De Luca. (1985). *Muscles Alive: Their Functions Revealed by Electromyography*. Baltimore: Williams & Wilkins.

Danskin, D., & M. Crow. (1981). *Biofeedback: An Introduction and Guide*. Palo Alto, CA: Mayfield Publishing.

Jonas, G. (1973). *Visceral Learning: Toward a Science of Self-Control*. New York: Pocket Books.

Pomerleau, O., & J. Brady. (1979). *Behavioral Medicine: Theory and Practice*. Baltimore: Williams & Wilkins.

Tiller, W. (1997). *Science and Human Transformation: Subtle Energies, Intentionality and Consciousness*. Walnut Creek, CA: Pavior.

Wickramasekera, I. (1976). *Biofeedback, Behavior Therapy and Hypnosis: Potentiating the Verbal Control of Behavior for Clinicians*. Chicago: Nelson Hall.

RESOURCES

Association for Applied Psychophysiology
   and Biofeedback
10200 West 44th Ave., #304
Wheat Ridge, CO 80033
(303) 422-8894

Biofeedback Certification Institute of America
10200 West 44th Ave. # 304
Wheat Ridge, CO 80033
(303) 420-2902

The Society for the Study of Neuronal
   Regulation (SNNR)
P.O. Box 160125
Austin, TX 78716
(512) 306-0406
www.ssnr.com

Training is available from some of the
following organizations:

Biofeedback Consultants of North America
128 South Monticello Drive
Syracuse, NY 13205
(315) 469-7296

Biomeridian International
12411 South 265 West, Suite F
Draper, UT 84020
(888) 224-2337, (801) 501-7517

Center for Applied Psychophysiology/
   Menninger Clinic
P.O. Box 829
Topeka, KS 66601-0829
(913) 273-7500 Ext. 5375

Heart Math Institute
14700 West Park Ave.
Boulder Creek, CA 95006
(831) 338-8700
info@heartmath.com

Micro Straight, Inc.
2709 Cherry Street
Kansas City, MO 64108
(816) 474-0144, (800) 238-2255

Sound Health Center
118 Wendover Road
Asheville, NC 28806
(825) 255-9688

Star Tech Health Services
1219 South 1840 West
Orem, UT 84058
(801) 229-2500
startech@itsnet.com

Thought Technology
2180 Belgrave Ave.

Montreal, Quebec, Canada H4A 2LB
(800) 361-3651, (514) 489-8251

Tools for Exploration
4460 Redwood Highway, Suite 2
San Rafael, CA 94903
(415) 499-9050

REFERENCES

Bartol G., & N. F. Courts. (1997). Psychophysiology of bodymind healing. In B. Dossey (Ed.), *American Holistic Nurses' Association Core Curriculum for Holistic Nursing*. Gaithersberg, MD: Aspen.

Crider, A. B., & A. G. Glaros. (1999). A meta-analysis of EMG biofeedback treatment of temporo-mandibular disorders. *Journal of Orofacial Pain, 13*(1), 29–37.

Flor, H., & N. Birbaumer. (1993, Aug.). Comparison of the efficacy of electromyographic biofeedback, cognitive-behaviorial therapy, and conservative medical interventions in the treatment of chronic musculoskeletal pain. *Consulting Clinical Psychologist, 61*(4), 653–658.

Gellman, H., & D. Nichols. (1997, Nov. 5). Reflex sympathetic dystrophy in the upper extremity. *Journal of the Academy Orthopedic Surgery, 6,* 313–322.

Goldberg, B. (1995). Biofeedback. In B. Goldberg (Ed.), *Alternative Medicine, the Definitive Guide*. Fife, WA: Burton Group.

Green, A., & E. Green. (1977). *Beyond Biofeedback*. New York: Dell.

Green, E., & A. Green. (1989). General and specific applications of thermal biofeedback. In J. V. Basmajian (Ed.), *Biofeedback: Principles and Practice for Clinicians* (3rd ed.). Baltimore: Williams & Wilkins.

Gupta, S., D. C. Mehl, A. K. Mehl, & S. Klein. (2000). Virtual interface therapy: Evaluation of a new therapeutic modality in the treatment of pediatric rehabilitation patients. Medical Information Research, University of Louisville School of Medicine, Louisville, KY.

Headley, B. (1994). Surface EMG: New rehab horizons. *Physical Therapy Products, 7,* 30–34.

Mauskop, A. (1991, Winter). Biofeedback and headaches. *National Headache Foundation Newsletter,* 3–4.

Mishra, K. D., R. J. Gatchel, & M. A. Gardea. (2000, June). The relative efficacy of three cognitive-behavioral treatment approaches to temporomandibular disorders. *Journal of Behavorial Medicine, 3,* 293–309.

Nolan, R. (2000). *Heart Rate Variability (HRV)*. Montreal, Canada: Thought Technology.

Parker, K., & H. Imbus. (1992). *Cumulative Trauma Disorders Current Issues and Ergonomic Solutions: A Systems Approach*. Chelsea, MI: Lewis Publishers.

Peper, E., V. S. Wilson, W. Taylor, A. Pierce, K. Bender, & V. Tibbetts. (1994). Repetitive strain injury: Prevent computer user injury with biofeedback: Assessment and training protocol. *Physical Therapy Products, 9,* 17–21.

Roy S., C. De Luca, & M. Casanvant. (1989, Sept.). Lumbar muscle fatigue and chronic lower back pain. *Spine, 14*(9), 992–1001.

Sabo, M. J., & J. Giorgi. (2000). Biofeedback. In D. Novey (Ed.), *Clinician's Complete Reference to Complementary and Alternative Medicine*. St. Louis: Mosby.

Sarafino, E. P., & P. Goehring. (2000, Winter). Age comparisons in acquiring biofeedback control and success in reducing headache pain. *Annals of Behavioral Medicine, 22*(1), 10–16.

Sella, G. E. (1995, June 10). *Workshop on Surface Electromyography (S-EMG)*. Martin's Ferry, OH: GENMED Publishers.

Tiller, W. (1997). *Science and Human Transformation*. Walnut Creek, CA: Pavior.

Wilson, P. N., N. Foreman, & D. Stanton. (1998). A rejoinder. *Disability and Rehabilitation, 20*(3), 113–115.

14

Craniosacral Therapy

Sherry Borcherding

CHAPTER OBJECTIVES

- Describe the goals and mechanisms of craniosacral therapy.
- State the benefits of craniosacral therapy.
- Describe the relevance and appropriate use of craniosacral therapy in occupational and physical therapies.
- Choose a credible training program in craniosacral therapy for further study.

Craniosacral therapy is a gentle, noninvasive, hands-on method of correcting imbalances within the body. The craniosacral system is a physiological structure that extends from the cranium via a system of membranes through the spine to the sacrum. It consists of

- the bones of the skull and face (cranium), spine, and the sacrum,
- the dural tube which surrounds these structures, and
- the cerebral spinal fluid which fills the dural tube.

Background and Development

Craniosacral therapy originates from the work of William Sutherland, D.O., and is based on the idea that the cranial bones move in relation to each other throughout life rather than ossifying in childhood. Sutherland discovered by palpation that the movement is regular and rhythmic (Smoley, 1991). From Sutherland's original work comes three different branches of treatment: cranial osteopathy, sacro-occipital technique (an aspect of chiropractic medicine), and craniosacral therapy.

The craniosacral system, based on Sutherland's original concepts, was later refined and expanded by John Upledger, D.O., who coined the term CranioSacral Therapy. Upledger has added theories and research about the origin of the cranial rhythmic impulse and the im-

Craniosacral therapy is a way of improving the environment in which the brain and nervous system live and work. It is an effective enabling activity for facilitating functional activities. Therapists use it to decrease pain and spasticity, increase range of motion, encourage optimal immune and parasympathetic nervous system functioning, facilitate autonomic flexibility, decrease tone and edema, break up scar tissue, balance the spinal and pelvic structures, relieve stress, and promote relaxation. It can also be used to find and eliminate emotional issues stored in the tissues.

portance of the reciprocal membrane system, as well as an extensive training program for allied health practitioners. There are other osteopaths who are less well known in the United States who also refined and expanded the work.

Craniosacral therapy is one of several techniques that fall under the general heading of manual or manipulative medicine and that are coming into the mainstream of allied health practice from the field of osteopathy. Craniosacral therapy is similar to, although not the same as, cranial osteopathy. It also shares many concepts and techniques with myofascial release. One primary difference between craniosacral therapy and cranial osteopathy is in the training of the practitioner. In the United States, cranial osteopaths are licensed physicians with special training in manual medicine. Craniosacral therapists, on the other hand, are health care practitioners such as occupational and physical therapists, massage therapists, and dentists who are licensed to touch the body and who have attended workshops in craniosacral therapy as a way of adding this skill to their existing repertoire of treatment techniques. A second difference between craniosacral therapy and cranial osteopathy is the pressure used in the touch. Craniosacral therapists use a very light touch, about 5 grams of pressure. The manipulations used in cranial osteopathy are often heavier and more directive. A third difference is in the focus of craniosacral therapy on the reciprocal membranes and the hydraulics of the craniosacral system rather than the bones and sutures of the skull (Upledger, 1995).

Mechanism and Action

Light touch coupled with intent and direction of energy is used to bring the cranial, spinal, and pelvic structures back into balance and to remove blockages that the body's own physiologic forces have been unable to overcome. One of the hallmarks of craniosacral therapy is the use of a very light touch. The amount of pressure used is seldom more than 1 ounce, and is often more on the order of 5 grams—the weight of a nickel. By using such a gentle pressure, the therapist assists the client's body to self-correct and avoids encountering resistance.

An experiential example can facilitate understanding of how light touch decreases resistance. For example, imagine a hard pull on one of your arms. Your immediate reaction is to resist by holding back against the pull, thus protecting yourself. The use of light touch is a way of not engaging the body's natural tendency to resist change.

Reliance on the inherent self-correcting mechanism of the body is another of the hallmarks of craniosacral therapy. This approach relies on the body's own wisdom and desire to move toward homeostasis to guide the treatment session (Milne, 1995). Treatment is a cooperative effort between the therapist who is trying to help the system work more effectively and the person receiving treatment. For this reason, treating the craniosacral system is not only useful for correcting dis-ease, but also for promoting a high level of wellness. According to John Upledger (n.d.),

> *Almost any recipient of CranioSacral therapy will benefit in terms of general health, function, and sense of well being. CranioSacral therapy restores autonomic nervous system flexibility and adaptability. It reduces accumulated physiological stress levels. It enhances the movement of blood and other fluids through the body tissues, increasing resistance to disease invasions. (p. 1)*

A third hallmark of craniosacral therapy is the understanding that trauma or other events that impact one part of the system can have adverse effects on other parts of the system. Normal function of the body is dependent on normal functioning of the craniosacral system (Upledger & Vredevoogd, 1983). The dura mater, which surrounds the brain and spinal cord, and the intracranial membranes, which separate the four quadrants of the brain, are parts of the fascial system. The fascia is like a net of fibrous tissue that goes throughout the body beneath the skin. It encloses all muscles, muscle groups, and organs. Thus, a restriction anywhere in the fascia can have far-reaching effects, even reaching inside the brain and causing twists and restrictions of neural and venous structures passing through the cranium. When the craniosacral system becomes dysfunctional, sensory, intellectual, or motor dysfunction can result. Improving the internal environment in which the brain and spinal cord reside is very helpful for disorders such as chronic pain (Upledger, 1988).

Theory and Terminology

There is a *craniosacral rhythm* (sometimes called a cranial wave or a cranial rhythmic impulse) that can be palpated anywhere on the body, but is most easily felt on the cranium or sacrum. Its two phases (called flexion and extension by Sutherland) alternate at a rate of 6 to 12 cycles per minute. This rhythm can be used therapeutically in several ways. Its amplitude, symmetry, quality, and rate at various locations on the body can provide diagnostic information about the type and location of restrictions. It can be brought to a gentle pause in a *stillpoint* to allow the system to relax and reorganize itself at a higher level. Although a stillpoint can be induced as a therapeutic event, it may also occur naturally as a spontaneous part of the homeostatic process (Upledger, 1987). The rhythm can be used as a *significance detector* (Upledger, 1990), allowing the therapist to know whether or not the body finds something important. The rhythm stops abruptly when the body is in the correct position or the emotion arising is significant, and returns when the release is completed, signaling the therapist to move on.

When the therapist's hands are correctly placed on the body, it may feel almost as though the body is "pulling them in." The hands are kept in position while the tissue is felt to move. Although these movements are very small and not visually apparent, they feel very clear to the therapist's proprioceptive sense. The hands follow the tissue in the *direction of ease,* or the direction it moves into naturally, as far as the tissue "wants" to go. The hands do not let the tissue "go back on itself," or return to its previous position. When it has shifted into the position it needs to be in for a release to happen, the position is held until the release is complete. A *release* can be felt under the therapist's hands in several ways. It may feel as though the tissue has softened. A feeling of heat may be given off. There may be a therapeutic pulse; there may be a feeling that the hands have been "released" from their position on the body.

A *therapeutic pulse* is one of the most common signs of release used by craniosacral therapists. It arises after the craniosacral rhythm has stopped, and subsides when the release is complete. It feels like the cardiac pulse in the wrist, except at a different speed. Sometimes therapists wonder whether it is a therapeutic pulse in the client or their own cardiac pulse that they are feeling. The answer is that one's own cardiac pulse does not arise and subside the way a therapeutic pulse in a client does.

Direction of energy and *intent* are used in craniosacral therapy in ways that are not commonly used in allopathic medicine. Energy is directed through the therapist's hands into the body to provide therapeutic benefit to the client. The therapist's intent as well as the hand position place the energy where it needs to go.

Indications and Contraindications for Craniosacral Therapy

Indications

- Headaches
- Back and neck pain
- TMJ
- Chronic fatigue/fibromyalgia
- Motor coordination
- Eye problems
- CNS disorders
- Autism
- Erb's palsy
- Chronic pain
- Traumatic brain injury
- Learning disabilities
- Stress and tension related disorders
- Posttraumatic stress disorders
- Orthopedic problems
- Scoliosis
- Tinnitis

Contraindications

- Elevated intracranial pressure
- Known or suspected intracranial hemorrhage or aneurysm
- Any condition for which it is ill advised to alter intracranial pressure
- Acute CVA
- Postsurgery nystagmus

Goals

Occupational and physical therapists who are just learning craniosacral therapy often begin by adding it to their existing "toolbox" of techniques and modalities, using pieces here and there to enhance traditional practice. For example, craniosacral therapy is an effective enabling technique to use before engaging in functional activities. The deep relaxation induced by some of the techniques is helpful in reducing tone and decreasing pain. The fascial releases are very useful in breaking up scar tissue and increasing active and passive range of motion. The fluid exchange is helpful in decreasing edema and facilitating immune system response. When used correctly (i.e., using no more than 5 grams of pressure and following the body's lead in a nondirective manner), craniosacral therapy techniques are safe even in the hands of a beginner.

Typical Treatment Session

Clients receiving craniosacral therapy are fully clothed with only belts and shoes removed. The therapist begins by "listening" to the body through palpation of the tissues, craniosacral rhythm, and energy forces at several locations to determine the primary location where intervention is needed. The parts of the body are intricately connected to each other, both in embryological development and in the web of the fascial system (Upledger & Vredevoogd, 1983). For this reason, the area of discomfort may not be the area where the primary problem lies.

Clients may be treated standing, sitting, or lying down. It is easiest to treat someone who is lying supine, but it is also possible to treat someone sitting in a wheelchair, squirming in the arms of the therapist, or moving about a room, as may be the case with young children. The more a client is moving about, the more skill is needed by the therapist to listen and treat effectively.

The treatment varies with the skill and experience of the therapist. In the beginning levels of craniosacral work, the therapist learns to feel and influence the craniosacral rhythm, to release fascial restrictions at the places where restrictions most commonly occur, and to use the bones of the skull as handles for palpating and influencing the intracranial membranes. Once direction of energy is learned, a change in the therapist's thinking about what is possible may result. To do this work, the therapist must believe that what is being felt under the hands is possible, is happening, and is able to have an influence on the body in spite of the light touch that is being used.

After completing the first level of training, a therapist will be able to provide limited craniosacral therapy. The therapist will understand the concept of therapeutic pulse, release, taking tissue into the direction of ease, and influencing the craniosacral rhythm. At this level, therapists should be able to provide balancing, encourage rhythmic flow of the cerebral spinal fluid, and release fascial restrictions by following a protocol of hand positions. Some dramatic results may occur with the use of this protocol, but a beginning therapist will probably not be able to replicate these because he or she does not yet fully understand the system and the process.

To provide a familiar analogy, imagine a new therapist working in a rehabilitation setting. A client with extensive injuries to the hand is referred for treatment. A new therapist has some tools for treating this client and will use those tools. However, after investing the time into advanced practice to become a certified hand therapist, this practitioner will have a much larger toolbox and much more expertise. Clients are likely to improve much faster, and the therapist is likely to be much more confident in his or her ability to facilitate healing at an optimal rate. Training in craniosacral therapy is much the same. A beginning craniosacral therapist will have some basic treatment skills, but will not have nearly the clinical expertise that comes with more coursework and many hours of experience.

Beyond the first course that teaches a basic protocol, training varies with the teaching institution. The ability to follow the cues provided by the body deepens, and there is an increased understanding of the movement of the cranial bones along with the ability to find and treat areas of primary concern within the body. Work inside the mouth is added to the protocol at this level if it was not a part of the original coursework, and the movements of the bones of the skull, particularly the sphenoid, are explored in more depth. The ability to use the hands to listen to the body in a sensitive way deepens along with the ability to follow cues the body offers to restore its balance and optimal functioning. Always, the body leads and the therapist follows. Osteopathy, which gave birth to craniosacral therapy, does not use force on the body. Forcing the body is an allopathic concept (Barral & Mercier, 1988). The therapist does not impose a predetermined treatment plan onto the body, which may be a shift in thinking for therapists. Consider the following case provided by a registered physical therapist who had completed the second level of Upledger training in craniosacral therapy:

Twyla is a 32-year-old woman with a history of a fall down some stairs 5 months prior. She had significant pain on the entire right side of her body and had also hit her head. She had no loss of consciousness, and there were no fractures. All injuries were soft tissue in nature, except for a bruised ego. The most persistent of her injuries was in her right ankle and leg, which continued to give her pain 5 months post injury. She had already received a full course of traditional physical therapy, including ice/heat, ultrasound, theraband exercises, and a stretching program, which she consistently performed.

Upon evaluation, she had a mildly antalgic gait, which would worsen with longer distances. She reported that she had been unable to participate fully in her walking exercise program since her fall. She had decreased active range of motion of the ankle in all ranges, especially inversion, eversion, and dorsiflexion. She had pain with passive inversion at her end range and pain with compression at the heel. She reported that her ankle felt "jammed." On palpation, there was a great deal of torsion around the right ankle and an area of tension in the right groin/pelvis.

Treatment began with some standard physical therapy interventions: manual distractions and mobilization of the ankle joint. While these felt good to the client while they were being performed, they did not help the problem. Next, a craniosacral technique was used. Both of the practitioner's hands were placed around the ankle joint and the torsional pattern was followed into the direction of ease until the cranial rhythm stopped. During the pause, some heat was released. Some slight softening of the tissue was felt, along with a line of tension strongly up into the right pelvis. One of the practitioner's hands was moved up to an area of tension that was superior and lateral to the right pubis and deep within the pelvis. Gentle pressure was applied until the tissue resistance barrier was met, and then 5 grams of pressure was used to engage the tissue. The cranial rhythm was still off. Movement was felt through the line of tension between the pelvis and ankle. A therapeutic pulse was felt in the ankle. When it subsided, the ankle and pelvic tissue felt softer. The cranial rhythm resumed.

When the client got up off the table and walked around, she was amazed. She said that her whole leg felt lighter and no longer had the feeling of being jammed at the ankle. No further sessions were necessary, and the client remained pain free after 2 months.

Emotional Aspects of Craniosacral Work

Upper levels of training provide a basis for dealing with the emotional issues that may be stored in the tissue and released with craniosacral treatment. Upledger (1990) calls this somato-emotional release, or regional tissue release. Therapeutic imagery and dialogue may also be used at this level to assist in finding the unconscious emotional holding patterns underlying the dysfunctional state. Upledger introduced the concept of an energy cyst that has been sealed off by the body as an adaptive response. This dysfunctional area, or energy cyst, does not cooperate with the fluid and tissue motion, costing the body extra energy for normal functioning (Upledger, 1990).

Emotional work may take one of several different forms. When contact is made with an energy cyst, it may reconnect the client with the original events, providing a cathartic experience. In other cases, the therapist may ask a client where an image is felt in the body. In this case, therapeutic dialogue or visual imagery may be used to assist in finding the emotional factors underlying the dysfunctional state and to open a dialogue with that part of the body, which will determine what it needs or what it is trying to do for the client. Or, the work may be silent, as the tissue seems to "unwind" itself from the original injury. The therapist acts as a facilitator by touching the body to allow it to assume the position it needs to be in to release the stored energy. The correct position is found by monitoring the craniosacral rhythm until it stops and holding that position as long as the rhythm is off. The emotional work in craniosacral therapy requires sensitivity and training on the part of the therapist guiding the experience. As the regional tissue release occurs, heat may be felt and the tissue can be felt to soften. The cranial rhythm, which has been off during the work, will be felt to resume.

The client may need to be referred to a psychologist or a psychiatrist to process the emotional content that comes up as the tissues release the stored emotions. Somato-emotional releases are not planned events. They occur as the tissues release stored emotions, and the therapist must be prepared to handle a distressed client in the moment, even if a referral is made after the session. What is appropriate in one practice setting may not be in another. It is important for the therapist to know his or her own limits, both personally and professionally, in helping clients who are processing emotions. In the following case, Sarah was seen in a private-pay situation, which allowed the treating occupational therapist the luxury of combining her practice skills in both physical dysfunction and mental health.

Sarah is a 50-year-old, Caucasian, married mother of two boys. She sought craniosacral treatment for a painful area midway between her scapula and spine at about the level of T6. The pain was of sudden onset, which she described as a "sharp knife." It was quite disabling and impacted all performance areas in Sarah's life. Prior to seeking craniosacral therapy, she had a neurological work-up, a 6-day series of oral steroids (which helped), massage, trigger point release, and a chiropractic adjustment. She had a TENS unit for home use, as well as a home traction unit that she did not know how to use and did not like. Although Sarah's husband is a physician, she had a strong preference for alternative care. Craniosacral therapy was used at her request.

Sarah was seen weekly for 2 months, then every other week for several more months. Therapeutic imagery and dialogue were used extensively with Sarah and were as much a part of the treatment as the physical manipulation and energy work. The painful area in her shoulder appeared in her visualization as a "clip" whose job it was to hold her together. At first, her image was of a solid wall of boards. With treatment, this changed to slats with room in between them, and later to a rubber band as the area softened. Finally, it changed to a new silver body suit that allowed for her expansion into a larger Self in a way that her old skin could not.

Sarah did not feel a need to see someone for psychological treatment. She used a journal to work with the images that occurred over the course of her treatment. The painful "clip" area resolved over a series of treatments. It has re-emerged twice since then, when events in Sarah's life have left her feeling not "together" enough to meet her own standards.

At more advanced levels, other nontraditional techniques may be used concurrently with craniosacral therapy. For example, Reiki energy may be called in, or the chakras may be balanced. Strain/counterstrain, muscle energy, therapeutic touch, relaxation, and visualization may also be used.

Sometimes craniosacral therapy is used as an enabling technique to facilitate the efficacy of more traditional forms of therapy. Consider the following case.

Abigail is a 10-year-old, Caucasian female in the fifth grade. She was first referred to OT for distractibility, learning and visual perceptual problems, and fine motor deficits. Her parents were concerned with her increasing difficulty with academic pursuits and homework, describing her as "messy, unorganized," and frequently "off task." Although Abigail received OT consultation through her school, her parents did not feel that Abigail was making significant progress within existing programs. At the request of her parents, the school psychologist referred Abigail to a private occupational therapist for an independent evaluation and follow up. Abigail's provisional diagnosis included attention deficit hyperactivity disorder–inattentive type and educational problems. No medication was prescribed pending trial of therapy services and reassessment.

Evaluation: Abigail presented as a pale child with a flat affect and minimal expression. Her parents reported that Abigail tended to be irritible when corrected and generally unresponsive toward suggestions. Homework and chores were an ongoing source of conflict. She had difficulty organizing, sequencing, or successfully completing middle-school-level activities. Abigail put forth good effort but gave very limited verbal or eye contact. She had an underlying low muscle tone and postural instability, as seen in her tendency to lean on her arms during sitting. Although visual deficits had been previously diagnosed and glasses prescribed, she did not wear her glasses and stated that they "didn't really help." She was unable to write the alphabet in cursive from memory.

Treatment: Abigail was initially seen one time weekly for one-hour sessions for 1 month. Craniosacral therapy was used each visit for the first 4 weeks as an enabling activity, to help her relax and explore home program suggestions. Upledger's early work at Michigan State indicated good success using this treatment approach with children with learning disabilities (Upledger & Vredevoogd, 1983). Craniosacral therapy was also used to allow the child to feel the postural corrections in herself. Postural changes allowed her to free the upper extremities for more skilled functions such as writing. Craniosacral therapy was used to work out restrictions in the dural tube and to decompress the occiput from C1 to permit clear passage of the neural and blood supply from the brain to the rest of the body. Other restrictions in the thorax were treated and released as they became apparent. The time spent in craniosacral therapy also allowed Abigail an opportunity to express her concerns and her feelings of frustration. Over the 4 weeks, Abigail more readily identified her problem areas and participated actively in developing solutions. Following these sessions, she was able to retain and apply strategies suggested, which she had been unable to do in the past. Abigail's increased ability to organize, problem solve, and communicate seemed to be the direct result of the craniosacral therapy. These results were sustained as evidenced by her improved academic scores, increased levels of initiation and participation, and decreased conflicts at home and school.

Abigail's home program was designed to facilitate postural stability, provide joint protection in activity, and increase tone. It contained alternate positions while doing homework and alternate materials to facilitate attention and to decrease physical exertion. It provided organizational and sequencing strategies, and incorporated visual motor integration along with a supplemental handwriting program emphasizing continuous movement of the hand. Her mother was shown how to encourage the home program, and consultation was given to the parents regarding the Individualized Education Plan (IEP). Abigail had a new optometry evaluation and was fitted with new glasses, which she began wearing, saying ". . . they work better." Following 1 month of treatment, frequency was reduced to 1 visit per month for an additional 5 months to include direct treatment and adjustments to the home program as appropriate to Abigail's progress.

Craniosacral treatment was phased out after the first 4 visits as new interventions evolved, including reassessment and functional strategies that enabled Abigail to take control of her own agenda for treatment. During her last 4 (monthly) visits, she identified her areas of concern and worked on these directly. By discharge, Abigail, her family, and school had established a mutually agreeable IEP, including reasonable expectations; Abigail was functioning successfully in her classes and at home; and she was discharged from OT services.

Appropriate Use Within OT and PT Practice

Craniosacral therapy can be used as an enabling activity, as it was with Abigail, or as a treatment technique, as it was with Sarah and Twyla. Sometimes a symptom can be treated effectively at its endpoint (e.g., using a TENS unit to control back pain) while at other times it is necessary to impact the system at a more basic level (e.g., using an exercise program to strengthen the muscles whose weakness is contributing to the back pain), or even at the level of prevention (e.g., making ergonomic corrections to a workstation so that back pain will not result from incorrect posture). Twyla's case illustrates the use of craniosacral therapy in relief of a symptom. Sarah illustrates the need to impact the system at a deeper level. Upledger (1996) has also used craniosacral therapy with newborns as a preventive measure, and has found it effective.

Discharge Indications

Ideally, clients are discharged when their symptoms abate. Since craniosacral therapy is done by practitioners from many disciplines in many and various settings, there is a wide latitude of discharge criteria. In a traditional hospital or rehabilitation setting, discharge may be based on short-term stay goals or payment status, regardless of remaining symptoms of imbalance within the craniosacral system. In a private-pay setting, a client may choose to continue being seen periodically as a part of a personal wellness program. Alternately, a client may decide to discontinue therapy due to dissatisfaction with the practitioner, the treatment, or the results.

Don is a 55-year-old man with severe back pain from a heavy machinery injury many years previously, involving multiple rib and vertebral fractures as well as soft tissue and crush injuries. He was being seen in a chronic pain program in an attempt to decrease his dependence on the heavy narcotics he had been using to manage his pain. After a number of days in the program, it was found that although he had received exercise-based physical therapy, he had not had much manual work done. He had not kept up with the exercise program, stating that it was too painful to perform. He was referred to physical therapy for a trial of manual therapy. Upon observation, he appeared to be in pain. His face was drawn, his shoulders were hunched, and his posture was guarded. He rated his pain as an 11 on a scale of 1 to 10. AROM of the spine was very limited. He was very irritible in manner and expressed doubts that anything could be done to help him. He did agree to a session of manual therapy. He had already begun a graded exercise program with his regular therapist and was tolerating it so far.

During the cranial portion of the protocol, especially during the work on the sphenoid and the temporals, the client was seen to show relaxation of his posture. His forward hunched shoulders dropped back onto the table. His breathing became much deeper and slower, and his color improved. There was

Training and Certification

As craniosacral therapy has emerged out of osteopathy and has been taught to allied health care practitioners, several disciplines have shown an interest in incorporating craniosacral therapy into their exclusive territory. In different states, physical therapists, massage therapists, and chiropractors have considered craniosacral therapy so closely related to their own discipline's knowledge base that only licensed practitioners within that discipline should practice. In order to keep craniosacral therapy pure and interdisciplinary, training and certification programs have been established to certify all qualified individual practitioners regardless of discipline.

There are at least three credible training programs in the United States:

- **The Upledger Institute** provides multiple levels of training worldwide. John Upledger is an osteopathic physician, and the Upledger Institute is the most widely known and utilized training program in the United States. There are four levels of basic coursework, plus three levels of advanced training. There are branches of training into specialty areas, such as pediatrics and process work. The Upledger Institute offers certification at two levels: techniques and diplomate. Training is conducted in a traveling seminar format, offered at various locations and times of the year.

- **The Milne Institute** provides a seven-level training program worldwide. Hugh Milne is also an osteopathic physician. While this program is less well known and publicized, training is equally rigorous and yields equally well-prepared practitioners. Certification requires successful completion of all seven levels of classes taught by the Milne Institute, along with completion of a required reading list and a final exam.

- **Dialogues in Contemporary Rehabilitation (DCR)** provides seven levels of cranial training as part of its program in integrative manual therapy. Sharon Weiselfish-Giammatteo, who directs this program, is a Ph.D. and registered physical therapist. This program requires a total of 62 credit hours, including the seven-part cranial series, to receive a diploma in integrative manual therapy through the International College of Integrative Manual Therapy in Connecticut. Further training can also lead to a bachelors, masters, or doctoral degree.

In addition to these three training programs, there are numerous training programs set up by individuals who do not have the background, expertise, and training offered by these three institutes. In many cases an individual will take a course or two from one of the major training institutes and decide he or she is qualified to teach and certify others in craniosacral techniques. It is wise to check the qualifications of the person or organization offering the training being advertised.

a softening of the tissues and a release of heat. At the end of the session, the client was assisted up. His posture was more upright and relaxed. He stated that maybe he felt a little better, but would not rate his pain. When he was seen the next day by his regular therapist, he stated angrily that nothing was going to help him. Later that day, he quit the program.

The role of occupational and physical therapy under managed care has changed dramatically. In addition, a client population that is more informed about the body-mind-spirit connection, less satisfied with the quality of traditional allopathic care, and more willing to pay out-of-pocket for treatments considered more effective is emerging (McCormack, 1997). As physical and occupational therapy evolve into the use of nontraditional therapeutic practices, it is important to remember that these are only tools for helping the client to increase function in the performance areas that he or she considers important. All therapeutic interventions must be client-based, leaving the client in charge of his or her own healing process (Parker, 1997). Nontraditional modalities need to be used in accord with practice guidelines and licensure regulations. When used in accord with practice guidelines, craniosacral work is truly a client-centered therapy.

Research

There has been some research done to prove the existence of the various parts of the craniosacral system (Upledger, 1995, 2000b), but there is a paucity of controlled studies on the effectiveness of craniosacral therapy as a treatment modality. With the exception of Upledger's studies on post traumatic stress disorder (PTSD) (Upledger, 2000a), most of the evidence for its effectiveness is anecdotal. It continues to be used by practitioners who see it work. As therapists move into evidence-based practice, and as this treatment modality moves more into the mainstream of health care, controlled comparative studies need to be done to prove or disprove its efficacy.

Summary

Craniosacral therapy is a gentle, noninvasive health care practice that comes to allied health from the field of osteopathy. To practice craniosacral therapy, therapists will need to seek education in the technique from a credible training program. Performing craniosacral therapy requires sensitivity to small movements in the human body. These palpation skills can be taught and learned, but it is important in doing this work that the therapist is willing to change paradigms from the traditional medical model to a willingness to believe and accept information that some mainstream practitioners still maintain is not present. One must also switch paradigms from the traditional therapy system of fixing things and be willing to wait patiently while the body self-corrects under your hands. A third paradigm change lies in believing that treatment can impact conditions that allopathic medical practice has considered to have reached a plateau or are "untreatable."

STUDY QUESTIONS

1. What is the quality of touch used in craniosacral therapy, and why is this important?
2. Where can good training in craniosacral therapy be obtained?
3. Define "energy cyst." How is it treated?
4. What is meant by the term *release*?
5. How do therapists use craniosacral therapy in a traditional practice setting?

SUGGESTED READING

Arnold, A. P. (1995). *Rhythm & Touch*. Albuquerque: Brotherhood of Life.

Chaitow, L. (1988). *Cranial Manipulation Theory and Practice*. London: Churchill Livingstone.

Cohen, D. (1996). *An Introduction to Craniosacral Therapy*. Berkeley, CA: North Atlantic Books.

Pronsati, M. P. (1991, May 27). Erb's palsy: Once considered incurable, now helped with NDT, craniosacral and manual therapy. *Advance for Occupational Therapists, 7*(21), 19–20.

Steiner, S. (1998, Nov. 26). CranioSacral therapy: Preparing for functional activity. *OT Week, 3*, 10.

TRAINING

Upledger Institute
11211 Prosperity Farms Rd.
Palm Beach Gardens, FL 33410
(561) 622-4334
http://www.Upledger.com

Milne Institute
PO Box 2716
Monterey, CA 93942-2716

(831) 649-1825
http://milneinstitute.com

Dialogues in Contemporary Rehabilitation
800 Cottage Grove Rd., Suite 211
Bloomfield, CT 06002
(860) 243-6571
http://www.DCRHEALTH.com

REFERENCES

Barral, J., & P. Mercier. (1988). *Visceral Manipulation*. Seattle: Eastland.

McCormack, G. L. (1997, Feb.). What is nontraditional practice? *OT Practice, 2*, 16–19.

Milne, H. (1995). *The Heart of Listening*. Berkeley, CA: North Atlantic Books.

Parker, J. S. (1997, Feb.). Our role as growth facilitators. *OT Practice, 2*, 20–23.

Smoley, R. (1991, May/June). Exploring craniosacral therapy. *Yoga Journal, 98*, 20–29.

Upledger, J. E. (n.d.). CranioSacral therapy. (Publication 000A) Available from Upledger Insitute, 11211 Prosperity Farms Rd. Suite D 325, West Palm Beach, Florida, 33410.

Upledger, J. E. (1987). *CranioSacral Therapy II: Beyond the Dura*. Seattle: Eastland.

Upledger, J. E. (1988, Winter). The therapeutic value of the CranioSacral system. *Massage Therapy Journal, 21*(1), 32–33.

Upledger, J. E. (1990). *SomatoEmotional Release and Beyond*. West Palm Beach, FL: UI Publishing.

Upledger, J. E. (1995). *Research and Observations Support the Existence of a Craniosacral System*. Palm Beach Gardens, FL: UI Publishing.

Upledger, J. E. (1996). *A Brain is Born*. Berkeley, CA: North Atlantic Books.

Upledger, J. E. (2000a, Spring). Post-traumatic stress disorder: Research soothes the skeptics. *Upledger UpDate*, 1–13.

Upledger, J. E. (2000b, Fall). The expanding role of cerebrospinal fluid in health and disease. *Upledger UpDate*, 6–7.

Upledger, J. E., & J. D. Vredevoogd. (1983). *CranioSacral Therapy.* Seattle: Eastland.

ACKNOWLEDGMENTS

The author wishes to thank Priscilla Douglas, R.P.T. and Meridith Jost, O.T.R. for contributing cases to this chapter.

15

The Feldenkrais Method®

Reuven Ofir

CHAPTER OBJECTIVES

- Understand the major concepts important in the Feldenkrais Method.
- Describe the difference between Awareness Through Movement and Functional Integration lessons.

Learning means acquiring the means to change one's behavior.

The Feldenkrais Method (FM) is a somatic educational method that employs movement and the sensory aspect of movement to generate new perceptions and new learning, which constitute the basis for new behavior. This learning process sharpens and expands perceptual awareness of our self-image in action (Schilder, 1950). The powerful effect of self-image over behavior is familiar when one thinks about how awkward and clumsy adolescents can feel. People are often less familiar with lapses in self-image, such as distortions of acture (i.e., posture in action), which can lead to pain and even disability. Enhancement of self-image and awareness produces therapeutic outcomes. The process by which such positive therapeutic outcomes emerge through FM is guided and propelled by the educational process of *learning to learn*, and not by a medically based paradigm.

Feldenkrais integrated two concepts originally developed by John Hughlings Jackson (1958) into his conceptual framework of function (1977). Feldenkrais, based upon Hughlings Jackson's work, stated that self-image is made up of four components: movement, sensation, feeling, and thought. Hughlings Jackson also stated, "Nervous centers represent movements, not muscles" (1958, p. 29).

Efficient function is contingent upon perfect congruence of the four elements in any action. The concept of *function* is central to FM, as is the concept of *awareness. Function implies integrated activity in numerous structures* (Jouvet, 1999). Efficiency of function demands full coordination and integration of multiple structures in the execution of any task. En-

150

The Feldenkrais Method uses an educational process to effect changes in movement behavior. Outcomes include alleviation and/or elimination of pain stemming from improper use of the self, improvement of postural alignment appropriate to any form of action, and acquisition of a sense of ease and joy of movement. The method has applications in numerous orthopedic and neurological conditions regardless of age.

hancement of perceptual awareness in function is the tool used in FM to achieve better integration. This can result in greater ease and improved pleasure and quality of life in all of life's domains.

Feldenkrais and the Method He Developed

Dr. Moshe Feldenkrais developed the Feldenkrais Method by questioning some very basic and established premises that had guided physical rehabilitation practices for many decades. His approach to helping people who suffered from movement disorders was counterintuitive, and as a corollary, was all embracing in the true sense of the word *holistic* (Feldenkrais, 1974).

Feldenkrais was born in Russia in 1904. At age 14, in the immediate aftermath of World War I, he traveled by cart, mule, and train to British-ruled Palestine. Several years later he was training Jewish youth in self-defense and Judo techniques, and he published a number of books on this subject. Because British authorities were suspicious of his activities, and since he wanted to continue his education, he discreetly left Palestine to complete his education in France, where he earned (first in order of merit) a master of science degree in mechanical and electrical engineering and a doctoral degree of science (with first class honors), which is a Ph.D., in engineering. His dissertation was titled, "Measurement of Very High Tensions" (voltages). While studying, he found time to open the first martial art school in France as a representative of Dr. Jigoro Kano, Japanese founder of Judo. Feldenkrais worked in Joliot-Curie's laboratory in France in research and construction of high-tension apparatus for nuclear fission work and collaborated in the design of the Van deGraaff generator.

As the Nazis entered France, Feldenkrais was spirited out and immediately recruited by the British Admiralty. While doing research for the British Admiralty, he fell and shattered his knee. Being of such high value to the British government, he had at his disposal the best orthopedic surgeons. All they could offer him was fusion of the knee at best, and at worst, amputation. He refused. Determined to heal himself, he embarked on an intense period of self-exploration to find out how he moved, how he could reduce the pain, reduce the tremendous tightness of his hamstrings in his injured leg, scratch his toes, wash them, get to the bathroom, roll over in bed, and so on. His self-exploration led to his developing his "work." Feldenkrais may have been the first man to wed the principles of Western scientific methodology with tenets developed over thousands of years in the Far East (1974) in developing a concrete method of improving quality of life through increasing self-awareness.

After the end of the World War II, Feldenkrais, at the behest of the late David Ben Gurion (the first Prime Minister of Israel), returned to Israel to lead the development of research and production of the fledgling new Israeli arms industry. He worked in the arms industry for a couple of years, but his passion for his own work consumed him, and he spent the rest of his life further developing and refining the work that has become known as the Feldenkrais Method. Feldenkrais died in Israel in 1984.

Application of the Method

The Feldenkrais Method is taught in groups or classes called Awareness Through Movement (ATM) and in individual sessions called Functional Integration (FI). In ATM a teacher verbally guides the students through a series of tightly constructed movement sequences, leading to improvement in generic functions—not specific skills per se, but improved organization of movement applicable across a whole array of basic activities such as breathing, walking, climbing, singing, working, dancing, and so on. Improvement in this context means greater efficiency of action: using less work to accomplish tasks or actions that previously required more effort. The result is that actions and functions become easier and therefore more pleasant. The same principles are applied in FI, but using manual contact as a communication tool with which to guide and teach the student. In FI, the hands do the talking—verbal interaction can be and is used, but usually minimally.

In both ATM and FI, the student remains dressed, removing only shoes, belt, and jewelry. Lessons are constructed in such a way that the participant can have no expectation or knowledge of where the lesson will lead or what the outcome will be. A learning structure such as this a priori neutralizes old habits and permits acquisition of new and possibly better habits. Moreover, it provides novelty (Langer, 1997) which stimulates innate curiosity and often is accompanied by expressions of joy, exuberance, contentment, and revitalization.

The pace of the lessons is generally slow, with frequent rest periods, which has been found necessary for optimal learning (Holcomb, 1997). Initially, lessons are done with students lying on mats on the floor or on a special wide plinth in FI (this is done as a means of neutralizing or minimizing the force of gravity as well as providing a sense of safety). As students progress and lessons become more complex, other postures are included, such as side sitting on the floor or on hands and knees, sitting on chairs, standing, and walking. The lessons are designed so that each student focuses upon himself or herself—on the *how* of doing—and the relationship of sensation to movement, movement to action, and action to function in relation to the environment. In other words, the focus is on the learning process, the exploratory process, not on the goal or outcome. Langer (1997) notes: "The teacher who tells students to solve a problem in a prescribed manner is limiting their ability to investigate their surroundings and to test novel ideas" (p. 121). The primary intention of the Feldenkrais instructor is to create conditions for novel sensations, leading to a changed and expanded perception of the student's self-image in action.

In order to be able to perceive differences, people need to compare one condition with another, one sensation with another. As a baseline for comparison, students are first guided to sense or perceive how they *habitually* organize themselves in preparation for executing a

Because the Feldenkrais Method uses an educational model as opposed to a medical one, indications and contraindications are not typically used to describe who should or should not participate in FI or ATM sessions. However, in order to benefit from FM, students will need to be able to follow verbal directions and be medically stable. Given that the method is learning-based, almost anyone, regardless of age, gender, or physical condition, can benefit from it. The only difference between people in these contexts would be their different rates of learning. Indeed, people from all strata of society turn to Feldenkrais practitioners for help and guidance. These tend to be people who are in pain or who experience limitations in their daily functions. Being dissatisfied with the quality of their lives, they seek to improve them.

task, one which, through misuse or abuse, had brought about the pain or dysfunction. The student is then cued to sense, feel, learn, and know several new ways of behaving in the course of their varied daily activities. No longer is such a person compelled by ignorance to act in one or, at most, only two possible ways. Now several options are available to that person, who can then select and choose the most appropriate one in accordance with the current circumstance.

Principles and Strategies Underlying the Feldenkrais Method

Organic Learning

Infants discover on their own how to roll over, sit, crawl, stand up, walk, and talk. They do so through an active exploration of themselves in relation to their environment, through an arduous process of observation and of trial, error, and success. Feldenkrais termed the way they learn "organic learning." He developed his method by striving to apply the exploratory processes of learning that a child goes through—of self-learning.

Efficient learning is a heuristic process, not by mindless rote, correction, imitation, or coercion of any sort. What people learn through this discovery process becomes their own creation. Such learning, if put to use, is permanent. It is "owned" by its discoverer, regardless of whether millions of people have discovered the same thing on their own.

Behavior Can Change Only When Perception Changes

If people do not know how they repeatedly hurt themselves through their own actions, they are destined to continue hurting themselves, and they gradually deteriorate further. In effect, they are simply committing an error that they do not know how to correct. Feldenkrais reasoned that since the largest proportion of brain cells are devoted directly or indirectly to movement, the most efficient way to effect the central nervous system would be through the medium of movement while methodically attending to the sensations accompanying such movements. Feldenkrais reasoned that executing efficient action requires a clear intention coupled with a precise orientation (direction) and timing. Not being clear about what one wishes to accomplish, not aiming precisely (i.e., not directing oneself in the precise manner in order to execute an action, or not carrying out the needed action in proper sequence and timely fashion) leads to failure to accomplish what one really wants to do, whether it is playing a musical instrument, driving a nail into a board, or pitching a baseball.

Feldenkrais developed hundreds of carefully constructed ATM lessons with structured movement sequences, leading his students to sense more distinctions: to see and hear more clearly, differentiating more and more subtle motor discriminations in order to help them refine their perceptual abilities. These lessons enable students to change behavior by gaining progressively greater precision and congruence between intention, orientation, and timing.

Creating Conditions for Efficient Learning

"Learning is the detection of a difference that makes a difference." (Bateson, 1972, p. 453)

Learning to differentiate our movements, sensations, and perceptions in FM requires using less effort. The sense of effort, or strain, is considered in this model as "noise"—interference with the ability to sense subtle sensory messages. If different mediums of communication are competing for the same channel, the clarity of the message is compromised. Concepts such as the Arndt-Schultz and Weber/Fechner laws are important to the creation of conditions for efficient FM learning. The Arndt-Schultz law states that physiological activity is excited by weak stimuli, optimal with moderate stimuli, and curtailed by strong stimuli (1989). Most people are aware of their ability to amplify weak signals when they are important: cocking one's ear, sniffing the air, sensing the slightest touch, and conversely covering one's ears when noise gets too loud, shutting eyes when the light shines too brightly, stiffening up when someone pushes too hard, and shutting down when overstimulated. These actions are people's efforts to optimize stimuli. The Weber/Fechner law describes the *just discernible sensory difference* in relation to effort, noting that the *threshold* of perceiving a difference in stimulus is a certain fraction of the overall stimulus already present (1989).

In the FM learning context, when an instructor, for example, instructs a student to raise an arm overhead and try to sense where the movement originates, the only way the student would be able to detect the origin and the trajectory of the ensuing movement would be by reducing muscular effort to a minimum. Lifting an arm in the air involves a subtle shift of weight through a trajectory that almost instantaneously is countered by an equal and opposite balance reaction. That upward reaching motion is also accompanied by an elongation of the trunk and a spreading of the ribs on the same side, as well as other changes in orientation. Increasing the muscular force results in the student being able to sense only muscular effort, overshadowing the subtle kinesthetic signals of movement originating in other areas of his or her body.

Another source of interference to learning that must be neutralized are the aches, pains and tensions that distract people from focusing attention on the learning process. Therefore, pain, discomfort, or anxiety are also considered noise. The instructor tries to create conditions of comfort and safety so that such distractions are eliminated, or at least minimized, thus enabling students to more clearly observe their sensations. It is also of vital importance that communication is clear and precise, and is *personally meaningful to the student*. For example, asking a student to straighten his or her elbow evokes a different level of attention and meaning, and consequently will change the way the student will organize that movement as opposed to asking the student to reach for the cup of tea on the table, to take the offered cake, or to push the teacher away. FM instructors also strive to communicate clearly so that there is no need to increase the volume and create noise. Quite the contrary, volume can and should be decreased—less is better in FM.

Differentiation

Differentiation is crucial to FM. Learning to differentiate movement means being able to simultaneously perform opposing movements, such as looking to the right while turning the head to the left, feining a jab with the left hand while punching with the right, playing rhythms on the piano with the left hand while playing the melody with the right. Furthermore, learning to differentiate enables us to reverse our actions at a moment's notice. Differentiation enhances reversibility. Reversibility enhances the ability to change one's actions appropriate to changed circumstances. For example, opening a closed hand to accept a gift, then closing to hold it; opening one's mouth to say something, then regretting it and immediately closing it; pouring a cup of tea, stopping midway, and deciding to have coffee instead—all of these actions require reversibility. Absent differentiation and reversibility, people could not play the violin, type with computers, eat, or procreate. In conditions such as spasticity, rigidity, or heightened tone, the ability to rapidly reverse a directional movement or to differentiate movement becomes difficult, slowed down, and in extreme cases impossible to execute, such as when an elderly person suddenly changes direction and ends up losing balance and falling, or when a person with spastic hemiplegia cannot unclench his or her hand and walks with a stiff lower limb as if there are no separate ankle, knee, or hip joints.

Learning to differentiate our movements requires a gradual increase of self-awareness in action. To be able to distinguish between 20 shades of white, as Inuits do, to differentiate the sound of a leaf rustling in the breeze from that of a tiger stalking, to appreciate the nuances of music, of good food, of fine wines, and to be able to tell whether one is working needlessly hard or with effortless grace can only be acquired through a learning process that uses comparison as its tool. FM uses hundreds of different lessons, successively contrasting different sensory experiences such as effort versus rest, slow versus fast movement, small versus large movement, contrasts between the left and right sides of the body, and visualizations of movement versus actual movement, all of which are designed to result in a change in one's perception of somatic self in relation to self and environment. In other words, the intention and the methods employed are designed to help the student to change his or her body image as a means of improving the accuracy and efficiency of function. Unique to this method is the use of exaggerated sensory differences in order to highlight contrast and the focus of attention on one side of the body so as to create heightened contrasts and distinctions.

For example, having a student perform a series of slow, sequential movements with a limb or a whole side of the body, while paying close attention to the accompanying sensations and feelings can be used as a template for the other side. The result is that the student often perceives the body part or side attended to in a different way—as being significantly clearer, larger, or longer. Subsequently in FM, if one side or part of the body has a movement deficiency or pain, the student can be guided to create an image of sequential movements using this "deficient" side, and asked to perform them. The result is often a quite significant improvement of function of that formerly deficient side within a far shorter time span than had been devoted to the original side. A remarkable similarity of such a process that tends to validate this technique in FM is the mirroring technique illustrated by Ramachandran (1996) in his work with phantom pain.

Attention and Learning

Without *active attention,* there is no learning. Lessons are therefore designed so that curiosity is constantly being stimulated by introduction of variation around the same theme. Students' introspective exploration of their own movements and sensations within the structure of a lesson stimulates their attention and self-motivation, similar to the way people might feel when trying to solve an interesting puzzle and being happily surprised when they find a solution. Such an approach in FM often results in an increase in creativity as well as physical flexibility.

Interactive Communication Between Instructor and Student

The most effective communication process is direct; it is not mediated through cognitive relay stations or multiple interpretations. Typically, in rehabilitation the primary intention of skeletal manipulation is to effect structures. With FM the intention is to communicate directly with the student's central nervous system. The practitioner giving an FI lesson uses tactile communication by cueing or guiding the student through the student's skeletal structures. These tactile communications are achieved by providing very gentle compressive and supportive forces applied through bony prominences.

Tactile communication between instructor and student during an FI lesson is mediated by a progressive series of questions and answers through application of slight, gentle, supportive pressures of the skeleton in a functionally oriented direction. The instructor basically poses the communication in the form of a tactile question: Are you organized, ready, willing, and able to move in this direction? The instructor waits for a response from the student before proceeding further. The response may be a *Yes, I am ready,* a *No, I am not,* or a *Maybe, but I need more time.* These responses are not verbal, nor are they instantaneous. The instructor is patient and waits for the response, sometimes for a few seconds, at other times maybe for a minute or two, while the student is processing the meaning of the communication. The instructor may sense a resistance to the proposal of movement, an accepting yielding, or a hesitation. Students can have a number of physical changes that act as indicators to the instructor—for example, they may pause in breathing or experience an increase in breathing depth or rate, eyes may flutter under closed eyelids, or they may become flushed. A cybernetic loop is thus established between student and teacher in the form of a communication more precise than verbal conversation, which can be plagued by inaccuracies, misunderstandings, and cultural differences.

When the instructor applies a very gentle manual cue through support of skeletal structures, the speed of communication is practically instantaneous, since hard and dense material such as bone transmits pressure information very efficiently. How is this done?

The instructor applies gentle compressive or supportive contact with the intention of eliciting in the student the perception of potential action through superior organization of his or her neuroskeletal muscular system in relation to gravity. Muscles organize themselves around bone in accordance with the direction of forces transmitted and congruent with the functional requirements for action. For example, the instructor might apply support to the sole of the foot by using a flat board while the student is supine; that is, using a pseudo floor. That support is perceived by the student as standing on the foot, and the central nervous system (CNS) will organize the motor apparatus in accordance with requirements for efficient standing, yet without the encumbrance of actual weight bearing. Since the student is supine, actual weight bearing with the accompanying habitual and reflexive distortions will be neutralized. Therefore, a new and more effective weight-bearing strategy is formed by the student, one which requires least effort. In other words, the CNS perceives a new way of standing, a more efficient way that requires less effort and is more pleasant.

In an ATM lesson verbal strategies are used to direct the student's learning process. The instructor uses many different strategies, such as voice modulation, changes of rate of delivery, appropriate pauses, multiple variations of saying the same thing, use of metaphors, visualization, imaging, varying complex instructions with simple ones, and applying constraints versus removing them. For example, the instructor might ask students to flex and extend a foot while paying attention to the sensations these movements evoke, tracing the emerging sensations along the skeletal path as more and more structures get involved, imagining and then performing the same movements with the other foot. The instructor might then instruct students to change their body configuration or orientation (for example, to turn from their backs to their fronts), bend their knee so that the leg will be vertical and upright, and do the same flexing and extending of the foot, and here tracing the emerging sensations and noting the differences.

The Value of Working Indirectly

Clear and direct communication does not mean that the work is locally directed. The location of discomfort or pain is usually the symptomatic area, but not necessarily the origin or the cause. Just as one would not tamper with an open wound in order to effect its healing, but would keep the wound clean, aerated, and if necessary provide antibiotic protection, in the Feldenkrais Method one does not delve into a painful area but views the system as a whole and approaches function from the point of view of the efficacy, or lack thereof, of interacting structures.

The Feldenkrais instructor would, when assessing a student's function, seek and determine where the self-image of the student is lacking or absent—in what aspect the student is unwittingly either not participating congruently in an action or, even worse, obstructing himself or herself. These inhibited areas will then be cued, "awakened" so to speak, to engage in the given activity at the appropriate sequence and in the proper direction for the same end as that of the whole organism.

Recalibration of Neuromotor Function

In traditional therapy, recalibration of the neuromuscular system can be attained using several techniques, such as proprioceptive neuromuscular function (PNF), elements of Jacobson's exercises (1965), or by multiple gentle, reciprocal movements such as described by Maitland

(1977). Traditionally, when one encounters a muscle overly contracted in one direction, for example, shoulders habitually held slightly elevated because of stress or tension, the therapist could, of course, ask that person to lower his or her shoulders. The therapist could even stretch those muscles to elongate them in the so-called proper direction. In the Feldenkrais method, the opposite course is taken; the student is verbally instructed (in an ATM class) or is manually guided (in a FI lesson) to further exaggerate what he or she is already doing. In other words, the instructor, by manually supporting the person in the pattern he or she is in, alerts the student to a habitual behavior pattern and then substitutes the instructor's effort for that of the student. The student perceives and interprets the sensation (often expressed as a sigh of relief) as being relieved of a heavy burden. The student can now let go and stop working. When that happens, students are surprised to discover that they had been working very hard, unnecessarily—meaning that their sensory/motor centers were discharging incessantly often even when they sleep, as often seen with the phenomenon of night bruxism.

"If you know what you are doing, you can do what you want." (Feldenkrais, 1974)

The work of FM is directed in such a way as to create the conditions enabling students to act in life with an awareness and knowledge of what they are doing. This means that instructors direct students to perform every action with congruent emotions, sensations, cognition, and physical execution. Action is performed with all structures cooperating simultaneously and in harmony.

Essential Variations as Prerequisites for Efficient Learning

Learning any task or function well requires that the learning involved be done in different configurations in relation to gravity and in different contexts. For example, walking does not improve beyond a certain basic skill level simply by walking more. Practitioners of FM believe that to really walk well demands acquiring basic skills of crawling, creeping, climbing, jumping, walking backwards, walking on one's back, and then changing the context in which all of these configurations are executed. Movements per se are meaningless. Writing at a desk and writing on a ceiling or a chalkboard are in the same basic category of function, and yet require very different motor organization. Climbing and descending a mountain requires different motor organization than climbing and descending stairs.

In FM, lessons are designed to provide students with multiple variations of executing the same movement patterns in such a way that the person thoroughly learns multiple patterns. Movement patterns are then integrated into actions by imparting meaning to them. This is done by applying them to normative activities of daily living with an emphasis on activities useful for and utilized uniquely by each individual, whether a plumber, a musician or a writer.

Lifelong Learning: The Function of the Brain is to Learn

Feldenkrais believed that our potential to learn, and therefore our potential to improve and grow, is enormous. He agreed with the popular notion that we effectively use only about 15 percent of our brain. This notion has recently been firmly criticized on the basis of PET scans and other measures demonstrating that we use all of our brain in our functioning. Feldenkrais's position was that indeed we do use all of our brain as a whole in all of our activities, but we have the potential to expand the use to which we put our brain, and that we sim-

Training programs in FM are offered around the globe. Training programs are accredited by training accrediting boards elected by Feldenkrais Guild members.[1] Minimum requirements for instructor accreditation is active participation in an accredited training program, which includes a minimum of 800 hours of instruction over a period of 3 to 4 years. This is primarily experiential and hands-on learning, but also includes a significant amount of lectures and demonstrations of the work. Material covered includes actual performance of some 300 ATM lessons, learning to perform FI lessons, and learning to teach ATM lessons. Topics embedded in the learning process include anthropology, evolution, anatomy, neurology, movement sciences, mechanics, physics, evolutionary and developmental psychology, and cybernetics.

Professional training programs are offered to the public and are advertised in the public media. Applicants come from all walks of life, and no specific prerequisites are required in order to be accepted as a student, although a significant portion of graduates have come from the ranks of physical and occupational therapy, nursing, physical education, the performing arts, and the behavioral sciences.

[1]The Feldenkrais Guild is the professional organization of North American Feldenkrais practitioners. Its headquarters are located in Portland, Oregon. Most countries in Europe have their own guilds, as does Australia, and the main governing bodies work closely with one another.

ply develop only about 15 percent of our innate capacity by arresting our development at a fairly young age. His assertion was that we can continue learning until the last days of our lives—learning additional languages, skills in arts and crafts, and in self-awareness and self-knowledge, thereby transcending and elevating ourselves on a constant basis.

Research

To date there are a few published research investigations of FM and one on the use of FM sensory imagery. Results suggest that FM produces subjective improvements in health and that the use of FM sensory imagery can increase efficiency of active movement. Gutman, Herbert, and Brown (1977) studied 32 senior citizens participating in either FM classes or a conventional exercise program. While no changes between the groups were noted in physical measurements, more FM participants reported subjective improvements in health, such as noting that their health was excellent or reporting better sleep. Johnson and colleagues (1999) studied the effect of individual FM sessions on individuals with multiple sclerosis. Significant differences for FM participants were noted in subjective measures of perceived stress and lowered anxiety, but not for functional ability or upper extremity performance. Stephens and colleagues (2001) found that subjects who participated in eight classes of ATM experienced significant improvements in certain measures of balance. And, Dunn and Rogers (2000) studied the effect of FM imagery on movement. They found that 8 out of 10 subjects who were able to successfully perceive a change with the FM imagery significantly increased active movement related to the imagery.

While physical improvements have not been found in research to date, more rigorous research methodology may facilitate validation. In addition, the author advocates using phenomenological models for researching FM as opposed to reductionist laboratory models. His Ph.D. dissertation (Ofir, 1993) suggests such an approach. The problem of applying straightforward scientific methodology for studying complex, multivariant systems such as human behavior was clearly elucidated by Lofti Zadeh, who was instrumental in developing the mathematics of fuzzy sets: "As the complexity of a system increases, our ability to make precise and significant statements about its behavior diminishes until a threshold is reached beyond which precision and significance or relevance become almost mutually exclusive characteristics" (McNeil & Freiberger, 1993, p. 43).

Case Studies

FM is a method stemming from an educational rather than a medical model; hence the following case studies are not medically oriented, but more descriptive in nature.

A Common Problem often Categorized as Orthopedic/Neurologic

Joe, who is a bit stiff, bends down to tie his shoelaces while standing or sitting. He is not aware that in reaching down to his shoelaces, he habitually contracts his abdominal musculature. Suddenly he freezes, grimaces in pain, and says "I've thrown my back again!" Such events are often accompanied by a rotational component and the inevitable excessive compression/tension forces resulting in herniated or even prolapsed disc. What happened here? Joe simply had no idea *how* he was bending down, whether to tie his shoelaces or to pick up a pen he had dropped onto the floor.

In bending forward and downward effortlessly, there is a fine orchestration of actions: looking down; lowering head; flexing of spine, hips, knees, and ankles; eccentric elongation of back extensors; a downward slide of the sternum; and continuous breathing. Joe was unaware that habitually he kept his sternum fixed and immovable. His back trouble was inevitable and was not a consequence of pathology but of innocent ignorance. He did not need to contract his abdominal musculature. Gravity should have been enough of a force assisting him to bend. His back muscles were "sensorily biased" to a certain habitual length and were prepared to relax and elongate just enough to permit him to reach his shoelaces in comfort. However, by habitually preventing the required downward motion of his sternum, he was short of reaching his shoelaces. Moreover, by habitually holding his breath whenever he performed an activity requiring even minimal physical effort, he constantly stiffened his torso, making it rigid. Striving to somehow accomplish his intended function, he now contracted his abdominal muscles and created a co-contraction of trunk flexors and extensors. This occurred because his brain interpreted the extra stretch imposed on the back muscles as a threat requiring a protective counter contraction. The message his brain received was at variance with the corollary discharge (Kelso and Stelmach, 1976). Joe reacted by overcontracting his back extensors, which produced a protective and painful spasm. Joe's interpretation ("I've got a bum back, same as my old man") implied that his fate was sealed and nothing much could be done about it.

In working with Joe, several strategies were employed: (a) reducing his spasm by substituting the effort of his contractions with manual, gentle compressions in the same direction of the muscular pull, (b) recalibrating the tone of his flexor/extensors in the direction of normalcy, and (c) using precise tactile cues, directing Joe to compare how he habitually bent down versus bending down or forward in a variety of new ways and in accordance with the environmental requirements. Bending forward to pick up a pen requires a somewhat different organizational strategy than bending under a bed to search for a lost shoe, and different from doing a somersault or a judo roll. Joe recovered fully and returned to his favorite pastimes of fishing and golf.

"What I am after isn't flexible bodies but flexible brains." (Feldenkrais, 1974)

Overspecialization and Common Misconception of the Effects of Stretching

Michele, a ballet dancer, spent many years perfecting her art. At age 35 she needed to have a hip replacement due to severe pain resulting from full destruction of the cartilaginous tissue of the hip joint. Why should this happen to a seemingly agile, fit young woman? One aspect of the aesthetic requirements of ballet is the ability to raise a long straight leg in flexion or abduction to between 135 and 180 degrees. To do so, one must stretch the hamstrings daily, year after year, while maintaining a fairly rigid and straight torso. Michele was not aware all of those years that while she thought she was stretching her muscles, what she was really doing was overstretching the whole complex of her connective tissue, fascia, tendons, and especially her hip joint capsule. Eventually, the compact structure of her hip joint was compromised and excessive joint play (McMennel, 1964) resulted in accelerated wear and tear of cartilaginous tissue.

Feldenkrais (1977) might have noted that Michele was a victim of two factors. One was the overspecialization of her art form, which resulted in overuse of certain parts of her body to the exclusion of others, and the second was her lack of awareness of the damage she was inflicting upon herself. Had she known what she was doing, she could have chosen other options, such as multiple forms of dance rather than strictly classical ballet, and refrained from excessive stretching. In FM Michele was taught to differentiate her torso from her hip joint (she already knew how to differentiate her hip from her pelvis, but not the converse). She experienced and learned to differentiate her 24 verte-

Exercise

In reference to high muscle tone, the reader can try a simple experiment: Clench one fist and try to pry open the fingers of that hand with your other hand while resisting with the clenched hand. Notice how the harder you try to pry the fingers open, the more the hand clenches. Now let go, rest a moment, and once again clench that fist; however, this time wrap the other hand around the clenched fist and very gently compress the clenched fist. Notice how the clenched fist tends to soften and relax.

brae and their 23 junctions one from another as well as to relate them one to another and to her extremities in her daily activities and in her dancing. She was encouraged to learn several additional dance forms, such as Latin and African, and she learned to maintain functional muscle length without the need to mechanically stretch them.

Nondivisibility of Body-mind

Sonia, a woman in her forties, is the child of a Holocaust survivor. Sonia worked as an executive secretary in a busy law firm. She suffered from fibromyalgia and repetitive stress injury. Two years of treatments, which included traditional physical therapy, myofascial release, massage, and ergonomic workstation efficiency, produced no discernible change. The Feldenkrais instructor Sonia consulted found that the salient point in her case was her embodied anxiety (as discussed in Levine, 1997). Fears she experienced as a child, hearing about the horrors of the Holocaust, produced a constant, habitual, partial startle reflex (Davis, 1984); posture with slightly forward hunched shoulders, forward head, and compressed abdomen; and a compromised breathing pattern, all of which reappeared as a full-conditioned reflex pattern (Babkin, 1974, Feldenkrais, 1974) and became exacerbated whenever she encountered anxiety-provoking situations of any kind.

The Feldenkrais work that was done with Sonia emphasized the use of slow, delicate movement patterns that enhanced pleasure sensations (Damasio, 1999) and helped recalibrate back to normalcy the balance between her overwrought sympathetic nervous system outflow and her decreased parasympathetic flow. Once that was achieved, the work progressed with the intention of assisting her to learn to sense the relationships between different body-mind states. She learned to sense the relationship of the coldness of her hands with the emotional feeling of anxiety as it would manifest itself in her contracted chest and shoulders, and in her shallow intermittent breathing. Through a process of approximations, she learned to discriminate between being in a habitual constricted/contracted state and having normal muscular tone. Tactics employed included visualizations as well as principles culled from Jacobson's (1965) relaxation exercises. Her gradual increasing sense and perception of self, her increasing awareness of herself as she lived at work, at home, and with her family, resulted in decrease of her symptoms and improvement in the overall quality of her life.

Postural Dysfunction Secondary to Misperception

John, a 63-year-old man, lost his balance, fell, and sprained his right ankle. He had been losing his balance with increasing frequency lately and was worried. John saw a Feldenkrais instructor, who observed him walk and who quickly ascertained that John was leaning to his left. When John closed his eyes, he leaned even more, but when asked to sense if he was vertically upright or biased to a side, John responded that he was straight. His proprioceptive/kinesthetic perception of verticality was at odds with his visual perception, as it was with objective data, but no amount of verbal correction changed his posture, nor did strengthening exercises, which he had tried for an extended period of time.

Within six FI sessions, John was standing and walking erect, with restored balance over all manner of terrain and a renewed sense of being grounded. The problem had been his biased perception. The muscle tone of the left side of his body was significantly higher than that of the right. This sensory bias resulted in a perception of being vertical even though he was tilted about 10 degrees off center, and this was only partially offset by his visual sense of the upright. John was acutely aware that he had been losing his balance, but he was completely unaware of the asymmetrical muscle tone between his left and right sides. To him, all was normal. The change in tone had occurred gradually and was too slow for his sensory apparatus to detect. Therefore, it went unnoticed and was simply incorporated into his usual feeling of normalcy. The first thing the FM instructor did with John was to have him stand and notice over which foot he bore more weight. The sensory baseline thus being established, the Feldenkrais instructor set about creating conditions in which the sensed difference would be further exaggerated. Once John could clearly sense how much he was leaning to one side, his own sensible system self-corrected, and no further loss of balance was reported.

Summary

The Feldenkrais Method is a unique educational approach that aims to introduce people to the means by which they can maximize their functional potential in life by progressively increasing the clarity of their self-image in action in relation to their environment. The education is based upon attaining higher states of perceptual awareness through the medium of movement and the associated sensory components of movement. The method teaches people to "learn how to learn," is process-oriented and experiential in nature, with a model of heuristics based upon organic learning, namely learning as infants and very young children learn. The application of the method is done in groups or classes, verbally directed or in a one-on-one manual mode directed by an accredited Feldenkrais teacher. There are no known contraindications to this method. Since this is an educational method, anyone can benefit from it and can access it through personal contact or by professional referral.

STUDY QUESTIONS

1. Describe four basic principles underlying the Feldenkrais Method of somatic education.
2. Is FM a subspecialty of medicine or an educational method, and why?
3. How does ATM differ from FI?
4. What does the *integration of function* mean to you?
5. What is the difference between training and learning?

SUGGESTED READING

Langer, E. J. (1997). *The Power of Mindful Learning*. Cambridge, MA: Perseus.
Reed, E. S. (1996). *Encountering the World*. New York: Oxford University Press.
Reed, E. S. (1997). *From Soul to Mind*. New Haven, CT: Yale University Press.

Rosenfeld, I. (1992). *The Strange, Familiar, and Forgotten*. New York: Alfred A. Knopf.

Rywerant, Y. (1983). *The Feldenkrais Method: Teaching by Handling*. New Canaan, CT: Keats.

Rywerant, Y. (2000). *Acquiring the Feldenkrais Profession*. Tel Aviv, Israel: El-Or Ltd.

Thelen, E., & L. B. Smith. (1994). *A Dynamic Systems Approach to the Development of Cognition and Action*. Cambridge, MA: MIT Press.

RESOURCES

Feldenkrais Guild of North America
3611 SW Hood Ave., Suite 100
Portland, OR 97201
(800) 775-2118
guild@feldenkrais.com
www.feldenkrais.com

International Feldenkrais Federation
30 rue Monsieur le Prince
75006 Paris, France
33 1 43 25 36 52
iff@peak.org

REFERENCES

Arndt-Schultz Law. *Churchill's Medical Dictionary*. R. Koenigsberg (Ed.). London: Churchill Livingston.

Babkin, B. P. (1974). *Pavlov, A Biography*. Chicago: University of Chicago Press.

Bateson, G. (1972). *Steps to an Ecology of Mind*. New York: Ballantine.

Beevor, C. E. (1904). *The Croonian Lectures on Muscular Movements and their Representations in the Central Nervous System*. London: Adlard & Son.

Damasio, A. R. (1999). *The Feeling of What Happens: Body & Emotion in the Making of Consciousness*. New York: Harcourt Brace.

Davis, M. (1984). The mammalian startle response. In R. E. Eaton (Ed.), *Neural Mechanisms of Startle Behavior*. New York: Plenum.

Dunn, P. A., & D. K. Rogers. (2000, Dec.). Feldenkrais sensory imagery and forward reach. *Perceptual Motor Skills 2000*, 755–7.

Feldenkrais, M. (1972). *Awareness Through Movement*. San Fransisco: Harper.

Feldenkrais, M. (1979). *A Study of Anxiety, Sex, Gravitation and Learning*. New York: International Universities Press.

Gutman, G. M., C. P. Herbert, & S. R. Brown. (1997). Feldenkrais versus conventional exercises for the elderly. *Journal of Gerontology, 32*(5), 562–572.

Holcomb, H. H. (1997, Sept. 19). Brain needs rest to store new skills. *Physical Therapy Bulletin*, 17.

Jackson, J. H. (1958). *Selected Writings*. Ed. James Taylor. London: Staples Press. Vol. 2.

Jacobson, E. (1965). *Progressive Relaxation: A Physiological and Clinical Investigation of Muscular States and Their Significance in Psychology and Medical Practice*. Chicago: University of Chicago Press.

Johnson, K., J. Frederick, M. Kaufman, & B. Mountjoy. (1999). A controlled investigation of bodywork in multiple sclerosis. *The Journal of Alternative and Complementary Medicine, 5*, 237–243.

Jouvet, M. (1999). *The Paradox of Sleep: The Story of Dreaming*. Trans. by Laurence Garey. Cambridge, MA: MIT Press.

Kelso, J. A. S., & G. E. Stelmach. (1976). Peripheral Mechanisms in Motor Control. In G. Stelmach (Ed.), *Motor Control: Issues and Trends*. New York: Academic Press.

Langer, E. J. (1997). *The Power of Mindful Learning*. Cambridge, MA: Perseus.

Levine, P. A. (1997). *Walking the Tiger*. Berkeley, CA: North Atlantic Books.

Maitland, G. D. (1977). *Peripheral Manipulation* (2nd ed.). London: Butterworths.

McMennell, J. (1964). *Joint Pain*. Boston: Little, Brown.

McNeil, D., & P. Freiberger. (1993). *Fuzzy Logic*. New York: Simon & Schuster.

Ofir, R. D. (1993). A heuristic investigation of the process of motor learning using the Feldenkrais Method in physical rehabilitation of two young women with traumatic brain injury. (Ph.D. dissertation, Union Institute, unpub.).

Schilder, P. (1950) *The Image and Appearance of the Human Body*. New York: International Universities Press.

Stephens. J., D. DuShuttle, C. Hatcher, J. Shmunes, & C. Slaninka. (2001). Improvements in balance and balance confidence resulting from the use of Awareness Through Movement, a structured, group motor learning process: A randomized, controlled study in people with Multiple Sclerosis. *Neurology Report, 25*(2), 39–49.

Weber/Fechner Law. *Churchill's Medical Dictionary*. R. Koenigsberg (Ed.). London: Churchill Livingston.

ACKNOWLEDGMENTS

My sincere thanks to Larry Goldfarb, Ph.D. and to Frank Wildman, Ph.D. for their gracious and valuable comments and guidance in preparing this manuscript; to Margaret Sabin, who in her generosity of spirit twice respectively, went over this manuscript in detail and extended much needed support, guidance, and valuable editing; and to Kathy Yates, who helped me to fine tune this chapter with her deft editing talent. Finally, my thanks and love to Michele, my wife, who patiently waited for me to conclude this project.

16

Myofascial Release

John F. Barnes

CHAPTER OBJECTIVES

- Understand the whole-body interrelationship of the fascial system.
- Describe the normal function of the fascial system.
- Understand the principles by which trauma, inflammatory process, or postural imbalance can contribute to strain and restriction in the fascial system.
- Appreciate the broad range of diagnoses and client populations for which MFR treatment is appropriate.
- Describe the basic principles of MFR treatment and how they are based on the biomechanic and bioelectric properties of fascial tissue.
- Describe a typical MFR treatment session.
- Understand how the current state of research into biomechanics and bioenergetics, combined with recent clinical inquiry, substantiates our understanding of the way in which MFR treatment affects tissue changes.

Myofascial Release (MFR) is a manual therapy which focuses on the fascial system. It is designed to complement traditional therapy approaches, which typically do not address the fascia system. Including MFR techniques in current regimens for evaluation and treatment allows therapists to provide a more comprehensive approach to client treatment that is safe, cost-efficient and effective.

Fascial restriction probably occurs each time we experience a trauma, an inflammatory process, or from poor posture over time. These restrictions can be conceptualized as the concentric layers of an onion—the layers slowly tightening until we begin to lose our physiologic adaptive capacity (see Figure 16–1). Myofascial restrictions can exert tremendous pressures, approximately 2,000 pounds per square inch (Katake, 1961), on neuromusculoskeletal and other pain producing structures. It is important to realize that myofascial restrictions cannot be visualized through standard diagnostic tests. For this reason it is possible that a large num-

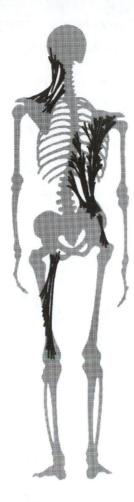

Figure 16–1   Schematic representation of multiple compensatory restrictions in the myofascial complex.

Reprinted with permission by John F. Barnes, PT.

ber of clients with various chronic pain complaints are being misdiagnosed while suffering the effects of myofascial restrictions. A number of these individuals have exhausted the full range of traditional medical avenues and have essentially been told that their problems are in their heads or that there is no real problem. The goal of MFR is to help return the individual's physiological adaptive capacity by increasing space and mobility, restoring three-dimensional balance, and returning the structure to a normal vertical orientation with gravity. This equilibrium allows the individual's self-correcting mechanisms to come into play, alleviate symptoms, and restore proper function.

MFR treatment techniques are utilized in a wide range of therapeutic settings and populations, and over a broad array of diagnoses including pain, movement restriction, muscle spasm, spasticity, neurological dysfunction, cerebral palsy, head injury, birth injury, cerebrovascular accidents, scoliosis, menstrual and pelvic pain and dysfunction, headaches, tem-

Myofascial release techniques give today's therapists the tools to significantly enhance their effectiveness in addressing a broad range of clinical challenges. MFR is built upon the idea that dysfunction involving the fascial system is the key causative factor in a vast number of commonly encountered diagnoses. This radical departure from traditional thinking leads the MFR therapist to assess and treat the body in its entirety, focusing on restrictions in the fascial system that are often the true source of problematic symptoms.

The use of MFR is appropriate across virtually all client populations. MFR techniques can be seamlessly integrated into therapeutic programs that employ both traditional as well as other complementary approaches. Importantly, as a manual therapy, the use of MFR techniques gives the practitioner the unique opportunity to provide clients with authentic healing through the power of touch.

poromandibular pain and dysfunction, chronic fatigue syndrome, fibromyalgia, myofascial pain syndrome, traumatic and surgical scarring, acute and chronic pain, and sports injuries.

Development

The body of MFR treatment techniques that have come to be known as the John F. Barnes Myofascial Release Approach represent a journey that began in Barnes's teens with a devastating weightlifting accident. That same journey continues today with over 40,000 Barnes-trained practitioners worldwide, working to shift generally accepted paradigms relating to pain and dysfunction away from a model focused on regional evaluation and treatment of musculoskeletal dysfunction. Nearly four decades of exploration and refinement have led to a widely practiced and increasingly accepted approach to the evaluation and treatment of pain and postural anomalies based on restrictions in the fascial system.

Barnes's initial back injury at age 17 led to over a decade of debilitating chronic pain. Surgery to remove a crushed vertebral disc provided improved function and lessened pain. However, his back continued to be problematic. Throughout this experience, Barnes began to experiment with self-treatment techniques to relieve his own pain symptoms. These techniques centered on the very prolonged holding of specific stretch positions. He began to successfully apply these techniques with his clients without an understanding of the mechanism by which they worked. Upon attending an osteopathic course dealing with connective tissue and soft tissue mobilization, Barnes realized that the techniques he had developed were very similar, but had several important differences. He found that he was holding the positions for much longer periods of time—at least 90 to 120 seconds. The time factor proved to be pivotal for releasing the entire elasto-collagenous complex, leading to permanent elongation of the tissues and relief of pain-producing pressure on other structures. Barnes' personal history with pain that "trapped" him in his body provided deep experiential lessons, enabling an enhanced appreciation of his clients' physical and emotional suffering.

The time component in the application of forces into treated tissues is one of the primary differentiating characteristics of the John F. Barnes approach, along with developing the sensitivity to find fascial restrictions and not forcing or sliding over the restrictions until complete release occurs. This is what distinguishes this approach from older forms of MFR in which forces were applied too aggressively and for too short a time. The prolonged application of light pressure permits the practitioner to feel the release of progressive myofascial barriers and "follow" the tissues as they release. The therapist's hands do not glide or slide over the skin, but maintain a continuous contact that allows the accurate monitoring of the releases and assessment of changes as they occur. Older versions of MFR only dealt with the elastic and muscular components and neglected the collagenous component. In addition, the treatment techniques tended to be applied regionally or symptomatically, and in a rough, mechanical way. This resulted in painful treatments that yielded only temporary results. Barnes's experience taught him that the fascial system could not be forced, but that permanent changes could be achieved by "finessing" the tissues, drawing upon a knowledge of their viscoelastic properties.

Building upon the foundation of self-taught techniques, Barnes began to visualize the body as an integrated whole through the complex interrelationships of the fascial network. He soon expanded this developing concept to include craniosacral therapy and myofascial movement facilitation, or unwinding, thus enabling treatment of the entire fascial system. The result is a body of refined concepts and treatment principles that can allow clients and therapists to accomplish true, authentic healing.

Treatment Principles

MFR aims to restore the body to a healthy and natural functional state by removing all fascial restrictions that may be causing pain and/or dysfunction. To achieve this healthy and natural state the therapist must first evaluate and assess what restrictions are present and then use MFR techniques to remove or "release" the restrictions, allowing the tissue to return to its normal healthy state.

After reviewing the physician's diagnosis and the client's subjective complaints, the therapist evaluates the client visually. The therapist is assessing for any asymmetries in the frontal, coronal and sagittal planes (see Figure 16–2). After the visual assessment, the therapist assesses the client manually. Palpation of the tissue for irregularities such as swelling, edema, changes in muscle tone, spasm, and so on, as well as an assessment of the craniosacral rhythm, is performed. Any irregularities can cause restrictions in the normal movement of tissue and must be addressed so that normal tissue movement can be restored. The findings of the assessment are used in determining where treatment should begin and in reassessing the client from treatment to treatment.

Treatment of tissue restrictions involves releasing all restrictions in both the elastic and the collagenous portions of the tissue. The therapist first applies gentle pressure in the direction of the restriction until it disengages or "releases." The therapist may find a series of restrictions, one on top of the other, in multiple directions, but ultimately the therapist will

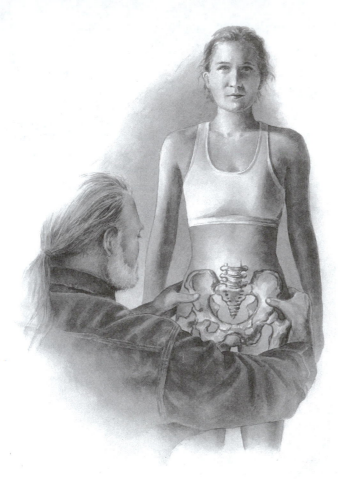

Figure 16–2 Therapists assess clients for assymetries in the frontal, coronal, and sagittal planes.

Illustration is used courtesy of John F. Barnes, PT.

Important Factors Relating to Fascia

- It supports and stabilizes, thus enhancing the postural balance of the body.
- It is integrally involved in all aspects of motion and acts as a shock absorber.
- It aids in circulatory economy, especially in venous and lymphatic fluids.
- Fascial change will often precede chronic tissue congestion.
- Such chronic passive congestion creates the formation of fibrous tissue, which then proceeds to increase hydrogen ion concentration of articular and periarticular structures.
- Fascia can be a major site of inflammatory processes.
- Fluid and infectious processes often travel along fascial planes.
- The central nervous system is surrounded by fascial tissue (dura mater), which attaches to the inside of the cranium, the foramen magnum, and at the second sacral segment. Dysfunction in these tissues can have profound and widespread neurological effects.

Indications

MFR techniques are safe and effective when used with clients with a broad range of diagnoses. Additionally, MFR can be applied to a full range of client populations, from neonates to geriatrics. The following list of indicated diagnoses is not intended to be exhaustive or comprehensive.

- back pain
- cervical pain
- chronic pain
- headaches/migraines
- temperomandibular joint dysfunction (TMJ)
- carpal tunnel syndrome
- fibromyalgia
- spasm/spasticity
- scoliosis
- cerebrovascular accident (CVA)
- neurologic dysfunction
- sports injuries
- restricted range of motion
- chronic fatigue syndrome
- head trauma

Contraindications

Contraindications for MFR treatment, such as malignancy, aneurysm, and acute rheumatoid arthritis, may be considered absolute, while others, such as hematoma, open wounds, and healing fractures, may be regional.

- malignancy
- cellulitis
- febrile state
- systemic or localized infection
- acute circulatory condition
- osteomyelitis
- aneurysm
- obstructive edema
- acute rheumatoid arthritis
- open wounds
- sutures
- hematoma
- healing fracture
- osteoporosis or advanced degenerative changes
- anticoagulant therapy
- advanced diabetes
- hypersensitivity of skin

reach a firm end-feel or barrier. These first releases are believed to be in the elastic component of the tissue. When the firm end-feel is felt it is believed that the collagenous component has been reached. The collagenous component is much stronger and usually requires more time and patience to work through. The pressure is maintained gently until the tissue is felt to "release" again. The therapist's gentle pressure moves along the direction of the tissue release until no further releases are felt.

As noted previously, when working on the collagenous component much patience is required. The tissue may not release very quickly and multiple restrictions may exist. In other words, a release may be felt and the tissue stops moving, but further restrictions are still felt on reassessment. The therapist must continue to maintain the gentle pressure until all restrictions have been released. Because of the inherent strength of the collagenous component of fascia, applying too heavy a force onto the tissue will cause it to resist, and therefore no releases will be attained.

As with many manual techniques the beginner therapist needs two things. One, a basic understanding of the physical nature of the tissues is required to achieve success in the technique, and two, practice makes perfect. Tissue work requires a "feel" for what is happening. The more times we place our hands on tissue the more we learn. Too much force is often applied when beginning to work with MFR techniques. Ultimately with practice the therapist learns when "more is less" and when "less is more."

MFR techniques can produce remarkable results in our clients. Because restoring normal, healthy tissue function often eliminates symptoms of pain and reestablishes proper movement patterns, it is an excellent technique with which to begin therapy. It is important to remember that other components of therapy such as modalities, exercise programs, stretching programs, and so on, may need to be incorporated into the treatment plan to achieve total health and function.

The Treatment Session

A typical MFR treatment session may last from 15 to 60 minutes. Upon presentation, the client is briefly screened for postural anomalies and is asked to describe the current state of symptoms. The client disrobes down to his or her underwear and lies on a treatment table. No oils or creams are used; they would impede the therapist's ability to assess tissue quality and would prevent the traction against the skin necessary to facilitate releases. Over the course of a session, the client may be positioned in prone, supine, sidelying, sitting, or standing as the treatment evolves. The therapist uses his or her fingers, palms, knuckles, elbows, and forearms to slowly stimulate and elongate the fascial tissues. Gentle but firm pressure is applied for at least 90 to 120 seconds for each therapeutic release. Often the positions are held for several minutes as the fascia continue to release. The course of a specific session is unpredictable, as the therapist will follow the releasing tissues and will be cued by vasomotor responses to other restricted areas. Thermal modalities such as moist heat or ice are frequently applied before the end of a session if indicated.

Manual techniques are augmented with instruction in self-treatment techniques, postural reeducation, motor reeducation, and strengthening and flexibility techniques. It is usually recommended that the client receive up to three treatments weekly in the initial phase of therapy. As the client's condition improves and he or she becomes more proficient with self-

Training in the John F. Barnes approach to MFR consists of a series of seminars offered in numerous locations throughout the United States and Canada every year. In general, the seminars build upon each other, moving from basic to more advanced techniques and seeking to help the therapist develop a progressively enhanced level of evaluative and treatment skills. The seminars combine lecture and discussion with hands-on training in specific techniques. Most seminars are instructed by John F. Barnes. Introductory level seminars are typically presented over a 3-day period with 20 hours of instruction. Workshops in myofascial mobilization, pediatric MFR, and equine MFR treatment are also offered. Therapists who have completed at least one seminar are able to participate in week-long skill enhancement seminars held at the MFR clinics in Arizona and Pennsylvania. It is important to note that while the seminars teach the required principles, philosophy, and techniques of MFR, conscientious practice in the clinical setting is required to enhance the practitioner's level of skill. At the present time, there is no state or nationally sponsored certification on MFR practice. There is, however, a worldwide network of MFR-trained therapists who communicate actively on the Internet and who organize study groups on the local level. Contact information regarding the seminar series can be found at the end of this chapter.

treatment techniques, the frequency of hands-on treatment is tapered off in preparation for eventual discharge. The overall length of treatment will be influenced by the complexity of the client's problems and by the level of compliance with self-treatment and management.

Research

Recent inquiries into the underlying scientific basis for healing through manual and energetic therapies are providing substantiation for the changes that bodyworkers and their clients have understood intuitively for ages. There have been a number of inquiries into the physiologic, biochemical, biomechanical, and piezoelectric characteristics of fascial tissue in situations of stress and injury. When subjected to microtrauma over time or to an acute injury, the fascial system tightens as a protective response. Fascial components lose their pliability and become restricted in their mobility, ground substance solidifies, collagen develops aberrant cross-links, and elastin loses its resiliency (Ingber & Folkman, 1989; Levin, 1990). Stauber and colleagues (1990) reported disruption in the extracellular matrix and a resultant inflammatory response with pain following posttraumatic eccentric exercise. Stauber, Knack, and colleagues (1996) later reported a 44 percent increase in noncontractile tissue (expansion of extracellular matrix and fibrosis) after 4 weeks of repeated muscular strain. Many researchers have identified the loose and dense connective tissue response to trauma (Hunt, Banda, & Silver, 1985), demonstrating the tendency of connective tissue to solidify, develop adhesions, and become less resilient both physiologically and mechanically.

Connective tissue demonstrates elastic, plastic, viscoelastic, and piezoelectric properties. Its morphologic state is determined by levels of energy input and temperature. The deformation of connective tissue is aptly described by Upledger's "spring and dashpot" model (Upledger & Vredovoogd, 1983) and Zachazewski's stress/strain curves (1989). Upledger's model describes the viscoelastic deformation of connective tissue over time (90 to 120 seconds). Stress/strain curves represent the same viscoelastic properties, but go on to depict the failure of the tissue when the rate of deformation exceeds the tissue's tolerance to the applied load. These studies suggest that the type of sustained application of force utilized in myofascial release can lead to changes in the ground substance (from sol to gel) and can break cross-links in collagen that made it fibrous and dense.

James Oschman (2000) provides a meticulously researched and highly detailed explication of the bioelectric, biomagnetic, and biomechanical underpinnings of manual and energetic therapies, including MFR. He builds upon the fact that the tissues of the body form a living matrix that is able to communicate information between and into every cell through the superconducting properties of many tissues, including the myofascia. Additionally, Oschman demonstrates that the human body generates its own biomagnetic fields and can be influenced by external magnetic field effects, including those generated by other humans. Zimmerman (1990) and Seto, Kusaka, and Nakazato (1992) demonstrated strong biomagnetic fields emanating from the hands of various types of manual therapists and healers. The frequencies of these fields varied from 0.3 to 30 Hz and were observed to sweep through the range of frequencies with most activity monitored in the 7 to 8 Hz range. This spectrum of observed frequencies from the hands of manual healers corresponds to known "frequency windows of specificity" for specific tissue healing effects (for example, frequencies of 2 Hz enhance nerve regeneration and frequencies of 10 Hz enhance ligament healing) (Sisken & Walker, 1995). These findings suggest that the changes seen with MFR treatment are produced by a number of means, not simply the influence of pressure and warming on fascial restrictions and the ground substance, but also through biomagnetic fields functioning at demonstrated therapeutic frequencies.

MFR treatment does not lend itself to rigidly controlled efficacy studies. The nature of each treatment is highly individualized to suit the client's specific needs. Research in the literature is scarce, underlining the need for additional work, including case studies and investigations comparing results of treatment utilizing MFR techniques with those achieved with traditional approaches. Sucher (1990a, 1990b) describes four individuals diagnosed with thoracic outlet syndrome (TOS) who were treated with MFR techniques. He suggests that the focus of treatment and the observed rapid reduction in symptoms support the presumed myofascial involvement of scalene and pectoral structures in the etiology of TOS. Another case study by Sucher (1993a) reported that an "aggressive, conservative approach" to treatment of carpal tunnel syndrome utilizing MFR techniques reduced pain and numbness and improved electromyographic measurements, lessening the need for surgery. In a follow-up study (Sucher, 1993b) of four subjects with carpal tunnel syndrome, magnetic resonance imaging (MRI) was used before and after treatment with MFR techniques. All subjects demonstrated clinical improvement. Nerve conduction velocities and electromyographic measures improved, as well. Anteroposterior and transverse cross-sectional area of the carpal tunnel increased significantly, as measured by MRI. Hanten and Chandler (1994) showed that the myofascial release leg pull technique produced significantly greater passive straight-leg raise ROM than controls in a study of 75 non-disabled females aged 18 to 29 years. Symptomatic relief was reported when MFR techniques were applied in the treatment of chest wall soreness in cancer patients who had undergone lumpectomy followed by radiation (Crawford, Simpson, & Crawford, 1996).

When viewed as a whole, the small body of clinical inquiry combined with basic research into tissue biomechanics and energetics, and evidence supporting the ability of trained practitioners to create changes in tissues, presents an emerging picture consistent with an understanding of the way in which MFR treatment effects changes.

Case Studies

The following case studies illustrate the effectiveness of MFR treatment techniques across a broad range of client populations. While these cases are drawn from diverse types of injuries and disorders, they share a strong common thread: A well-intended, "local" or symptomatic approach to treatment is not effective when dealing with symptoms that arise from myofascial restrictions. A whole-body approach to evaluation and treatment, mindful of the three-dimensional complexity and the incredible tensile strength of the myofascial/osseous complex, must be applied in order to address the root of chronic pain complaints and their accompanying functional limitations. In addition, the third case serves to demonstrate the manner in which MFR techniques can be used as an integral component of a comprehensive program that includes other treatment regimens.

Rotator Cuff Tendonitis

A 37-year-old male psychologist was referred for evaluation and treatment with a diagnosis of right rotator cuff tendonitis. He had fractured his left clavicle in 1981 while playing touch football. Treatment of that fracture included immobilization in a "figure 8" sling, resulting in damage to the right long thoracic nerve with subsequent winging of the right scapula. The neuropathy resolved over a 6-month period; however, right scapular pain and weakness persisted. The client experienced an acute exacerbation of his symptoms in 1987 while moving a coal stove. Acromioplasty of the left shoulder was performed in February 1989, with the shoulder again immobilized in a sling, resulting in additional loss of range of motion.

The client had received several courses of traditional physical therapy treatment over the years since his original football injury, experiencing only temporary improvements in his symptoms. The program immediately preceding his treatment with MFR consisted of 60 traditional physical therapy treatment sessions from March through November of 1991. These sessions included the use of heat, ultrasound, strengthening exercises, and extensive use of mobilization and muscle energy techniques. Despite this extensive treatment regimen, the client continued to lose range of motion and strength, and continued to experience constant, severe pain in both scapulae. He experienced progressive deterioration of his functional capacity, finding himself unable to reach for objects due to limited range and unable to carry items greater than one pound due to severe pain. As a result, the client reported that he was very depressed, feeling hopeless, and perceived that he was wasting away.

When he initially presented for evaluation, the client demonstrated only 90° of bilateral shoulder flexion and abduction, and moderate loss of bilateral glenohumeral internal rotation. Strength at the shoulders was assessed as "fair minus to fair." The client was treated with a combination of MFR techniques, stretching exercises, moist heat, and neuromotor reeducation techniques. MFR techniques emphasized upper extremity releases, as well as deep fascial releases throughout the pectorals, axillae, thoracic inlet regions, respiratory diaphragm, lateral scapular and thoracic regions, and into the posterior thoracolumbar region.

Following a 2-week intensive treatment program employing MFR treatment techniques, this client gained 129° of passive range of motion in both shoulders. Right shoulder flexion alone improved from 90° to 161°, an increase of 71°. Bilateral shoulder strength increased to "fair to good minus." The client reported

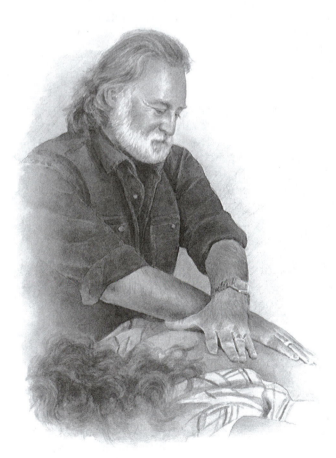

Figure 16–3 Myofascial releases at the shoulder area. Illustration is used courtesy of John F. Barnes, PT.

a 60-percent reduction in pain and greater ease in movement. He was instructed in a progressive home program for enhanced stabilization, strengthening, and stretching to maximize range of motion and strength and to maintain the beneficial structural changes that had been achieved through treatment.

His newfound freedom from myofascial dysfunction allowed this client to move away from his life of chronic pain and to greatly improve his functional level. He was discharged from treatment feeling much freer physically and emotionally. His extensive home program provided him with a sense of control and hope that he could be pain-free and living a much more functional life.

This case is illustrative of the failure of narrowly focused symptomatic treatment approaches to comprehensively address the causes of chronic pain syndromes. Years of extensive therapeutic efforts directed at this client's shoulders and scapulae in isolation had been unsuccessful. One key to the success of this client's treatment with MFR techniques was the recognition that restrictions of anterior thoracic structures were severely limiting his motion and comfort. Addressing these anterior restrictions was pivotal in achieving the overall success of his program.

Periodic Back Pain

A 19-year-old female presented for treatment with complaints of periodic back pain brought on either by rapid movements or by prolonged periods of sitting or standing. These complaints had been present for 18 months. More recently, she had been plagued by increasingly frequent left shoulder and neck pain that spread into her head, causing headaches and discomfort in the temperomandibular region. Over the 6 months leading up to treatment, her neck and shoulder pain had become more severe, increasing to daily frequency. The client provided historic information revealing a series of injuries over a 3-year period, beginning with a fall from a horse in which she landed on her sacrococcygeal region and sprained her left ankle. In addition, she reported that the horse stepped on her chest. She sustained a second fall 7 months prior to treatment, during which she landed on her left hip and resprained her left ankle. A third fall occurred 1 month prior to treatment, impacting her right hip.

Postural evaluation as part of the initial assessment process highlighted numerous asymmetries and other postural anomalies. Evaluation of her pelvis revealed an elevated right posterior superior iliac spine (PSIS), a low right anterior superior iliac spine (ASIS), and a high right iliac crest, possibly indicating an anterior torsion of the right ilium. Spinal assessment demonstrated an increased lumbar lordosis, excessive low thoracic kyphosis, and a severe forward head position. This client's right shoulder was depressed, both scapulae were widely abducted, the left scapula was winged, and both shoulders were positioned forward and in internal rotation. Additionally, her right tibia was externally rotated and both knees were positioned in genu recurvatum. This combination of postural imbalances literally extending from head to foot contributed to functionally very inefficient posture and was an indication of severe myofascial restrictions throughout the client's body. In conjunction with the postural abnormalities, the client

Table 16–1 Range of Motion

Joint Motion	Initial ROM	After Three Sessions
Thoracolumbar spine		
Flexion	Smooth, symmetric	Smooth, symmetric
Extension	Occurred only in lumbar spine	Thoracic and lumbar spine extend
Right sidebending	Smooth, symmetric	Smooth, symmetric
Left sidebending	Unable to bend laterally	Smooth, symmetric
Right rotation	Limited 50%	Within normal limits
Cervical spine		
Flexion	0°–70°	0°–65°
Extension	0°–45°	0°–65°
Right sidebending	0°–35°	0°–36°
Left sidebending	0°–38°	0°–35°
Right rotation	0°–65°	0°–65°
Left rotation	0°–75°	0°–74°
Shoulder		
Right flexion	0°–160°	0°–170°
Left flexion	0°–150°	0°–168°
Right abduction	0°–145°	0°–155°
Left abduction	0°–128°	0°–158°
Right internal rotation	0°–30°	0°–40°
Left internal rotation	0°–30°	0°–55°
Hip		
Right internal rotation	0°–10°	0°–30°
Left internal rotation	0°–7°	0°–30°
Right external rotation	0°–37°	0°–37°
Left external rotation	0°–27°	0°–40°

demonstrated limited range of motion in her spine, shoulders, and hips, and remarkable loss of strength in her proximal musculature.

MFR treatment commenced with transverse fascial plane releases focusing on the thoracic inlet, respiratory diaphragm, and pelvic floor. In addition, upper extremity releases were performed, as well as deep myofascial releases over the psoas, abdominal, and anterior thoracic regions, and throughout the back and thighs. Cranial base and lumbosacral decompression techniques were performed to address restrictions at both ends of the vertebral column. Soft tissue mobilization techniques were used bilaterally on both pectoralis major and minor, and throughout the back musculature.

After only three treatment sessions, the client's pain complaints had disappeared and dramatic postural changes were evident. Table 16–1 shows changes in active assisted range of motion in the cervical spine, shoulders, and hips between the initial assessment and after the third treatment session.

Table 16–2 illustrates strength changes that occurred in key musculature after three treatment sessions. As a true strengthening program had yet to be added to her home program, these changes more accurately reflect the enhanced ability of muscles to generate power when in proper postural alignment and when appropriately lengthened.

Observed postural changes included a dramatic reduction of previously excessive spinal curvature, forward head position, and forward, internally rotated shoulders. The client's knees were no longer held in recurvatum and both the pelvic and shoulder girdles demonstrated improved symmetry. Subjective complaints of pain in the low back, neck, right shoulder, TMJ, and head all ceased.

Attention to the major myofascial restrictions throughout this client's body led to a rapid resolution of her pain syndrome. This enabled a dramatic improvement of her postural alignment in gravity. Once the described corrections were achieved, the client was ready for intensive muscular reeducation and strengthening, followed by postural awareness training. A home program was recommended as an integral part of this process. With continued strengthening of weak musculature and more efficient movement patterns, the client was able to maintain and improve upon the changes already achieved and to significantly improve her functional performance.

This case illustrates the whole-body effects of repetitive trauma and the progressive debilitating nature of symptoms from myofascial restrictions when

Table 16–2 Strength

Strength	Initial Strength		After Three Sessions	
Lower abdominals	2/5		3/5	
Psoas	4−/5 R	4+/5 L	4/5 R	4/5 L
Lower and middle trapezius	3+/5 R	3−/5 L	4−/5 R	4−/5 L
Shoulder medial rotators	3−/5 R	3−/5 L	3−/5 R	3−/5 L
Shoulder lateral rotators	4/5 R	4/5 L	4/5 R	4+/5 L
Hamstrings	4+/5 R	4/5 L	5/5 R	4/5 L
Hip abductors	4/5 R	5/5 L	4/5 R	4/5 L
Gluteus medius	4−/5 R	4+/5 L	4/5 R	4/5 L
Gluteus maximus	3+/5 R	3+/5 L	4+/5 R	4/5 L

they are not aggressively addressed. Long-term postural compensations from improper pelvic alignment, for example, can produce severe symptoms elsewhere, such as headaches, neck pain, and temperomandibular dysfunction.

Hypertonicity and Associated Structural Deformities

A 7-year-old male with cerebral palsy was presented for treatment after extensive medical and surgical care to address severe hypertonicity and associated structural deformities. Born 1 month beyond full-term, this child sustained prolonged anoxia during stress-testing procedures 1 week prior to delivery and again during delivery. Chest tubes had to be inserted immediately after birth to treat pneumothorax. This young boy's cerebral palsy manifested itself as spastic quadriplegia with athetosis, further complicated by a seizure disorder and microcephaly. His high tone predisposed him to muscle and tendon shortening, resulting in contractures and associated deformities. Tendon lengthening procedures were performed at ages 2 and 4. He underwent fundoplication surgery with insertion of a G-tube at age 4, two surgical interventions for strabismus, and a procedure for undescended testicles.

The client's family rejected suggestions that they should institutionalize this very involved child. He was enrolled in early intervention programs in which he

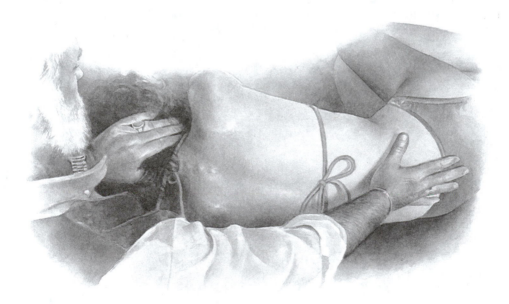

Figure 16–4 Sidelying dural tube stretch.   *Illustration is used courtesy of John F. Barnes, PT.*

received traditional therapies. A program of patterning was also pursued. These therapies produced very limited results. At age 2, client and family were introduced to neurodevelopmental therapy (NDT) during a 5-week long hospital admission. NDT comprises a specialized set of techniques that focus on changing muscle tone, lengthening muscles, and improving postural alignment in order to facilitate improved functional movement. NDT proved to be very productive for this client, and he was referred to a specially trained therapist after discharge from the hospital.

During this client's subsequent prolonged hospital admission at age 4, he was introduced to MFR techniques. His initial intervention using MFR techniques yielded rapid and significant results. Treatment of severe fascial restrictions in the chest and psoas musculature, scarring from his G-tube insertion, and restrictions about the hip joints, allowed a drastic improvement in this client's sitting position. Strong spastic pulling into left side-bending was notably reduced. His positional scoliosis was significantly improved. The degree of rapid, positive improvement experienced by this client motivated his family to pursue intensive treatment with MFR techniques.

Intensive MFR treatment built upon the work that had brought such positive changes and also focused increasingly on the client's cranial and dural tube restrictions. Following his first treatment, the client vocalized and laughed the entire evening. His level of arousal and attention span were dramatically improved. His tendency toward "scissoring" of his lower extremities reduced greatly. This problem recurred following the surgery for undescended testicles, but disappeared following resumed MFR treatment. The postsurgical regimen of eye-patching following the two strabismus surgeries was eliminated following MFR treatment. The release of cranial restrictions and the resumption of movement of the cranial bones appeared to lead to the elimination of seizure activity and the ability to discontinue use of antiseizure medications. A subsequent growth spurt created renewed tightening of the dural tube and cranial structures, and a resumption of seizure activity. Medications were reintroduced temporarily but were stopped again after two myofascial/cranial treatments addressed the new restrictions. The client is now able to communicate that he feels cranial tightness, signaling his mother to perform release techniques to relieve the restrictions and prevent the return of symptoms.

The benefits of treatment using MFR techniques with this client had far-reaching effects that were both structural and behavioral. This case demonstrates the way in which MFR techniques can work hand in hand with other effective treatment regimens to provide a powerful therapeutic result. The overall goal of MFR treatment is to reduce fascial restrictions affecting the length of muscles and tendons, providing improved osseous and ligamentous alignment. The end result is to allow for enhanced movement and function. This is completely consistent with and complementary to other recognized treatments such as NDT and sensory integration (SI). Myofascial release techniques can be utilized alone or in creative synergy with other approaches.

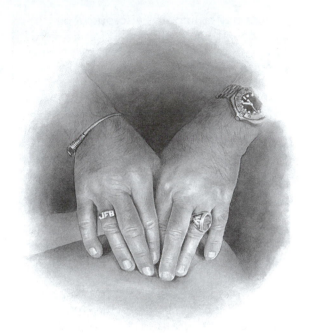

Figure 16–5 A myofascial release hand position.

Illustration is used courtesy of John F. Barnes, PT.

Summary

The therapist skilled in MFR techniques is concerned with releasing and reorganizing the body's fascial restrictions mechanically and reorganizing the neuromuscular system. This reorganization occurs by supplying the central nervous system with new input (awareness), allowing for change and improved potential and consciousness. It is important for those providing treatment to realize that the body is a repository of information. The body can be used as a biofeedback system for the master therapists' finely trained, sensitive hands. It can then be used as a handle or lever to allow for structural and biomechanical change.

The biomechanical, bioelectrical, and neurophysiological effects of MFR represent an evolutionary leap for our profession and our clients. This is a total approach, incorporating a physiologic system that, when included with traditional therapy, medicine, or dentistry, acts as a catalyst and yields impressive, clinically reproducible results (Barnes, 1990).

STUDY QUESTIONS

1. Fascial restrictions can exert approximately _____ pounds per square inch of pressure on neuromuscular/skeletal structures?
   a. 2500 lb/sq. in.   c. 1000 lb/sq. in.
   b. 2000 lb/sq. in.   d. 500 lb/sq. in.

2. The MFR therapist is taught to find the cause of symptoms by evaluating the fascial system by _____.
   a. reviewing the physician's diagnosis
   b. visually analyzing the structure of the human frame, palpating tissue texture, and observing the craniosacral rhythm
   c. considering patients' subjective complaints
   d. A and B
   e. all of the above

3. Identify two goals of MFR treatment:
   1.
   2.

4. Fascia creates interstitial spaces at the cellular level and has extremely important functions. List three of these functions:
   1.
   2.
   3.

5. In which of the following settings/client populations is myofascial release treatment appropriate?
   a. geriatrics/neurologic   d. chronic pain
   b. sports clinic   e. all of the above
   c. pediatrics

6. List five types of diagnoses that would benefit from myofascial release treatment:
   1.
   2.
   3.
   4.
   5.

7. Briefly describe why a myofascial release therapist takes a whole-body approach to both assessment and treatment.

SUGGESTED READING

Barnes, J. F. (1990). *Myofascial Release: The Search for Excellence.* Paoli, PA: MFR Seminars.
Barnes, J. F. (2000). *Healing Ancient Wounds: The Renegade's Wisdom.* Paoli, PA: MFR Seminars.
Levine, P. A. (1997). *Waking the Tiger: Healing Trauma.* Berkeley, CA: North Atlantic Books.
Oschman, J. L. (2000). *Energy Medicine: The Scientific Basis.* London: Churchill Livingstone.
Talbot, M. (1991). *The Holographic Universe.* New York: HarperCollins.
Travell, J. (1983). *Myofascial Pain and Dysfunction.* Baltimore, MD: Williams & Wilkins.
Zukav, G., & D. Finkelstein. (1979). *The Dancing Wu-Li Masters: An Overview of the New Physics.* New York: Bantam.

RESOURCES

International Myofascial Release
  Seminars
1–800-FASCIAL
www.myofascialrelease.com

The Paoli Myofascial Release Treatment
  Center
222 West Lancaster Ave.
Paoli, PA 19301
(610) 644–0136

Sedona's Myofascial Release Treatment
  Center ("Therapy on the Rocks")
676 North Highway 89A
Sedona, AZ 86336
(520) 282–3002

REFERENCES

Barnes, J. F. (1990). *Myofascial Release: The Search for Excellence*. Paoli, PA: MFR Seminars.

Crawford, J. S., J. Simpson, & P. Crawford. (1996). Myofascial release provides symptomatic relief from chest wall tenderness occasionally seen following lumpectomy and radiation in breast cancer patients [letter]. *International Journal of Radiation Oncology, Biology, Physics, 34,* 1188–1189.

Hanten, W. P., & S. D. Chandler. (1994). Effects of myofascial release leg pull and sagittal plane isometric contract-relax techniques on passive straight-leg raise angle. *Journal of Orthopedic Sports Physical Therapy, 20,* 138–44.

Hunt, T. K., M. J. Banda, & I. A. Silver. (1985). Cell interactions in post-traumatic fibrosis. *Clinical Symposia, 114,* 128–149.

Ingber, E., & J. Folkman. (1989). Tension and compression as basic determinants of cell form and function: Utilization of a cellular tensegrity mechanism. In W. Stein & F. Bronner (Eds.), *Cell Shape: Determinants, Regulation and Regulatory Role*. San Diego: Academic Press.

Katake, K. (1961). The strength for tension and bursting of human fasciae. *Journal of the Kyoto Prefecture Medical University, 69,* 484–488.

Levin, S. M. (1990). The myofascial-skeletal truss: A system science analysis. In J. F. Barnes, *Myofascial Release: The Search for Excellence*. Paoli PA: MFR Seminars.

Oschman, J. L. (2000). *Energy Medicine: The Scientific Basis*. London: Churchill Livingstone.

Seto, A., C. Kusaka, & S. Nakazato. (1992). Detection of extraordinary large bio-magnetic field strength from human hand. *Acupuncture and Electro-Therapeutics Research International Journal, 17,* 75–94.

Sisken, B. F., & J. Walker. (1995). Therapeutic aspects of electromagnetic fields for soft-tissue healing. In M. Blank (Ed.), *Electromagnetic Fields: Biological Interactions and Mechanisms*. Advances in Chemistry Series 250. Washington, DC: American Chemical Society.

Stauber, W. T., P. M. Clarkson, V. M. Fritz, & W. J. Evans. (1990). Extracellular matrix disruption and pain after eccentric muscle action. *Journal of Applied Physiology, 69,* 868–874.

Stauber, W. T., K. K. Knack, G. R. Miller, & J. G. Grimmett. (1996). Fibrosis and intercellular collagen connections from four weeks of muscle strain. *Muscle & Nerve, 19,* 423–430.

Sucher, B. M. (1990a). Thoracic outlet syndrome—A myofascial variant: Part 1. Pathology and diagnosis. *Journal of the American Osteopathic Association, 90,* 703–704.

Sucher, B. M. (1990b). Thoracic outlet syndrome—A myofascial variant: Part 2. Treatment. *Journal of the American Osteopathic Association, 90,* 810–812, 817–823.

Sucher, B. M. (1993a). Myofascial release of carpal tunnel syndrome. *Journal of the American Osteopathic Association, 93,* 92–94, 100–101.

Sucher, B. M. (1993b). Myofascial manipulative release of carpal tunnel syndrome: Documentation with magnetic resonance imaging. *Journal of the American Osteopathic Association, 93,* 1273–1278.

Upledger, J., & J. Vredovoogd. (1983). *Craniosacral Therapy.* Seattle, WA: Eastland Press.

Zachazewski, J. E. (1989). Improving flexibility. In R. M. Scully & M. R. Barnes (Eds.), *Physical Therapy.* Philadelphia: J.B. Lippincott.

Zimmerman, J. (1990). Laying-on-of-hands healing and therapeutic touch: A testable theory. *BEMI Currents, Journal of the Bio-Electro-Magnetics Institute, 2,* 8–17.

ACKNOWLEDGMENT

The author wishes to thank Maury Malyn, M.S., P.T., for his assistance in the preparation of this chapter.

17

Noncontact Therapeutic Touch

Guy L. McCormack

CHAPTER OBJECTIVES

- Differentiate and define noncontact therapeutic touch and therapeutic touch as forms of intervention.
- Provide information about the history and development of noncontact therapeutic touch.
- Review the strengths and weaknesses of using noncontact therapeutic touch in occupational therapy and physical therapy practice.
- Review relevant research to support the rationale for noncontact therapeutic touch.
- Describe the application of noncontact therapeutic touch in respect to classic case studies.

Therapeutic touch (TT) is a form of intervention that has been practiced since ancient times. Noncontact therapeutic touch (NCTT) is defined as an alternative, complementary technique that is similar to laying-on of hands but is not performed within a religious context, nor does it require a proposed faith (Samarel, 1992; Sayre-Adams, 1995). Today TT and NCTT are used interchangeably.

Background and History

Noncontact therapeutic touch was developed in the early 1970s by Dolores Krieger, a nursing professor at New York University. Dora Kunz, who was a well-known healer, worked with Krieger to study the effects of laying-on of hands and therapeutic touch.

The practice of NCTT bears resemblance to some of the practices of Franz Anton Mesmer (1734–1815), who claimed that humans possess a form of energy called *animal magnetism* (Hilgard & Hilgard, 1975). In a typical treatment session, Mesmer's hands were slowly moved over the patient's head, placed on the shoulders and down the extremities (proximal to distal) toward the fingers, until the hands moved along the entire length of the

Noncontact therapeutic touch is the intentional direction of energy to effect client health. Its four phases, centering, assessment, unruffling, and treatment, can be taught to anyone who is motivated to learn and is open to the concept of centering. Many times clients who receive NCTT early in the recovery period require less pain medication and sleep more peacefully. It is used in therapy practice to facilitate typical treatment goals by preparing clients for purposeful activities, decreasing anxiety and pain, and increasing relaxation.

patient's body along the longitudinal axis. He would also pass his hands over the patient perpendicular to blood vessels and shake his hands to expel the magnetic forces (Rogo, 1992; Zimmerman & Hinrichs, 1995). Mesmer believed his hands possessed electrical properties and that the presence of his hands could produce a cure.

Today, more than 200 years later, we know that the human body possesses paramagnetic qualities (Birla & Hemlin, 1999; Cohen, 1975; Desmedt & Tomberg, 1989; Marty, Sigrist & Wiler, 1994). For example, scientific studies in recent years have verified that constituents of the blood and the tissues of the skin contain electrical potentials that have been associated with tissue healing (Foulds & Barker, 1983; Illingworth & Barker, 1980). Such electrical and magnetic properties suggest that there is a physical mechanism occurring when NCTT is performed.

Basic Concepts

NCTT practitioners develop their ability to use their hands to detect barely perceptible differences in the energy field. To achieve this ability, practitioners must learn to alter their mental state, a process called *centering* (Krieger, 1979). Centering is a voluntary meditative act whereby one learns to calm the mind and focus on the moment. Practitioners seek to perform NCTT in a nonjudgmental way with the intent to help or heal. Furthermore, NCTT practitioners believe that the human energy field can be manipulated to promote healing (Benor, 1994; Krieger, 1979).

Touch and Energy Transfer

Human touch can take on many different forms of stimulation and communication. However, in NCTT there is no physical contact between the client and the practitioner. The technique is performed by holding the hands about 2 to 4 inches away from the surface of the body of the person receiving the treatment. Thus, inherent in the therapeutic touch process is the belief that the hands influence a human energy field.

Most therapists have been prepared for their professions under the biomechanical model, which has a high reliance upon principles of anatomy, physiology, chemistry, and Newtonian physics (Wilson, 1991). The biomechanical model has contributed to the understanding of orthotics, kinesiology, and assistive technology in the rehabilitation setting. NCTT is rooted in the fields of quantum physics and systems theory. In this model, no system functions in isolation. All systems interconnect and influence one another (Davis, 1994; Dossey, 1991; Gerber, 1988; Rossi, 1986).

In NCTT there is the belief in the transfer of energy from the practitioner to the client. According to Heidt (1991), subtle energy is linked to the belief that all living organisms are part of a greater order or whole. According to field theory, all matter is energy and all living systems produce vibrating fields of energy (Capra, 1984). Braud (1992) believes that mental processes such as strong positive emotions, imagery, visualization, and relaxation training can influence the presence of the energy field. In this chapter, it will be proposed that the human energy field is the same as the electromagnetic field produced by the heat generated by body metabolism.

Universal Energy

In Krieger's theory of NCTT (1979, 1981, 1993), the practitioner must subscribe to the belief in "universal energy," or *prana* (a Sanskrit word meaning "vital force"). This universal energy is believed to flow through the body and is transformed by energy centers called *chakras* (Sanskrit for "wheel" or "circle") (Fish, 1996; Karagulla & Kunz, 1989). The quality and flow of *prana* or universal energy is associated with wellness. If the universal energy is blocked, it will result in a condition of ill health. Krieger's followers (Doherty & Jackson, 1986; Heidt, 1981; Macrae, 1988; Quinn, 1989) have insisted that the flow of energy can be perceived or intuitively assessed and directed through the hands of a practitioner in the absence of any physical contact.

Typical Treatment Session

In the technique delineated by Dolores Krieger (1979, 1981, 1993), the therapist must learn to perform four steps: centering, assessment, unruffling, and treatment. *Centering* is the most critical phase and occurs throughout the process. Krieger describes centering as awareness and the ability to be fully present in the moment. The practitioner consciously induces a meditative or trance-like state by visualizing an image, by focusing on the breath, or by repeating a simple phrase (mantra) in his or her mind. When the practitioner learns to center, he or she reaches a state of mind that presumably enables the capacity of *intentionality,* or the intent to help or heal.

In the second phase, *assessment,* the practitioner holds the palms of his or her hands at a distance of 2 to 4 inches from the participant's body with the palms of the hands facing the surface of the skin. The participant can be fully clothed or under covers. Clothing does not seem to impede the process, although practitioners prefer natural materials, such as cotton or wool, as opposed to synthetic garments such as polyester. Synthetic garments are believed to impair the transmission or conduction of energy (Borelli & Heidt, 1981).

In the process of assessment the practitioner uses sweeping or scanning hand motions over the body of the recipient. In this phase, the practitioner assesses the "energy field" that is presumably emitted from the participant's body. Independent anecdotal studies conducted by Macrae (1980) and McCormack (1991) suggest that the practitioner can perceive waveforms of different frequencies as the hands pass over different segments or quadrants of the body. These different sensations may be associated with activity of the autonomic nervous system, muscle tension, areas of pain, decreased blood supply, inflammation, infection, and a variety of painful orthopedic disorders. Many practitioners who subscribe to Krieger's philosophy believe that the energy field exists beyond the boundaries of the skin and reflects disturbances, blockage, or imbalances in the passage of energy that normally passes through the soft tissues of the body.

The third phase the process is called *unruffling* or *clearing* (Krieger, 1979, 1990). The energy field is described as possessing a "texture" and it is perceived as being rough, agitated, uneven, wrinkled, or disorganized (Krieger, 1990). During this phase, the practitioners use their own energy of both hands with palms facing toward the person's body and move toward the periphery in long sweeping strokes and circular motions to "decongest" the participant's energy field.

In the fourth phase, which is considered the *treatment*, the practitioner uses his or her hands to modulate energy to reestablish a balance. Thus, the last step is often called modulation. In this phase the practitioners hold their hands in a stationary position to *redirect* or *transfer* energy from one part of the body to another (Krieger, 1979). Many practitioners use imagery to conceptualize imbalances and direct the flow of energy.

Smith (1990) has criticized the terminology of therapeutic touch, arguing convincingly that the operational definitions used by Krieger (1979) are metaphorical and ill conceived. However, the procedure for performing NCTT is consistently described in the literature (Heidt, 1990; Krieger, 1979; Macrae, 1983; Quinn, 1989). To achieve this consistency in protocol and achieve best results, therapists should follow the four steps (centering, assessment, unruffling, and treatment).

To perform NCTT, the therapist should stand on the side of the bed where the client has discomfort or where surgical procedures have been performed. The practitioner must utilize universal precautions and take appropriate measures to protect the client and himself or herself. The procedure is conducted by first centering to achieve a relaxed state and then performing an assessment of the human energy field with particular attention to the area where the discomfort is experienced. The assessment is documented on an anatomic chart, marking areas of the body that "give off" different sensations. Depending on how the client is positioned, the therapist will hold his or her hands near the site where the surgery was performed. The hands will move in a slow, circular, clockwise direction about 4 inches away from the area of pain. As the hands dwell on areas, they may sense some heat or a prickly sensation.

Collectively, the literature has shown that NCTT has produced the following benefits:

1. *To produce a relaxation response.*
2. *To provide pain relief.*
3. *To reduce anxiety and emotional stress.*
4. *To augment tissue healing.*
5. *To improve sleep patterns.*
6. *To enhance the immune response.*
7. *To comfort clients who are dying from a terminal illness.*

Therapeutic touch can be learned and applied effectively in clinical settings if one is motivated to learn and open to concepts such as centering. In a study conducted by McCormack (1999), two graduate occupational therapy students were trained with standard lessons on the performance of NCTT according to the procedure described by Krieger (1979). Post-surgery clients who received NCTT from the students reported a statistically significant reduction of pain on objective measures.

In the past 20 years, the field of nursing has developed a substantial body of knowledge encompassing the theory of, clinical practice of, and research on NCTT (Astin et al., 2000; Mulloney & Wells-Federman, 1996). Conservative estimates suggest that close to 10,000 nurses have been trained to perform NCTT, and the technique is either required or an elective part of the curriculum for over 80 nursing departments in colleges and universities throughout the United States (Fish, 1996). NCTT is practiced around the world by an estimated 100,000 people, including at least 43,000 health care professionals in hospitals, rehabilitation centers, hospices, and community health centers (Kauffold, 1995; Maxwell, 1996; Mulloney & Wells-Federman, 1996). Practitioners can take workshops to become certified as a therapeutic touch practitioner, but there are no formal degrees offered at this time from accredited colleges and universities. To inquire about training and certification requirements contact the Nurse Healers-Professional Association (see "Resources").

Potential Use with OT and PT Practice

In occupational therapy practice NCTT can be used as an adjunctive method under the occupational performance frame of reference. Adjunctive methods are preliminary procedures that prepare clients for purposeful activities (Pedretti, 1996). In this frame of reference there is a continuum of treatment that may begin with adjunctive methods such as positioning, splinting, sensory or motor facilitation, the use of physical agent modalities, relaxation training, and a host of traditional or alternative techniques. The application of NCTT reduces the perception of pain and enables clients to relax. In addition, clients who have muscle spasms or hypertonicity (spasticity or rigidity) may benefit clinically in that they show gains in range of motion and voluntary movement because the skeletal muscles become more compliant after NCTT. Clinical experience has also shown that children with learning disabilities who exhibit hyperactive behavior tend to calm down after an NCTT session.

In physical therapy practice NCTT can also be used to modulate pain and anxiety before manual exercises or activities such as gait training in clients who may have balance problems. The use of NCTT is also very helpful as a precursor to manual stretching, joint mobilization, wound management, myofascial release, and other manual interventions.

A skilled NCTT practitioner may use the NCTT assessment prior to performing palpation, passive range of motion, manual muscle testing, and sensorimotor evaluations. Many times, the skilled NCTT practitioner gains insight about regions of pain and discomfort that cannot be achieved through biomechanical techniques.

Research

Research on NCTT has ranged from collections of purely anecdotal reports to true experimental design methodology. The literature review will suggest that the clients who receive NCTT have reduced anxiety, have a greater relaxation response, and experience statistically significant decreases in pain intensity when compared to groups who receive the sham and control treatments. Based on these findings, the performance of NCTT may be cost-effective in many clinical settings.

Mechanism

There have been few attempts to identify the actual mechanisms responsible for the effects of NCTT. One of the problems with determining both mechanism and cause and effect relationships (outcomes) of NCTT has to do with problems authors have had in operationally defining study terms and in describing study subjects (Winstead-Fry & Kijec, 1999) and procedures. This makes replication of results difficult. For example, the process of NCTT has been described metaphorically as a manipulation of the human energy field and as a transfer of universal energy. The term "energy" is not operationally defined by most authors (Capra, 1984; France, 1991; Glickman & Burns, 1996).

The transference of electricity and/or use of magnetic fields may explain the mechanism of NCTT. The electromagnetic properties of skin can be measured with sensitive instruments to track the direct currents (DC) involved in tissue healing (Baker, Jaffe & Vanable, 1982; Becker, 1962; Becker & Selden, 1985; Cohen, 1975; Edelberg, 1977; Foulds & Barker, 1983; Illingworth & Barker, 1980; Zimmerman, 1989). Results of endogenous biocircuit studies have provided substantial evidence that both superficial and deep layers of the skin generate DC and alternating currents (AC) (Foulds & Barker, 1983). It is also well known that electrocardiograms, electroencephalograms, and electromyography units monitor measurable frequencies of alternating currents generated by specific tissues of the body (Guyton, 1991). Magnetic fields have been measured over the heart, brain, eye, and skeletal muscles (Braud, 1992; Brenner, Lipton, & Kaufman, 1978; Reite & Zimmerman, 1978). Small electrical currents have been recorded in superficial wounds and reported to be an important element in tissue healing (Alverz, 1993; Becker & Selden, 1985; Illingworth & Barker, 1983; McCulloch, Kloth, & Feeder, 1995).

In studies of the transcutaneous potentials of the human body, it has been found that the hands and feet are negatively charged when compared to the rest of the body (Baker, Jaffe, & Vanable, 1982; Becker & Selden, 1985; Foulds & Barker, 1983). It is also known that tumors and skin wounds contain a concentration of positively charged ions. Based on this knowledge, it possible that the negatively charged hands "pull off" or dissipate the accumulation of positively charged ions in painful tissue sites through NCTT. Smith (1972) found that NCTT produced a magnetic field equivalent to a 13,000 gauss electromagnet.

The production and transfer of heat may also explain, in part, the mechanism responsible for NCTT. Scientists have demonstrated that the rate at which the body produces electrical activity appears to be influenced in part by body temperature (Guyton, 1991). During NCTT, capillaries dilate, causing the skin to warm up. Heat emitted from the body gives off waveforms that operate within the electromagnetic spectrum. It is conceivable that heat can be transferred from the practitioner's hands at a short distance to the body of the participant by means of heat conduction (Guyton, 1991).

Outcomes

NCTT is one of the better studied "energy" therapies with regard to outcomes. Winstead-Fry & Kijek (1999) conducted a meta-analysis of NCTT studies and found that of the 29 studies that met criteria for analysis, the researchers' hypotheses were supported in 19 and rejected in 10. This reflected positive, statistically significant outcomes in almost two-thirds of the studies. Austin and colleagues (2000) also conducted a systematic review of the available data on NCTT and found that 7 of 11 of the studies showed positive treatment effects. In addition these authors concluded that NCTT is more effective than mock therapeutic touch.

Much of the research on NCTT is notable for its rigor in scientific method. Most studies compare NCTT with sham NCTT or other control groups, and a substantial minority utilize double-blind methodology, randomization, or both. Research on NCTT has primarily tested pain, anxiety, and stress reduction outcomes. Other significant related studies are on wound healing and the effect of a healer's hand presence on plants.

Research supports the use of NCTT in treatment of pain. Subjects studied include elderly adults with degenerative arthritis (Eckes Peck, 1997), adults with tension headaches (Keller & Bzdek, 1986), and adults with burns (Turner, Gauthier, & Williams, 1998). Adults with postoperative pain did not experience significantly less pain than the sham control group but did wait significantly longer before requesting pain medications and received significantly fewer doses of analgesic medication (Meehan et al., 1990).

While one study was performed that did not detect significant differences in anxiety (Parkes, 1985), overall research also supports using NCTT in stress reduction and treatment of anxiety. Simmington and Laing (1993) found that elderly institutionalized subjects who received NCTT and a 3-minute massage had statistically significant reductions in anxiety scores when compared with other groups. Turner, Gauthier, and Williams (1998) found significant reductions in anxiety scores when using NCTT versus sham NCTT with burn patients, and Gagne and Toye (1994) found that psychiatric patients who received NCTT or relaxation training experienced anxiety reduction. NCTT also produced significant reductions in physiological measures of stress as well as in the time required to calm children after stressful experiences (Kramer, 1990) and in anxiety after a natural disaster (Olsen et al., 1992).

Research on NCTT also supports its use in wound healing. Krieger (1975, 1976) found that hospitalized patients who received NCTT had a statistically significant increase in hemoglobin values when compared with controls. Wirth (1992) found that adults with skin biopsies who received NCTT experienced accelerated healing as compared with controls, and Quinn and Strelhauskas (1993) found that suppresser T-cell counts dropped dramatically in both subjects and NCTT practitioners after NCTT. Grad, Cadoret, and Paul (1961) found that mice treated by a healer who held his hands over them healed significantly faster when a surgical incision was made on their backs. The study also showed that iodine-induced goiters grew significantly more slowly on mice that were treated by a healer than on mice that were not.

Finally, Grad (1965) found that when a healer held his hands over them, barley seeds grew significantly taller and greater in number and produced more chlorophyll than barley seeds without the healer intervention.

The Placebo Response

Critics have argued that the benefits of NCTT are due primarily to the placebo effect (Fish, 1996; Glickman & Burns, 1996; Jaroff, 1994). The placebo effect cannot be ignored while discussing the efficacy of NCTT, because any process that is performed with the intent to help or heal may set up the conditions for a nonspecific placebo response. Clinically, placebo is defined as a presumably inert or neutral substance or procedure, such as expectations, that elicits a therapeutic response (Evans, 1974; Shapiro, 1971; Wickramasekera, 1980). Placebo effects are poorly understood and regarded as a "nuisance" by medical researchers (Raj, 1992).

If NCTT does have a therapeutic effect due to a placebo response, clients in a state of ill health are ideal candidates for it. Placebos can reliably attenuate a range of health and illness behavior (Ader, 2000), and they have been shown to alleviate pain. In 26 double-blind placebo studies, consisting of a total of 1,991 participants, it was shown that approximately 35 percent of those participants who received a placebo reported that their clinical pain was reduced by at least half of its original intensity (Wickramasekera, 1980).

On the other hand, research demonstrating the electrical properties of the body support the notion that NCTT could act as an active therapeutic agent, and the research presented above supports the use of NCTT in pain management, anxiety, and wound healing. Additionally, animal and plant studies are important because there is little chance of the placebo effect as an intervening variable. Each of the animal and plant studies described above, while not performed by a NCTT practitioner but by a healer whose actions were similar to NCTT, showed positive treatment effects. The use in research of control and/or sham treatment groups controls for placebo effects such as positive expectations. Because of the rigor in NCTT research designs overall, it is unlikely that the treatment effects noted above occurred purely from expectation.

Perception of the Human Energy Field

A study published in the *Journal of the American Medical Association* by Rosa and colleagues (1998) has challenged whether NCTT practitioners can actually perceive a human energy field (HEF). Twenty-one NCTT practitioners were tested under blinded conditions to determine whether they could correctly identify which of their hands was closest to the investigator's hand. Placement of the investigator's hand was determined by flipping a coin. Fourteen practitioners were tested 10 times each, and seven practitioners were tested 20 times each. Based on probability, 50 percent correct would be expected by chance alone. The results showed that the NCTT practitioners identified the correct hand in only 123 (44 percent) of 280 trials, slightly less than would be expected by chance alone.

There were several methodological flaws in this study. First, the investigator was a 9-year-old child who was a conducting an experiment for school under the guidance of her mother. As it turns out, her mother is a registered nurse who has been known to dispute the practice of NCTT. Therefore, the study may have been conducted and written with some bias and intent to discredit the practice of NCTT. Second, the practitioners' vision was occluded while their hands were held in a stationary position with the palms up. Meanwhile, the young investigator randomly positioned her hand 8 to 10 cm above either the participant's right or left hand. One problem with this method is that the practitioners' hands are usually moving, palms down in a slow manner, over the body of a person who is ill or experiencing pain. The field generated by regions of a body that are infected, inflamed, or deprived of blood supply are very different than that generated by the hand of a healthy 9 year old. It is difficult to argue with the simplicity and statistical probability of the procedure, but the method did not replicate the actual conditions and protocol of NCTT.

The literature suggests that NCTT be based on the belief that healing can occur through interactions with the human energy field (HEF). The healing powers of physical touch in general is well established (Schoenhafer, 1989). However, a scientific explanation of NCTT healing has yet to be revealed. To date, clinical studies on therapeutic touch have provided evidence that NCTT can decrease pain intensity, anxiety, elicit a relaxation response, and accelerate tissue healing.

Case Studies

Total Hip Replacement

Jake is a 64-year-old male who had a right total hip replacement secondary to complications of a hip fracture due to osteoporosis. Jake appeared to have a low threshold for pain and was very anxious about participating in rehabilitation. He has worked in construction most of his life, is not married, lives alone, and has few friends. Jake was uncertain about his future in construction and employment opportunities. For his postsurgical pain, he was prescribed Vicodin, a drug that is a combination of opiod and nonsteroidal anti-inflammatory agents. The pain medication was not sufficient to alleviate his pain and anxiety. He was not cooperative with the progression of bearing weight on his hip joint and the degree of movement he was asked to perform by the physical therapist. Jake was referred to occupational therapy to review his psychosocial adjustment and precautions for positioning, and to evaluate his independence in activities of daily living and provide assistive devices to enable him to perform personal hygiene activities.

During the initial interview, it became evident that Jake was hypersensitive to touch and did not believe his hip would be stable enough to ambulate. Given informed consent and educational information to assure him that he was ready to proceed in rehabilitation, the therapist obtained permission to perform NCTT at the beginning of each session. For 5 days, 10 minutes of NCTT preceded the conventional occupational therapy interventions. Jake reported he felt more relaxed after the NCTT and trusted the therapist's judgment to move forward with the rehabilitation program. By the fourth day he willingly participated in mobility and activities of daily living training. Work simulation assessments suggested that he could resume employment in a modified capacity. A home program was recommended along with vocational counseling.

Evidence-based practice has shown that NCTT can be used as an adjunctive method to alleviate pain and anxiety. Studies have suggested that NCTT can alleviate pain and augment the effects of pain medication in patients who have undergone surgery (Ekes Peck, 1997; McCormack, 1999).

Low Back Pain

Pam is a 51-year-old female who was referred to occupational therapy for vocational exploration and chronic low back pain. She sustained a back injury while lifting a heavy box on an assembly line. She has been seen in physical therapy and has taken various pain medications but has not received sufficient relief. She is receiving psychological counseling at the request of her physician. Pam was referred to occupational therapy for vocational exploration, body mechanics, and energy conservation training. The therapist conducted a brief pain inventory assessment and discovered that pain was the primary obstacle to a productive lifestyle. Pam was evaluated with NCTT as an adjunctive method before each treatment session. The assessment was documented on an anatomic chart, marking the areas of the body where the energy field gave off different sensations. NCTT was performed by holding the hands near the lumbar vertebrae and pelvic girdle on the side where the pain was most pronounced. The practitioner's hands were moved in a slow, circular, clockwise direction about 4 inches away from the area of pain. As the hands dwelled over the pain site, there was a perception of heat and a prickly sensation.

The sensation arising from low back pain was perceived as a deficit or a sensation that the field was hollowed out or drawing inward. As the practitioner's hands slowly moved over the waistline, a deficit was found beneath the blocked areas in the field. The hands were held close together over the site of pain to transfer energy as if the hole in the field was being filled (Feltman, 1989).

The next procedure was to allow the hands to come in contact with the low back area. The left hand was placed about 2 inches below the navel and the right hand was placed at about the L4–L5 vertebrae to elicit a therapeutic release of soft tissues. The simultaneous presence of the hands in contact on both the anterior and posterior surfaces was intended to increase blood supply to the low back area, improving circulation and releasing muscles tension.

This technique was applied for the duration of 20 minutes each day for 10 treatment sessions. Pam reported considerably less pain on the pain scale and other objective measures. On a daily self-reported activity configuration, Pam reported an increase in activity levels and returned to part-time employment.

Summary

NCTT, or TT, is classified as an energy therapy by NCCAM. Developed by Dolores Krieger and Dora Kunz, it resembles in theory and practice the healing process practiced by Franz Anton Mesmer over 200 years ago as well as some practices of laying on of hands. Most NCTT practitioners believe in universal energy and intend to direct this energy to clients for positive healing effects. Studies support the use of NCTT in pain and anxiety management, wound healing, and relaxation. Therapists can use NCTT for these purposes, and to prepare clients for therapy and to gain insight about clients that traditional testing procedures typically do not provide.

STUDY QUESTIONS

1. Describe the differences between NCTT and direct contact touch such as massage.
2. Describe two mechanisms that may play a role in the effects produced by NCTT.
3. Outline and explain the four steps of performing NCTT.
4. According to the literature, what are the primary benefits of NCTT?

Resources

Nurse Healers-Professional Association,
   Inc.
175 Fifth Ave., Suite 2755
New York, NY 10010

References

Ader, A. R. (2000). The placebo effect: If it's all in your head, does that mean you only think you feel better? *Advances in Mind-Body Medicine, 16,* 7–46.

Alverz, O. M. (1993). The healing of superficial skin wounds is healed by external electrical current. *Journal of Investigative Dermatology, 81,* 144.

Astin, J. A., K. R. Pelletier, A. Marie, & W. L. Haskell. (2000). Complementary and alternative medicine: One year analysis of a Blue Shield Medicare supplement. *Journal of Gerontology, 55*(10), 4–9.

Baker, A., L. Jaffe, & J. Vanable. (1982). The glabrous epidermis of cavies contains a powerful battery. *American Journal of Physiology, 242,* 360–365.

Becker, R. O. (1962). The direct current control system: A link between environment and the organism. *New York State Journal of Medicine, 40,* 1169–1176.

Becker, R. O., & A. Selden. (1985). *The Body Electric: Electromagnetism and the Foundation of Life.* New York: William Morrow.

Benor, D. (1994). Hands-on help . . . healing is being increasingly applied in clinical practice. *Nursing Times, 90*(44), 28–29.

Birla, G. S., & C. Hemlin. (1999). *Magnet Therapy.* Rochester, VT: Healing Arts Press.

Borelli, M. D., & P. Heidt. (Eds.). (1981). *Therapeutic Touch: A Book of Readings.* New York: Springer.

Braud, W. G. (1992). Human interconnectedness: Research indications. *Revision: A Journal of Consciousness and Transformation, 5*(10), 19–25.

Brenner, D., J. Lipton, & L. Kaufman. (1978). Somatically evoked magnetic field of the human brain. *Science, 180,* 745–748.

Capra, F. (1984). *The Tao of Physics.* Toronto: Bantam Books.

Cohen, D. (1975). Magnetic fields of the human body. *Physics Today, 28,* 34–43.

Davis, C. M. (1994). Solid objects are not solid: And other ruminations on atoms, energy, and therapeutic presence. *Magazine of Physical Therapy, 2*(9), 61–65.

Desmedt, J., & C. Tomberg. (1989). Mapping early somatosensory evoked potentials in selective attention: Critical evaluation of control conditions used for titrating by difference the cognitive P30, P40, P100 and N140. *Electroencephalography and Clinical Neurophysiology, 74,* 321–346.

Doherty, C., & N. Jackson. (1986). Therapeutic touch. *AARN Newsletter, 42*(6), 11–13.

Dossey, L. (1991). *Meaning and Medicine.* New York: Bantam Books.

Eckes Peck, S. D. (1997). The effectiveness of therapeutic touch for decreasing pain in elders with degenerative arthritis. *Journal of Holistic Nursing, 15*(2), 176–198

Edelberg, C. (1977). Relation of electrical properties of skin to structure and physiologic state. *The Journal of Investigative Dermatology, 69,* 324–327.

Evans, F. J. (1974, Apr.). The power of the sugar pill. *Psychology Today, 7,* 32.

Feltman, J. (1989). *Hands-on Healing.* Emmaus, PA: Rodale Press.

Fish, S. (1996). Therapeutic touch: Healing science or metaphysical fraud? *Journal of Christian Nursing, 13*(3), 4–10.

Foulds, I. S., & A. I. Barker. (1983). Human skin battery potentials and their role in wound healing. *British Journal of Dermatology, 109,* 515.

France, N. E. M. (1991). A phenomenological inquiry on the child's lived experience of perceiving the human energy field using therapeutic touch. University of Colorado Health Science Center, 234P (University Microfilms No. PUZ9215316).

Gagne D., & R. C. Toye. (1994). The effects of therapeutic touch and relaxation training in reducing anxiety. *Archives of Psychiatric Nursing, 8*(3), 184–189.

Gerber, R. (1988). *Vibrational Medicine*. Santa Fe, NM: Bear.

Glickman, R., & J. Burns. (1996). If therapeutic touch works, prove it. *RN, 59*(12), 76.

Grad, B. (1965). Some biological effects of the laying on of hands: A review of experiments with animals and plants. *Journal of the American Society for Psychological Research, 59*(2), 95–129.

Grad, B., R. J. Cadoret, & S. Paul. (1961). The influence of an unorthodox method of treatment on wound healing in mice. *International Journal of Parapsychology, 3,* 5–24.

Guyton, M. A. (1991). *Textbook of Medical Physiology* (8th ed.). Philadelphia: Saunders.

Heidt, P. (1991). Helping patients to rest: Clinical studies in therapeutic touch. *Holistic Nursing Practice, 5*(4), 57–66.

Heidt, P. (1990). Openness: A qualitative analysis of nurses' and patients' experiences of therapeutic touch. *Image: Journal of Nursing Scholarship, 22*(3), 180–186.

Heidt, P. (1981). Effect of therapeutic touch on the anxiety level of hospital patients. *Nursing Research, 30*(1), 32–37.

Hilgard, E. R., & J. R. Hilgard. (1975). *Hypnosis in the relief of pain*. Los Angeles: William Kaufmann.

Illingworth, C. M., & A. T. Barker. (1980). Measurement of electrical currents emerging during the regeneration of amputated finger tips in children. *Clinical Physiological Measures, 1,* 87.

Jaroff, L. (1994, Nov.). A no-touch therapy. *Time, 144*(12), 88–89.

Karagulla, S., & D. Kunz. (1989). *The Chakras and the Human Energy Field*. Wheaton, IL: Theosophical Publishing House.

Kauffold, M. P. (1995). TT: Healing or hokum? Debate over energy medicine runs hot. *Chicago Tribune Nursing News, 11,* 1.

Keller, E., & V. M. Bzdek. (1986). Effects of therapeutic touch on tension headache pain. *Nursing Research, 35*(2), 101–106.

Kramer, N. A. (1990). Comparison of therapeutic touch and casual touch in stress reduction of hospitalized children. *Pediatric Nursing, 16*(5), 483–485.

Krieger, D. (1993). *Accepting Your Power to Heal: The Personal Practice of Therapeutic Touch.* Santa Fe, NM: Bear.

Krieger, D. (1990). Therapeutic touch: Two decades of research, teaching and clinical practice. *NSNA/Imprint, 37*(3), 83, 86–88.

Krieger, D. (1981). *Foundations of Holistic Health and Nursing Practices: The Renaissance Nurse.* Philadelphia, PA: J. B. Lippincott.

Krieger, D. (1979). *The Therapeutic Touch: How to Use Your Hands to Help or to Heal.* Englewood Cliffs, NJ: Prentice-Hall.

Krieger, D. (1976). Healing by the "laying on" of hands as a facilitator of bioenergetic change: The response of in vivo human hemoglobin. *Psychoenergetic Systems, 1,* 121–129.

Krieger, D. (1975). Therapeutic touch: The imprimatur of nursing. *American Journal of Nursing, 75*(56), 784–787.

Macrae, J. (1988). *Therapeutic Touch: A Practical Guide*. New York: Alfred A. Knopf.

Macrae, J. (1983). Therapeutic touch as meditation. *The American Theosophist, 71*(10), 338–348.

Macrae, J. (1980). Therapeutic touch in practice. In J. Jackson (Ed.), *The Whole Nursing Catalog.* Philadelphia: Saunders.

Marty, W., T. Sigrist, & D. Wiler. (1994). Measurement of the skin temperature at the entry wound by means of infrared thermograpy: An investigation involving the use of .22 to .38 caliber handguns. *American Journal of Forensic Medical Pathology, 15*(1), 1–4.

Maxwell, J. (1996). Nursing's new age? *Christianity Today, 40*(3), 96–99.

McCormack, G. (1999). The effects of non-contact therapeutic touch, absorption, health belief and pain in the elderly population. Unpublished dissertation. Saybrook Institute, San Francisco, CA.

McCormack, G. (1991). *Therapeutic Use of Touch for the Health Professional*. Tucson, AZ: Therapy Skill Builders.

McCulloch, J. M., L. C. Kloth, & J. A. Feeder. (1995). *Wound Healing Alternatives in Management*. Philadelphia: FA Davis.

Meehan, T. C., C. A. Mersman, M. E. Wiseman, B. B. Wolff, & D. Malgady. (1990). Therapeutic touch and surgical patient's reactions. Abstracted. *Journal of Pain, 5,* 149.

Mulloney, S. S., & C. Wells-Federman. (1996). Therapeutic touch: A healing modality. *Journal of Cardiovascular Nursing, 10*(3), 27–49.

Olsen, M., N. Snead, R. Bonadonna, J. Ratcliff, & J. Dias. (1992). Therapeutic touch and post-Hurricane Hugo stress. *Journal of Holistic Nursing, 10*(2), 120–136.

Parkes, B. (1985). Therapeutic touch as an intervention to reduce anxiety in elderly, hospitalized patients. *Dissertations Abstract International, 47,* 573B (University Microfilms No. 8609563).

Pedretti, L. W. (1996). *Occupational Therapy: Practice Skills for Physical Dysfunction* (4th ed.). St. Louis, MO: Mosby.

Quinn, J. F., & A. J. Strelhauskas. (1993). Psychoimmunologic effects of therapeutic touch on practitioners and recently bereaved recipients: A pilot study. *Advances in Nursing Science, 15*(14), 13–26.

Quinn, J. F. (1989). Future directions for therapeutic touch research. *Journal of Holistic Nursing, 7*(10), 19–25.

Raj, P. P. (1992). *Practical Management of Pain*. St. Louis: Mosby Year Book.

Reite, M., & J. E. Zimmerman. (1978). Magnetic phenomenon of the central nervous system. *Annual Review Biophysiological Bioengineering, 7,* 167–188.

Rogo, D. (1992). *Techniques of Inner Healing*. New York: Paragon.

Rosa, L., E. Rosa, L. Sarner, & S. Barret. (1998). A close look at therapeutic touch. *Journal of the American Medical Association, 279*(13), 1005–1010.

Rossi, E. L. (1986). *The Psychobiology of Mind-Body Healing*. New York: W. W. Norton.

Samarel, N. (1992). The experience of receiving therapeutic touch. *Journal of Advanced Nursing, 17,* 651–657.

Sayre-Adams, J. (1994). Therapeutic touch: a nursing function. *Nursing-Standard, 8*(17), 25–28.

Shapiro, A. (1971). Placebo effects in medicine, psychotherapy and psychoanalyis In A. Bergin & S. Garfield (Eds.), *Handbook of Psychotherapy and Behavior Change*. New York: Wiley.

Shoenhafer, S. O. (1989). Affectional touch in critical care nursing: A descriptive study. *Heart and Lung, 18*(2), 146–154.

Simmington, J. A., & G. P. Laing. (1993). Effect of therapeutic touch on anxiety in the institutionalized elderly. *Clinical Nursing Research, 2*(4), 438–450.

Smith, J. A. (1990). Therapeutic touch: A critical appraisal. In T. Barnard & E. Braqilton (Eds.), *Therapeutic Touch: The Foundation Experience*. Madison, CT: International University Press.

Smith, M. J. (1972). Paranormal effects on enzyme activity. *Human Dimension, 1,* 15–19.

Turner, J. G., D. K. Gauthier, & M. Williams. (1998). The effect of therapeutic touch on pain and anxiety in burn patients. *Journal of Advanced Nursing, 28,* 10–20.

Wickramasekera, I. E. (1980). A conditioned response model of the placebo effect: Predictions for the model. *Biofeedback and Self-Regulation, 5*(1), 5–18.

Wilson, J. (1991). *College Physics*. Boston: Allyn and Bacon.

Winstead-Fry, P., & J. Kijec. (1999). An integrative review and meta-analysis of therapeutic touch research. *Alternative Therapies in Health and Medicine, 5*(6), 58–67.

Wirth, D. (1992). The effect of noncontact therapeutic touch on the healing of full thickness dermal wounds. *Nurse Healer Professional Associates, 13*(3), 4–6.

Zimmerman, J. (1989). Biomagnetism attracts diverse crowd. *Research News, 245*(8), 1041–1043.

Zimmerman, J., & D. Heinrichs. (1995). Magnetherapy: An introduction. *Newsletter of the Bio-Electro-Magnetics Institute, 1*(1), 3–6.

18

Reflexology

Gretchen Schaff

CHAPTER OBJECTIVES

- Understand the history of reflexology.
- Describe the concept of maps.
- Describe zone theory and its relationship to reflexology.
- Understand how reflexology can be used to augment traditional therapy.
- Understand indications and contraindications for reflexology.

Welcome to the world of lilliputians in the shape of feet, hands, and ears. Reflexology posits that in these parts of our bodies lie the whole of us—the macrocosm reflected in a microcosm. Upon understanding the concepts of reflexology in this chapter, readers will no longer view the feet, hands, and ears as only organs for locomotion, activities of daily living, or hearing. Indeed, they represent a powerful door of opportunity to gain ready access to the entire person in front of the therapist, for the purpose of aiding the client's healing process.

Reflexology is a healing modality that uses physical pressure applied to the feet, hands, and ears to effect changes on the whole body. Through the use of specific finger and hand techniques, psychological, physiological, and physical changes can occur to assist the body to heal. The use of tools is not part of traditional American reflexology, although some are used in Taiwan, China, and elsewhere. The goal of reflexology is to maintain or improve client homeostasis. While reflexologists do not treat for specific illnesses, often physical symptoms can be relieved by the reflexologist's provision of a graded stimulus to the whole body via the "reflex points" (points of contact) and by relaxing the feet and hands themselves. Results of the technique may include general changes, such as a decrease in physical and mental tensions, which is a factor in reducing many symptoms, and specific changes, such as improved blood and lymph transport, nervous system function, and motor output.

Reflexology is part science and part art. The science is based on the study of the human body. The art is based on the practitioner's manual skills and knowledge.

Reflexology is both a body of knowledge and a manual therapy that complements many other therapies and treatment techniques. The technique involves the use of thumbs, fingers, and hands to stimulate reflex points within zones of the body. Reflexology is differentiated from massage in several different ways, including specific manual techniques. It can be used to address targeted physical symptoms as well as to facilitate homeostasis and enhance client health.

Theory and History

What is the basis for the belief that the feet, hands, and ears are connected in a unique way to the rest of the body? It is now understood that every cell in the body, from the moment of conception, carries an imprint of the entire being, via the DNA "blueprint" (Frandsen, 2000). Reflexologists use "maps," or charts, that show how the entire body relates to the feet, hands, and ears. While maps vary in specificity, in general (in the foot) the pads of the toes correspond to the cranial cavity, the forefoot to the thoracic cavity, the midfoot to the abdominal cavity, the heel to the pelvic cavity, and the spine to the medial border of the foot (Issel & Rogers, 2000). See Figures 18–1 and 18–2.

In the late 1500s the concept of zones of energy in the body was introduced. This theory presented 10 longitudinal zones, going from the tips of toes and fingers to the top of the head, that energetically unite everything in that zone. The theory of zones is similar to that of meridians (energy pathways that traverse the body) in Traditional Chinese Medicine (Dougans, 1996; refer to Chapter 8, "Introduction to Asian Medical Systems," which has a detailed discussion of and resources for TCM and meridians). The concept of zones of energy has been greatly expanded upon since the early 1900s.

It is thought in zone theory that an area of pathology in the body will eventually show up as pain in the feet, hands, or both. Conversely, if one has an abnormal condition of the feet or hands, there will be an effect through the zones into the body itself. Like treating "root" problems in TCM, the focus of reflexology is treatment of the entire individual by assisting in the balancing of all body systems. Reflexologists use the term *reflex points* to refer to the points of contact of the hand, feet, and ears that connect through energetic zones to the musculoskeletal system, the nervous system, and all organs, glands, and other body parts. Reflexologists manually stimulate reflex points to effect this change throughout the body. Crane (1997) explains the "reflex" in reflexology, noting that the body responds in a reflexive (involuntary, unconscious) way to reflexology stimuli.

Eunice Ingham is considered the mother of modern reflexology. Ingham, a therapist practicing with Dr. William H. Fitzgerald, transformed Fitzgerald's treatment utilizing zone theory in the early 20th century. Ingham is credited with extensively focusing on and mapping the foot. She developed a method of alternating compression, and she widely promoted and taught her version of this treatment technique, dubbed reflexology (Eastman, 1991).

Reflexology on the ear is called auriculo therapy. Many types of pain and forms of muscle spasm can be reduced with work on the ears. Due to the small surface area of the ear, au-

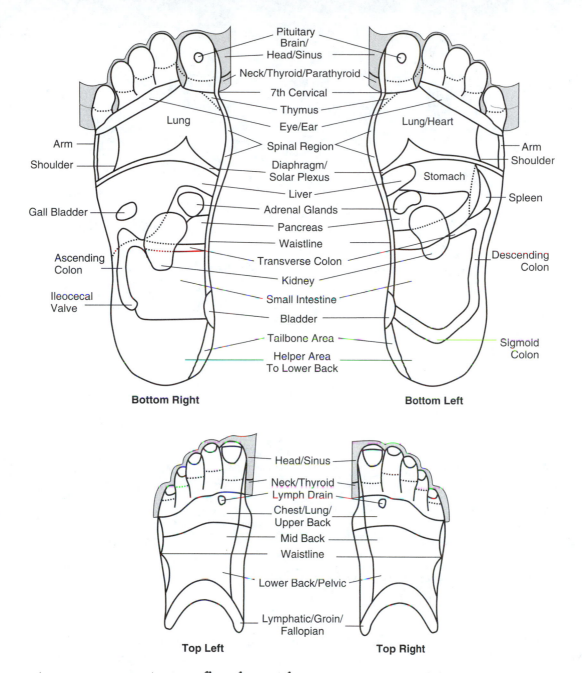

Figure 18–1 Foot Reflexology Charts *From Kunz,* Hand & Foot Reflexology, A Self-Help Guide. *Fireside Press, 1992.*

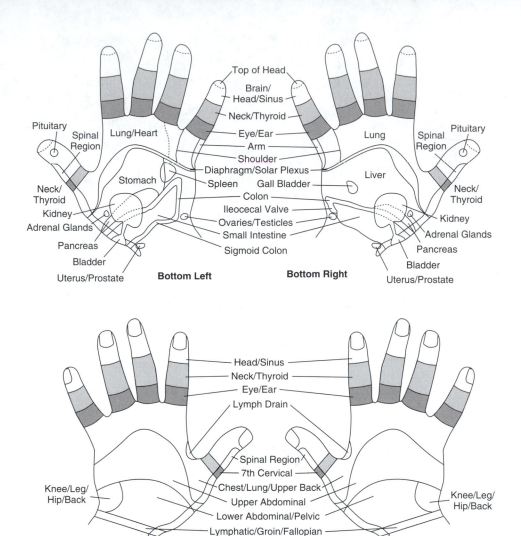

Figure 18–2 Hand Reflexology Charts *From Kunx,* Hand & Foot Reflexology, A Self-Help Guide. *Fireside Press, 1992.*

riculo therapy may be performed with a tool, usually an auricular probe, which is smaller than a finger and allows a more precise touch. Advanced techniques, requiring specific training, include electro-acupuncture and needle acupuncture as well as electrical stimulation with equipment compatible with auricolo therapy.

The theoretical basis for the use of reflex points in the ears is based on neurophysiological principles as well as energetic and embryological theories from Traditional Chinese Medicine. The relationship between specific parts of the ear to the other body parts was initially developed in modern times in France by Dr. Paul Nogier in 1957. In America, the first basic ear chart was drawn in the early 20th century by Dr. J. S. Riley as part of his technique for

A professional reflexologist will

1. Take a health history, including medications, and update it periodically.
2. Ascertain occupation and recreational activities, particularly as they relate to feet and hands.
3. Inquire about emotional status and stress levels.
4. Ask the client to state his or her expectation for the visit.
5. Observe gait pattern and wear pattern of shoes.
6. Make a visual and palpatory assessment of body parts to receive treatment: feet, hands, and ears, comparing right and left.
7. Make referrals to appropriate health care professionals for any significant deviations from normalcy.
8. Note any possible contraindications or precautions. Ask to speak to the client's physician if he or she has questions.
9. Explain what the session will entail, alert clients to possible reactions and explain self-care procedures.

zone therapy (Crane, 1997). An increasing number of reflexology schools and practitioners are incorporating ear reflexology points in their curriculums and in client sessions, with the encouragement and training of Bill Flocco, a master reflexologist.

Differentiating Reflexology and Massage

The significant differences between working on hands and feet for reflexology versus massage lie in theory, manual techniques, and a philosophy about lubrication. The reflexologist approaches the hands and feet as a microcosm representing the whole body, while the traditional massage therapist focuses on directly treating the tissue under his or her hands. Some reflexology techniques may look similar to those used in Swedish massage, as both techniques work on the feet and hands to affect the musculoskeletal system. Unique to American reflexology, as devised by Eunice Igham (1998), is a discrete method of finger and thumb "walking" using primarily the distal-lateral corner of the thumbs; that is, the therapist maintains an abducted position of the carpal/metacarpal and a neutral one of the metacarpophalangeal joints while flexing and extending the thumb's interphalangeal joint to effect a creeping or caterpillar-like motion. This thumb walking is the primary method used to assess and treat all areas of the feet and hands in reflexology. Ingham initially labeled this *compression massage,* but later settled on the term *reflexology* to more accurately represent the theoretical premise for which the techniques is used.

Reflexologists also use techniques such as direct pressure on a point of contact, a hooking in and pulling back, and rotating on a point with the tip of the thumb or index finger. Most reflexologists also employ a variety of techniques to release tension in the joints of the

The American Reflexology Certification Board (ARCB) is a national nonprofit corporation established to certify reflexologist competency. The ARCB offers a national certification program. In 1999 ARCB's prerequisites to sit for the professional reflexology test included 110 hours of classroom instruction and 90 hours of post-classroom documented sessions, to be recorded on the organization's forms. The test, for which ACRB provides a study guide, has both a written and practical component. ARCB board members travel to various U.S. cities to administer the test.

The American Commission for Accreditation of Reflexology Education and Training (ACARET) is a national, independent, nonprofit board to set standards for professional reflexology curriculums and has initiated an accreditation process for those schools seeking recognition of their high standards. Curriculum requirements of 300 hours include specific hours of study on anatomy and physiology, with an approach that emphasizes the integration of body systems and in-depth study of leg/foot and forearm/hand, including biomechanical aspects, skin conditions and common pathologies, and reflexology theory, techniques, and history. There are sections on ethics, business practices, sanitation, CPR, and some electives. Students are expected to offer unsupervised practice sessions outside the classroom to expand their experience and proficiency, to reciprocate sessions with a reflexology teacher for 5 hours, and receive supervision for 10 sessions in a clinic.

Interested therapists can contact the Reflexology Association of America (RAA), ARCB, or state reflexology organizations for training opportunities. Some massage schools offer brief (25 to 50 hours) programs that can be taken separately from their massage diploma. Information about such programs or independent reflexology schools can also be found in national massage magazines (*Massage & Body Work* and *Massage*) or local publications listing course offerings in a variety of holistic health practices. As in most of the healing arts, one will find a variety of ideas about reflexology—some rigid, some eclectic, some encouraging innovation. Reflexology theories and techniques have traditionally evolved through educated opinion, and will continue to evolve. The reader is urged to seek out a program that meets both ACARET standards and one's own needs.

A therapy student or practitioner may be able to find a program that will credit previous education, such as anatomy and physiology, so that these courses are not repeated and the student can focus on reflexology theory and practical skills. Finding a seasoned practitioner as a tutor will be helpful, and a great deal can be learned from the books noted at the end of this chapter, as well as from videos on the subject. However, since the practice of reflexology involves many tactile and manual skills, it is best to have some classroom or tutorial instruction.

There is a difference between calling oneself a professional reflexologist and utilizing some ideas from reflexology in a therapy practice. Just as other people may use some skills taught to occupational and physical therapy practitioners but cannot call themselves an OT or PT without appropriate training, so too, unless one has undergone a full reflexology training program, one must not use this professional title.

hands and feet, especially fore and mid sections, as well as wrists and ankles (Issel & Rogers, 2000). In recent years Sandi Rogers, of Australia, has encouraged reflexologists to also learn techniques to address the muscles of the forearm and leg in order that any tension there can be released so that the hands and feet can function more freely.

Another significant difference between reflexology and massage is that reflexologists generally eschew any form of lubrication during a treatment, with the exception of corn starch to absorb sweat or a light lubrication creme on very dry feet, because they have found that one can have more precise contact with discrete areas of hands and feet without lubrication. Lotion is often applied at the end of a session as an added benefit to the client's skin. However, recently introduced in the United States by Father Joseph of Taiwan is a technique (referred to as the Father Joseph Method or FJM) that requires lubrication because of the deep penetration and gliding moves utilized.

Possible Reactions

A reflexology session is a healing session and as such some uncomfortable reactions are possible. The more common are generalized or local discomfort; flu-like symptoms as the body experiences some cleansing and rebalancing: nausea, headache, fatigue, dizziness; increased output of organs of elimination (skin, bladder, bowel), emotional release (e.g., crying); changes in sleep patterns; or temporary exacerbation of a disease or commencement of symptoms from a subclinical illness. All of the above are often temporary. If they persist, some adjustment in parameters of the reflexology session must be made, and the client should be referred to a more appropriate clinician.

Practice

In both traditional and integrative health care settings, reflexology can be used as an informal assessment tool. The feet especially will often reveal areas of congested tissues that may correspond to areas of congestion in the corresponding body parts. Reflexology techniques also quickly initiate an overall (whole-body) state of relaxation. Reflexology can be used by a trained therapist along with other appropriate techniques when there is an order for manual care as part of, or the total of, the treatment plan. Therapy notes should reflect the use of reflexology (DeDomenico & Wood, 1997).

Incorporating reflexology techniques, the therapist can work both indirectly and directly on the effected area(s), increasing client comfort and hastening the recovery process. Work on one or more of the microcosms can be focused on specific areas in the macrocosm to initiate increased blood flow and decreased nerve irritation to that area. Techniques can be used to *indirectly* address any region of the body that cannot be touched directly for therapeutic intervention, such as a burn, an ulcer, Kaposi's sarcoma, an unhealed surgical scar, a section that is encased in a cast, or a body part that cannot tolerate touch, such as where there is intense nerve or muscle pain (e.g., neuralgia or myositis).

How long a client is treated with reflexology techniques depends on several factors. How ill or frail is the client? Short sessions of 5 to 15 minutes are appropriate for those who are acutely ill, very young, frail, or elderly. An appropriate approach is "less is more," which

Indications for Reflexology

- Pain relief
- Relaxation of muscle spasms
- Reduction of nerve irritation/pain
- Stimulate flow of blood and lymph
- Stimulate or sedate all glands and organs
- Introduce self-help management techniques
- Effect systemic/overall relaxation
- Enhance sense of well-being and reduce effects of stress

Contraindications/Precautions for Reflexology

Some authors and instructors state that there are almost no contraindications for reflexology. As with any therapeutic intervention, however, one must assess each individual client and treat him or her accordingly. If not used judiciously, a modality which is powerful enough to have the potential for good also has the potential for harm. Thus, depending on degree of severity of symptoms, possible contraindications or precautions to consider are

- Any condition of feet, hands, or ears that would preclude touching that part: skin that is not intact, infection, gangrene, athlete's foot, unhealed fracture, or significant osteoporosis, including Sudeck's atrophy.
- Phlebitis or lymphangitis.
- Acute infection or diseases, especially with fever, or if the client is contagious.
- High risk pregnancy, especially first trimester of first pregnancy (consult obstetrician). *Note:* Many women report anecdotally that reflexology can assist in becoming pregnant and maintaining good health during pregnancy as well as helping them have a comfortable delivery. Caution must be observed with high-risk pregnancies. Discuss benefits versus possible adverse reactions. Also be aware that there are some meridian points (i.e., SP6, GB40, B160) to avoid until the woman is ready to deliver (Reid & Enzer, 1997).
- Premature infants until they have stabilized; treatment should be carefully monitored by nursery staff.
- Unstable blood pressure. *Note:* Reflexology often helps normalize blood pressure, but one must be cautious when blood pressure has great swings.
- Severely psychologically disturbed clients, unless the client is in a supportive mental health facility.
- Clients with multiple diagnoses and/or multiple medications: Be very cautious.
- Recent heart attack or organ transplant, until stable and approved by doctor.
- Lymph-borne cancers, unless reflexology done for pain relief in a hospice situation. *Note:* Reflexology has the potential to stimulate the immune system along with all the glands and organs, thus providing support for the body to facilitate health and healing.
- The first few days after chemotherapy.

refers both to duration and intensity of techniques, so that the body is not overstimulated and pushed into a healing crisis.

It is best to treat the whole two feet (or hands or ears) for the whole body, as it is believed everything in the body is interconnected and the therapist may not know for sure what that particular body needs to stimulate healing for a specific problem area. The reality of most PT and OT departments is that time is rather constrained. Even 5 minutes spent on the ears, the smallest or most compact microcosm, the fingers or toes to loosen all joints, or the pads of the thumbs or great toes, where all five zones for that side of the body are represented, is seen as being of great benefit.

A typical session by a professional reflexologist for an overall "tune-up" usually lasts 30 to 45 minutes in the United States. A client receiving the FJM may have his or her feet worked on for 10 minutes, very intensely and firmly, and may be seen for a series of 10 daily sessions at a minimum.

Frequency varies according to the problem being addressed. As long as the duration of sessions and the intensity of technique work are carefully graded to monitor the client's reactions, a person can receive reflexology techniques daily. Closely spaced sessions are especially appropriate for musculoskeletal problems, including self-care with hand techniques or the use of tools such as a foot roller or small bumpy ball (e.g., "goosebumps" ball) for the hands. Brief sessions once, twice, or three times a day of self-care are also appropriate for issues of edema and pain management. As with most any other therapy, sessions are typically closely spaced initially, then gradually scheduled less frequently as symptoms decrease and the client's ability to manage self-care increases. Ideally, sessions are daily or at least three times a week for the greatest benefit. Once symptoms have diminished, clients can continue with self-care techniques and have periodic "tune ups" from a reflexologist. Acute conditions generally resolve more quickly than chronic conditions.

There are many opinions about intensity of technique application. As mentioned earlier, for those clients whose health is fragile or unstable, "less is more" definitely applies. Care must be taken to observe reactions, as with any other therapeutic intervention. It is usually best to start with some joint loosening techniques for the digits, metacarpals/wrist or metatarsals/ankle. This begins to soften tension in the tissues. The reflexologist uses light palpation for an assessment of the foot, hand, and ear. Once the most tender or sensitive areas have been identified, then moderate to firm pressure can be applied to effect a change in the sensitivity and thus address the macrocosm target area.

One of the advantages of working on a microcosm (i.e., feet, hands, ears) is that the areas are small, allowing for efficient treatment. While reflexology has many benefits, it does not replace other forms of hands-on care, such as trigger point and myofascial release, traditional Swedish massage, and so on, which are done directly on the areas in need of help and are not based on the concept of microcosms or a map and zones.

Reflexology can be combined with other healing arts, such as Reiki, Jin Shin Jyutsu, polarity, and chakra balancing. These energy-based techniques can be performed on the microcosm to affect the macrocosm. For example, one can give a person a Reiki session by only addressing the map of the body on the feet. Many polarity therapy techniques involve the feet, hands, and ears, but if all one had access to were the microcosms, one could theoretically address the whole body through those areas by incorporating reflexology techniques.

Reflexology techniques of thumb-walking and joint loosening can be of great benefit to a nonambulatory client in that they will serve to mimic some of the sensory-motor aspects of walking by keeping the feet flexible as well as by stimulating the myriad of sensory end organs, including proprioceptors, found in the feet especially, but also in the hands.

Research

Outcome, mechanism (how and why the method works), and sociological (e.g., what problems reflexologists typically treat, the duration of and reimbursement for treatment) studies on reflexology, while in their infancy, reflect promising results.

Outcome Studies

The earliest American reflexology research using modern medical research protocols was performed by Oleson and Flocco (1993). Thirty-five women with previous premenstrual syndrome (PMS) were randomly assigned to receive either reflexology or placebo reflexology. These researchers found that reflexology significantly reduced PMS for the 8 weeks of the study and for 2 months after treatment versus placebo reflexology.

Eriksen (1995) studied the effect of reflexology on 220 patients who had either migraines or serious tension headaches. The study did not report findings in terms of significance, but at follow up after 6 months, 25 percent of the tension headache group and 20 percent from the migraine group reported being "cured." Seventy-six percent of migraine subjects reported positive effects since reflexology treatment, and 19 percent of subjects were able to cease using headache medication.

Zhen-shen and Xue-zhen (1998) treated 38 people with cerebrovascular accidents (CVA), using reflexology. The authors note 74 percent ($n = 28$) of the subjects experienced significant relief of symptoms (i.e., returned to walking independently). Because there was no control group, however, it is difficult to attribute the clinical change to reflexology.

The China Reflexology Association has collected data on the efficacy and effects of reflexology on many types of diseases and dysfunction. This data includes detailed descriptions of reflexology interventions for specific problems. By far the most published research on reflexology is from the Chinese, although obtaining a full English translation of the reports is an issue. Refer to Flocco (1999) and Kunz and Kunz (1999); in both, a comprehensive list of U.S. and international reflexology research has been compiled.

Mechanism

Research done to explain the relationship of human body cavities to the feet is underway in Australia by Rogers (1993). A preliminary study suggests that there are relationships between foot disturbances (deviations from normal) and zone-related conditions. For example, it was noted that if the calcaneus deviated significantly from neutral, the subject almost invariably reported some sort of pelvic cavity discomfort, such as bowel, bladder, reproductive, or sacroilliac and lower lumbar problems. Rogers plans further studies to validate the correspondence of the midfoot to the abdominal cavity and the forefoot to the thoracic and cranial cavities.

Investigations of some physiological changes one might expect with reflexology sessions were reported by Dalal (1999). This researcher measured skin impedance at areas corresponding to reflex areas on the feet and found that impedance decreases at reflex areas when a corresponding organ or system is malfunctioning, in proportion both to the extent and duration of system dysfunction. This study is important because it gives credence to the "maps" reflexologists use to address illness.

Uebaba (1999) studied the effect of reflexology on the circulatory system with a total of 30 subjects. After reflexology, subjects had significant changes in heart rate (which decreased), metabolic rate and CO_2 excretion/O_2 uptake (which increased), and no significant changes in blood pressure, EEG activity, cardiac output, and muscle blood flow output.

Frankel (1997) compared measures of baroreceptor reflex sensitivity (BRS) (e.g., blood pressure and sinus arrhythmia) on groups of subjects who had reflexology ($n = 10$), foot massage ($n = 10$), or no treatment ($n = 4$). Decreases in BRS are typically experienced with relaxation. He found that the reflexology and foot massage groups experienced reduced BRS more, though not significantly more, than the control group. While the sample size in this study was small, it suggests that reflexology with foot massage is clearly differentiated from no treatment. More research is needed to distinguish how traditional foot massage differs from reflexology.

Sociological Studies

Reflexology is the most frequently used CAM in Denmark (Rasmussen et al., 1988; Andersen, 1990; Launso, 1992, as cited in Launso, 1993), and the Danish Organization of Reflexologists, with other CAM organizations, have studied reflexology practice in Denmark thoroughly (Launso, 1993). Launso found, for example, that Danish reflexologists use it mostly for muscle/body pain (39 percent), stomach pain/digestive problems (14 percent), asthma/bronchitis/allergy (8 percent), headache/migraine (7 percent), and hormonal problems (5 percent). The majority of reflexology clients complained of a minimum of two health problems (53 percent), have chronic health problems (more than 5 years duration; 56 percent), and have seen a doctor prior to beginning reflexology (77 percent).

Case Studies

Spastic Pyloric Sphincter

One of the author's early confirmations of the power of reflexology involved a nurse in her mid-30s who had developed liver cancer. She was in urgent need of a transplant and was put on a waiting list. Apparently brought on by tension, her pyloric sphincter became so spastic that she vomited any liquid or solid she tried to ingest. This continued for 2 months, at which time a compatible liver became available. Despite her stomach problem, her doctor decided to proceed with the transplant, as compatible donor organs are hard to find. A month after her successful surgery, she was still unable to drink or eat. A mutual friend suggested that reflexology might help her. Using Hanne Marquardt's book *Reflex Zone Therapy of the Feet* as a guide, techniques that would help relax her whole body as well as ones focused on her digestive tract were chosen. As she was in the hospital and in serious condition, a light and short (15 to 20 minutes) session was performed. She seemed to tolerate the work well and slept better that night. A second treatment was given 4 days later. This time, reflexology was performed a little deeper and somewhat longer, again planning the session to focus on the digestive "map" on her feet as well as addressing the whole two feet to facilitate healing in the whole body. When the author called a few days later to set up a third appointment, the client replied, "You can come *if you want to,* but I just had pizza and coke. Thank you very much!" Apparently she had been dreaming of the day she could resume eating and drinking her favorite foods. No further reflexology was indicated after this dramatic resolution to the client's complaint.

Limited Motion in Neck and Shoulder

While driving his SUV on a country road, Al was rear-ended by an 18-wheel truck. When this 38-year-old man came to an outpatient physical therapy department a few weeks later, the range of motion in his neck was extremely limited in all planes, as was range of motion in the shoulder girdle. Al rated pain in this area as a 10 out of 10. Previously, he had been in excellent health, performing vigorous outside work as a landscape architect and owner of horses. Initially, it was hard for him to tolerate clothing, especially jackets, as he was very sensitive to any pressure on his skin and muscles. He could not be treated by hot packs, ultrasound, or electrical stimulation because of his extreme sensitivity. Al was seen 3 times weekly for 45 minutes each session. For the first 2 weeks that the author saw the client, reflexology was used to decrease his overall tension and pain as well as to decrease pain and prepare him for effleurage to the neck and shoulders. Techniques included extensive work, loosening interphalangeal, metatarsal-phalangeal and tarsal and metatarsal joints, and thumb-walking, especially over the pad and stem of the great toe as well as the long medial arch. Also, both feet were worked on to enhance immune functioning and overall health, since he was under severe stress. As discomfort in his feet and hands diminished, so did the sensitivity in his neck and shoulder region, to the point where he could tolerate and benefit from other modalities (e.g., direct massage) and also begin an exercise program. The author continued to work with the client for manual sessions, using reflexology as a preparatory treatment and progressively incorporating more massage as well as myofascial and trigger point releases. After 8 weeks of treatment, the client was discharged from therapy. Range of motion was restored to half of "normal," with low to moderate pain (4 to 5 out of 10) occasionally spiking to a higher degree (7 or 8). He was able to return to work, performing light duty, supervisory tasks as a landscaper.

Charcot Joints

Miriam is a 58-year-old artist who has diabetes type II and breast cancer, for which she had a mastectomy and now undergoes chemotherapy. Additionally, she was told in 1991 that she had charcot joints (joint disease marked by bony overgrowths) of the left foot, especially around the navicular bone. The left foot is markedly pronated, with resultant near-ulceration, approximately ½-inch diameter, of the plantar surface, midway along medial side. She reported that the resultant foot pain was debilitating, and clinical examination revealed 75 percent range of motion limitations in the toes, forefoot, and ankle. The client was able to ambulate with a cane only limited distances (200 to 300 feet).

Miriam was referred to physical therapy for foot pain, upper extremity lymphedema, and pain secondary to shingles. The client was seen in outpatient physical therapy 1 to 2 times a week by the author for manual care and by a physical therapist who specialized in exercise programs. She was referred for reflexology to address the foot pain and lymphedema. Manual lymphatic drainage (MLD) techniques were used to address mild lymphedema of limbs, and light to moderate effleurage and petrissage were used for reconditioning. Reflexology usually encompassed about half of the allotted 30 minute session on her feet, incorporating gentle joint mobilization and a variety of specific reflexology techniques to address the vascular and lymphatic circulation of the feet and entire body.

Gradually, over a course of 4 months, Miriam's feet became more flexible, her circulation improved to the point where her skin was fully intact, and she reported an improved sense of well-being as well as significantly less pain. She was discharged, able to ambulate around the block and while shopping, and used the cane only for long walks of three blocks and over. At a recent visit to her orthopedic physician, who had been contemplating a major foot reconstruction, Miriam was told that not only could he see that her skin was well-healed but also that the x-rays showed her navicular bone and surrounding joints were greatly improved, with no evidence of charcot damage.

Summary

Ingham wrote "Reflexology in any form is only a means of exercise, a means of equalizing the circulation; we all know circulation is life, stagnation is death. Everything around us that is alive is in motion" (1998, p. 104). This healing method is based on the concept of mapping—guides that detail the relationship between the feet, hands, and ears to the whole body. The therapist stimulates reflex points, or points of contact, on the feet, hands, and ears to effect change both locally (to the directed area) and at corresponding body areas. Reflexology can be used as an adjunct to traditional therapy practice or provided as a standalone holistic practice.

STUDY QUESTIONS

1. Define the concept reflexologists refer to as a map.
2. Where on the foot are the following body cavities represented: cranial, thoracic, abdominal, and pelvic?

3. How does reflexology differ from massage?
4. How can reflexology be used to augment traditional therapy for specific conditions?
5. What is the research support for reflexology use?
6. Consider a client you have seen in a clinical internship. Discuss which reflex points a reflexologist might aim to address and why. Are you seeking to address specific illnesses or overall homeostasis? Also discuss two discharge options one might use with such a client.

SUGGESTED READING

Dougans, I. (1996). *Complete Illustrated Guide to Reflexology*. Rockport, MA: Element Books.

Issel, C. (1990). *Reflexology: Art, Science & History*. Sacramento, CA: New Frontier Publishing.

Kunz, K., & B. Kunz. (1993). *The Complete Guide to Foot Reflexology* (rev. ed.). Albuquerque, NM: Author.

Kunz, K. J. B. (1996). *The Parent's Guide to Reflexology*. New York: Three Rivers Press.

Marquardt, H. (1984). *Reflex Zone Therapy of the Feet*. New York: Thorsons.

Oleson, T. (1996). *Auriculo Therapy Manual* (2nd ed.). Los Angeles, CA: Health Care Alternatives.

RESOURCES

Associated Bodywork & Massage
   Professionals, Inc. (ABMP)
1271 Sugarbush Drive
Evergreen, CO 80439-7347
(800) 458-2267
www.abmp.com

Reflexology Research Project
Kevin Kunz
PO Box 35820, Station D
Albuquerque, NM 87176
www.reflexology-research.com
www.foot-reflexologist.com

REFLEXOLOGY ORGANIZATIONS

State Organizations

Contact RAA to see if your state has one.

National Organization

Reflexology Association of America (RAA)
4012 South Rainbow, Ste. KPMB#585
Las Vegas, NV 89103-2059
(702) 871-9522
www.reflexology-USA.org

International Organization

International Council of Reflexologists (ICR)
PO Box 30513
Richmond Hill
Ontario L4C OC7 Canada
icr.samek@sympatico.ca

National Certification for Professional
   Reflexologists

American Reflexology Certification Board
   (ARCB)
PO Box 740879
Arvada, CO 80006-0879
(303) 933-6921

National School Accreditation for
   Professional Reflexologists

American Commission for Accreditation
   of Reflexology Education and Training
   (ACARET)
PO Box 9111
Seattle, WA 98108
(206) 284-8389
lhensell@netzero.net

REFERENCES

Andersen, J. G. (1990). Overtro eller nytænkning. Befolkningens brug af og holding til alternative be-handlingsformer. In Danish. (Superstition or innovation. The population's use of and attitude towards alternative treatment.) Center for Cultural Research, Arhus University, Arhus.

Crane, B. (1998). *Reflexology: A Basic Guide*. Rockport, MA: Element Books.

Crane, B. (1997). *Reflexology: The Definitive Practitioner's Manual (Feet, Hands, Ears)*. Rockport, MA: Element Books.

Dalal, K. (1999). A quantitative estimation of reflex areas/points and management of different ail-ments through reflexology. *International Council of Reflexologists 1999 Conference*, 70–73.

DeDomenico, G., & E. Wood. (1997). *Beard's Massage* (4th ed.). Philadelphia: Saunders.

Dougans, I. (1996). *The Complete Illustrated Guide to Reflexology*. Rockport, MA: Element Books.

Eastman, Y. (1991). *Touchpoint: Reflexology, The First Steps.* Campbell River, B.C., Canada: Ptarmigan Press.

Eriksen, L. (1995). Reflexology is an effective treatment for headaches. *Danish Reflexologists Associa-tion Research Committee Report.*

Flocco, B. (1999a). *Reflexology Articles.* Burbank, CA: Sanford.

Flocco, B. (1999b). *Reflexology Research.* Burbank, CA: Sanford.

Frandsen, (2000). Why does Reflexology work? Is the explanation found in the embryo? *ICR Newslet-ter, 9*(4), 10–12, 14.

Frankel, B. S. M. (1997). The effect of reflexology on baroreceptor reflex sensitivity, blood pressure, and sinus arrhythmia. *Complementary Therapies in Medicine, 5*, 80–84.

Ingham, E. (1998). *Stories the Feet Can Tell and Have Told Thru Reflexology.* St. Petersburg, FL: Ingham Publishing.

Issel, C., & S. B. Rogers. (2000). *Reflexognosy: A Shift in Paradigm.* Sacramento, CA: New Frontier Publishing.

Kunz, K., & B. Kunz. (1999). *Medical Applications of Reflexology: Findings in Research about Safety, Efficacy, Mechanism of Action and Cost-Effectiveness of Reflexology.* Albuquerque, NM: RRP Press.

Launso, L. (1993). *A Description of Reflexology Practice and Clientele in Denmark.* Copenhagen, Den-mark: The United Danish Reflexologists' Association Research Committee.

Oleson, T., & W. Flocco. (1993). Randomized controlled study of premenstrual symptoms treated with foot, hand, and ear reflexology. *Obstetrics and Gynecology, 82*(6), 906–911.

Rasmussen, N. Kr., M. V. Groth, S. R. Bredkjær, M. Madsen, & F. Kamper-Jørgensen. (1988). Sund-hed og sygelighed i Danmark i 1989. In Danish. (Health and morbidity in Denmark in 1989.) A report from DIKE's study. Dansk Institut for Klinisk Epidemiologi, Copenhagen.

Reid, L., & S. Enzer. (1997). *Maternity Reflexology.* Bowen Mountain, N.S.W., Australia: Born to Be Free & Soul to Soul Reflexology.

Rogers, S. (1993). Reflexology on trial. *LifeWise Magazine, 1*(4), 17–20.

Uebaba, K. (1999). Physiological changes by reflexology: Modification of circulatory system by reflex-ology. *1999 China Reflexology Symposium Report*, 84–85.

Wills, P. (1996). *The Reflexology Manual.* Rochester, VT: Healing Arts Press.

Zhen-shen, W., & L. Xue-zhen. (1998). Treatment of 38 cases of ischemic apoplexy with reflexology. *1998 China Reflexology Symposium Report*, 1–4.

19

Reiki

Ann Marie McClintock

CHAPTER OBJECTIVES

- Define Reiki.
- Discuss theories about Reiki's mechanism of action.
- Describe a typical Reiki session.
- Explain the relevance of Reiki to rehabilitation practice.
- Understand related research.
- Describe Reiki training.

The Japanese word *Reiki* refers both to a "universal life energy" and a gentle, noninvasive healing technique used to promote healing through the transferring of this energy. *Rei* refers to "universal spiritual guidance" and *ki* to "vital life force." Reiki is classified by the National Center for Complementary and Alternative Medicine (NCCAM) as a biofield medicine that uses the subtle energy fields in and around the body for medical reasons. Usually described as a hands-on healing method, Reiki can also be given without physical touch and in long distance work without physical proximity to the client. Reiki has even been referred to as "nontraditional prayer" (Wirth & Cram, 1994).

Reiki is an example of an "ancient wisdom" healing method that was rediscovered and developed in Japan in the early 20th century. The exact mechanism of Reiki healing is not known, yet Reiki literature abounds in anecdotal stories of personal healing. As Reiki is scrutinized by science, evidence of its healing effects is emerging.

Reiki is a simple healing method to learn in that one is empowered through a unique system of "attunements," or energy transfer processes. The attunements consist of energy transfer from Reiki master to student and are accomplished through an "initiation" through which the intentions of both are aligned with the Reiki source for the empowerment to take place. Attunement and healing effects, while subjective, are palpable. Common experiences of Reiki energy are heat, vibration or tingling, and sharper perception of colors and bodily sensations.

Reiki's most frequent claim is that it is a gentle, noninvasive, holistic healing method that can be used in pain and stress reduction; it works by restoring mental, emotional, and physical balance. With advanced use, Reiki is a way to restore wellness and to grow in mind, body, and spirit, developing talents and personal potentials. For one who has embraced Reiki as a "way," there is no ending point to its use, but a continuation through all of life. Pursued daily and for life, Reiki becomes the vitality of the spiritual journey.

As a complementary healing method, Reiki connects universal life energy with the body's innate self-healing wisdom. Reiki is as equally useful in community wellness, preventive medicine, and health promotion programs as it is in treatment of disease. Reiki attunements are available to all persons, including children. All levels of human development and human frailty can be found among its practitioners. To become a Reiki master is accomplished through the master attunement, although mastery by Reiki is realized through dedication and daily practice of Reiki principles. While Reiki is a spiritual and not a religious healing practice, it is sometimes accompanied by ritual or prayer in a variety of community and personal interpretations. Although Reiki is an unusual modality to the scientific mind, its effects can be felt, observed, described, and quantified.

Historical Background

There are many types and variations of Reiki, but the word Reiki by itself usually refers to, and is used here to refer to, the Usui tradition of natural healing. Many ancient cultures have healing traditions utilizing the universal life force and laying-on-of-hands. Mikao Usui, Japanese scholar and theologian, influenced by Buddhist teachings and keenly interested in healing, dis-

Therapy Focus

Reiki is an energy therapy. It can accompany conventional therapy practice or alternative health techniques, such as craniosacral therapy, therapeutic touch, and others, before, during, or after a usual therapy session. Reiki can be offered prior to a treatment or procedure that causes anxiety or discomfort for a client. Reiki can be provided post-therapy for relaxation, pain reduction, and enhancement of natural healing. As an adjunct in the therapy clinic, Reiki is offered as a brief period, perhaps 10 minutes, of hands-on healing. Reiki can also be integrated with a therapy method; it is simply activated by thoughtful intention. This involves intending (sending) Reiki energy at the same time one is treating a client.

Reiki can be used as a health-promoting "partner" to any treatment modality—physical, psychological, or spiritual. A Reiki clinic can be an adjunct to rehabilitation and other hospital services and can serve both inpatients and outpatients. Use of volunteers allow for this service to be both inexpensive and convenient. Staff as well as clients can receive Reiki "stress-reducing" sessions in the workplace. Reiki can also be part of an aftercare plan. Interested family members, caregivers, and clients can be attuned to Reiki and continue to provide Reiki after discharge.

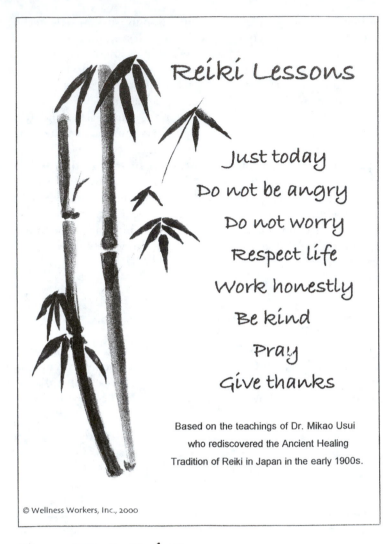

Figure 19–1 Reiki Lessons   *Used with permission of Wellness Workers, Inc.*

covered the ancient Reiki healing art in the early 1900s. Following 21 days of fasting and meditation on secluded Mount Kurama in Japan, he had a mystical experience of enlightenment and attunement with the Reiki source. A humble and compassionate man and a "teacher," described on the Usui memorial as one "who uses the 'great spirit' for social purposes, to teach the right way to many people and do collective good," he began using this system and passed his knowledge on to others (Petter, 1997, p. 28). Other notable persons in Reiki lineage are Dr. Chujiro Hayashi and Mrs. Hawaya Takata. Before her death in 1980, Mrs. Takata initiated 22 students as Reiki masters. She and her students are largely, but not exclusively, responsible for bringing Reiki to the United States and into the world. Reiki teachings were handed down orally by Mrs. Takata to her students. As recently as 1997, *Usui Reiki Ryoho Hikkei,* a manuscript written by

Dr. Mikao Usui as a handbook for his Reiki students, was discovered in Japan and translated into English (Petter, 1999).

The principles of Reiki as taught by Dr. Usui to his students are equally guidelines for and outcomes of Reiki healing practice: daily meditation, an attitude of gratefulness, integrity in work, emotional and mental balance, and kindness to all living things.

How Reiki Works

The exact mechanism of Reiki is unknown. Because of observed effects of behavioral or physical change and subjective reports of felt changes, such as reduced anxiety, lessened pain, brightened mood, increased energy, and spiritual and existential change, the following is a frequently offered hypothesis:

Reiki infuses the human energy field with vital life force. This is guided by the innate and unconscious cellular wisdom of the body-mind itself, which draws upon *ki* according to its needs. This is experienced in practice as being drawn or "pulled into" the body, as if by cellular demand. A healthy and balanced physical state is characterized by high ki, or free flow of vital life force.

Pert (1997) describes "biochemicals of emotion," which exchange information between the neural, endocrine, immune, and other systems of the body. Disturbances in people's vitality, as expressed in physical illness, are concomitantly to be found in their emotional and thinking lives. These disturbances exist in the biofield, or energy field, that surrounds and penetrates the physical body. The character of energy flow in the body is first electromagnetic and then ionic before it becomes molecular. As a result of this flow from subtle to dense, disorders in the physical body appear to result from imbalances in the subtle energies or biofield. That is, biofield disturbances precede the manifestation of disease. Reiki energy works to dissolve these blocks to restore balance, working at the "cause" rather than the symptom.

While concepts such as psychoneuroimmunology (PNI) partially explain healing phenomenon, the precise mechanism of how the *mind of a person in intention of healing* can bring about healing, physiologic effects in the bodies and minds of people is not known. Even more challenging is the mechanism of long-distance healing and how this can result in healthful changes in another person. Ancient traditions and present-day theorists hold that the human body is made up of energy systems. The unified energy foundation of the universe theory presumes a consciousness-mediated interconnectedness that permeates everything and is able to influence energetic and material events. Reiki healing could occur by way of this energy connection. The study of quantum physics and unified field theory probe for answers to these questions. Refer to Rubik (1995), Gerber (2001), and Dossey (1999) for further readings on possible mechanisms.

In addition to theorized mechanisms, research in the biomagnetic human energy field points to scientific basis of energy healing. Instruments such as the SQUID (superconducting quantum interference device) magnetometer, Kirlian photography, tensometers, and nuclear magnetic resonators have been used to detect extremely subtle energy fields emanating from objects. Electrical conduction and electromagnetic field studies measure the flow of this energy via energy healing techniques such as therapeutic touch and Reiki (Wirth & Cram, 1994; Brewitt, Vittetoe, & Hartwell, 1997; Benor, 2001; Becker & Seldon, 1985).

Indications

- Enhance relaxation
- Support the body's natural healing process
- Support the immune system
- Manage stress and tension
- Reduce anxiety or fear
- Combat fatigue
- Alleviate depression
- Calm the mind
- Alleviate acute or chronic pain
- Enrich lifestyle
- Balance mind, body, and spirit
- Provide spiritual comfort

Contraindications

- Reiki should not be provided if clients do not want it

A Reiki Session

A typical Reiki session has formal hand positions and is often done with the client lying down on a massage table. Reiki does not require assessment, although an energy technique called "scanning" can be used, which is helpful in sensing energy field differences. There is great variation in the length of a Reiki session: An average session is likely to be about an hour. Hand positions taught for Reiki vary from complex and specific to basic positions simple enough to be learned by children. These positions occur along the energy centers of the spine, known in Eastern thought as the chakras; these parallel the glands of the endocrine system and major nerve plexuses of the body. Time spent on an energy center may be 3 to 5 minutes; an experienced practitioner will usually feel the energy flow as it is "drawn" by the body, and the sensation itself will provide guidance to the practitioner in when to move on to another area. Energy techniques frequently used with Reiki include scanning, smoothing, lifting negative energy off of, and energizing the energy field. Sometimes techniques employing breath, tapping, sound, visualization, color, crystals, and other vibrational healing tools assist the movement of energy. Many books provide excellent instruction on Reiki (Baginski & Sharamon, 1988; Barnett & Chambers, 1996; Horan, 1992; Severino, 1995; Rowland, 1998). Lubeck, Petter, and Rand (2001) present recently discovered Japanese Reiki techniques.

Reiki can be offered with great flexibility. Distant healing, sent by intention, usually while in a meditative state and with the use of sacred symbols, is most easily described as a nonlocal healing method similar to prayer. While this seems unusual to the "Western" mind, as science investigates prayer, it is demonstrating that prayer makes a healing difference (Byrd, 1988; Dossey, 1999). It is the writer's belief that Reiki, like prayer, engaged by clear healing intention and without directedness towards specific outcomes, may be found to have its greatest power.

The initial experience of Reiki is usually one of relaxation. Although initial sessions may alleviate symptoms, continuation with Reiki works at the level of "cause." Physical symptoms or emotional reactions such as tearfulness may occur as energy blocks are cleared and cleansed. Mental and emotional issues come "up" for clearing as Reiki deeply impacts the body-mind. Attunements to Reiki and intensive Reiki healing work bring about a change in the person's energy field to a higher vibration. This is sometimes accompanied by physical detoxification symptoms as negative energy is released. Other possible outward signs of this process are dreams and emotional changes (Horan, 1992). Some Reiki teachers suggest dietary changes and quiet meditative time to assist the body in the purification process that accompanies attunement (Rand, 1998) and deeper healing work.

Reiki supports the body's natural healing process. Practitioners have found that superficial problems can be alleviated in one session and that chronic issues may be gradually lessened through Reiki-supported lifestyle change. Dramatic healing effects such as cancer remission (ICRT, 1990–2001) and spiritual change (Mansour et al., 1998) are also reported anecdotally.

Reiki does not have a "typical" practice. It is widely applicable and can accompany just about any therapy or helping session. Present applications are found in hospitals, community clinics, prisons, schools, nursing homes, hospices, wellness centers, health and fitness centers, spiritual retreat centers, and perhaps most importantly, the home.

Health care workers can suggest Reiki to clients as a relaxation technique that enhances physical healing by helping the body to relax. Reiki is a gentle healing touch that may reduce pain and lessen anxiety or fear of a procedure. The client's approval should be sought, although a simple explanation or demonstration is often all that is needed. Reiki must usually be experienced to be appreciated, and so a "sample" session might be offered to help a person decide whether to pursue it further. With children and confused elderly, it may be as simple as a demonstration of touch, requesting approval first, because it often makes a person feel better. It should be clear that Reiki is meant to be supportive of and not to replace any traditional medical care.

Reiki can be quietly incorporated into the conventional therapy session (Behar, 1997) or can be integrated into healing sessions using other hands-on alternative techniques, such as Shiatsu, trigger point, and massage. While Reiki is often given on a massage table, a quick treatment in a chair or wherever the client is can also occur. Reiki can be integrated into psychosocial or mental health therapies as well as bodywork therapies. It can be given "by intention" with no touch required. The effects of Reiki may be felt or subjectively reported immediately or may become evident only with cumulative contacts. When Reiki is given with repeated client contacts on a long-term basis, and observations of psychosocial or behavioral changes are recorded, cumulative effects should be noted.

Reiki in Wellness and Healthy Lifestyle Programs

Because the body may have accumulated disease and unhealthy energy blocks over years of living, the clearing away of blocks often occurs as a gradual, natural healing process over years of improved living. Reiki supports clear intention in the client to "do the work" of healing, which means to choose to care for the self through a balanced lifestyle, good nutrition, and balance in activities and rest, self-care, work, recreation, and mental and spiritual activities. As one pursues Reiki on a daily basis, healthy lifestyle and personal development of talents and abilities is promoted. Reiki does this by breaking through the emotional issues or negative mental attitudes that prevent growth from occurring. This method has application in health promotion and wellness programs in which an individual seeks to work towards lifestyle changes that support health on all levels. Gleisner (1992), Upczak (1999), and Narrin (1998) provide delightful personal accounts of the process of Reiki lifestyle change.

Reiki is an inexpensive technique to teach clients and families to carry out at home. It enhances care given to the elderly and to those with chronic illness. It is a caring technique for caregivers in a family to give and receive. Some interesting applications of Reiki are the training and attunement of prison inmates to Reiki (Stanley, 1999), and of police officers and firefighters (Kahne, 1998). It has also been used with pain (Olson & Hanson, 1997), in palliative care (Bullock, 1997), during pregnancy and childbearing (Hebner, 2000), and to support surgical patients (Alandydy & Alandydy, 1999). Reiki is used with pastoral care with HIV/AIDS (Stevens, 2001), and often as a complementary therapy for nursing practice (Nield-Anderson & Ameling, 2001; Rivera, 1999). A study in process is the use of Reiki with teenagers struggling with stress and substance abuse (Terry Anderson of California Institute of Integral Studies, June 18, 2001, personal communication). Descriptions of innovative Reiki applications developed in several hospitals have been gathered by Rand (1998); many of these allow large numbers of patients to receive Reiki at little cost. Barnett and Chambers (1996) describe hospital Reiki rooms where staff and patients come to receive Reiki sessions staffed by volunteers. Reiki Web sites offer long-distance healing for personal requests. International long-distance Reiki healing organized through the Internet focuses group intention on world peace, human rights, and the healing of the earth itself.

Research

Abundant anecdotal examples of Reiki healing effects in health care are provided by Barnett and Chambers (1996), Eos (1995), and Rivera (1999) as well as in a myriad of books and articles recounting personal stories of healing. Few rigorous research studies have been conducted on Reiki. Subtle energy and spiritual healing methods such as Reiki have been criticized for lack of scientific validity, yet changes in attitudes towards energy healing is occurring at this time (Ai et al., 2001). Benor (2001) has extensively reviewed over 191 controlled studies in the area of spiritual and energy healing, with two-thirds of these demonstrating significant effects.

Reiki Outcome Studies

Olson and Hanson (1997) conducted a pilot study to explore the usefulness of Reiki as an adjunct to opioid therapy in management of pain. This study involved 20 volunteers experiencing pain at 55 sites for a variety of reasons, including cancer. Pain was measured using a visual analogue scale and a Likert scale before and after the Reiki treatment. Both instruments showed a highly significant ($p < 0.0001$) reduction in pain following the Reiki treatment.

Unique to Reiki is the attunement through which one becomes empowered to access universal life force energy consistently. Unlike other therapy disciplines and skills, the ability to practice Reiki is opened through this process rather than through "education" in the academic or skills-training sense. Attunement links the student with the Reiki source and empowers him or her to become a conduit for universal life force energy. The attunement also fine-tunes and balances the energy system and has clearing and cleansing effects for a time afterwards.

Reiki certification programs typically involve three levels. In First Degree Reiki, practitioners learn about the history of Reiki, the concepts involved, and hand positions on the self and others. The practitioner becomes empowered through a series of attunements; sacred symbols are generally not revealed. Second Degree empowers healing at deeper levels of the energy field, including emotional and mental balancing and long-distance healing, and teaches and uses sacred symbols. Third Degree further enhances healing energies and prepares the practitioner to teach and attune others. Third Degree is generally taught after a person has had some experience in practice and application.

There is considerable variation in the training, the number of attunements, the length of the training, and the content of programs. Despite these differences in programs, Reiki energy is always transferred, by intention, from master to student during an attunement. Certification is provided by the Reiki master who has provided the initiation. A student who wishes to appreciate the history and practice of this healing tradition should seek a teacher or training institute of good reputation and practice. A teacher that practices and embodies Reiki principles in daily life may be sought by reputation and personal recommendation. Health care professionals may opt to "shop around" for classes that offer college credit, CEUs, or professional contact hours. One can seek referral for a Reiki teacher through the American Holistic Nurses Association, which awards contact hours for Reiki educational programs they have approved. Some Reiki teachers who have developed a health care focus in training may offer guidelines on how to implement a Reiki service within a health care setting, suggest an education plan for introducing clinical staff to Reiki, offer a review of Reiki literature, and provide clinical policy, referral, and service delivery ideas for different settings and client populations. All of this is not essential to the empowerment to Reiki healing, but it may go a long way in convincing an administrator of Reiki practicality and help ease the implementation of a Reiki program in a particular agency or department.

Wardell and Engebretson (2001) examined physiological and biochemical correlates after 30 minutes of Reiki in a pilot study with a group of 23 healthy subjects using a single-group repeated measure design. Comparing before and after measures, there were significant reductions in state anxiety and systolic blood pressure, and significant rises in salivary immunoglobin-A (IgA). There were no significant changes in salivary cortisol. Skin temperature increased and electromyography readings decreased during the Reiki session, but these measures were not significant. Findings suggest that a single Reiki session has an effect on decreasing perceived anxiety, increasing signs of relaxation and increasing humoral immunological functioning. The salivary IgA finding warrants further study to explore the relationship between Reiki and immune response.

Wirth and colleagues studied effects of Reiki in combination with other complementary modalities such as Qi Gong, LeShan, therapeutic touch, and intercessory prayer. These include the use of LeShan and Reiki with dental pain (Wirth et al., 1993); the use of LeShan, therapeutic touch, Reiki, and Qi Gong on hematological measures such as blood glucose and urea nitrogen (Wirth et al., 1996); and the use of therapeutic touch, Reiki, LeShan, and intercessory prayer with wound healing (Wirth, Richardson, & Eidelman, 1996). While some results are favorable for complementary therapies, the studies did not consider Reiki in isolation or contrast it with other energy methods; thus it is not possible to draw conclusions about Reiki efficacy.

Wirth and Cram (1994) conducted a study on the psychophysiology of Reiki and LeShan distant healing, considering them to be "nontraditional prayer." This study utilized a randomized double-blind, within-subject, crossover design to examine the effect of Reiki and LeShan distant healing upon autonomic and central nervous system (CNS) parameters, using the electromyogram (EMG) to measure electrical activity in muscles. Twenty-one subjects were randomly assigned to treatment and control conditions. The treatment provided was simultaneous Reiki and LeShan distant healing, with no contact between healers and subjects. Combined Reiki and LeShan healing were found to show highly significant reductions in EMG activity of paraspinal ($p < .0002$) and lumbar ($p < .001$) muscles. The significant decrease in overall EMG activity for the treatment condition suggests that subjects actually became more comfortable during this session. This well-designed study confirms that EMG measures can validate subjective reports of relaxation with healing treatments and suggests that Reiki and LeShan distant healing may be helpful in reducing neuromuscular pain. Healers reported subjective experience of prayer states, which they felt accessed deeper states of healing.

It is felt that Reiki affects change towards a state of physical balance. Wetzel (1989) studied changes in the hematocrit and hemoglobin values in response to Reiki attunements for 48 nonrandomized subjects; a control group of 10 did not receive Reiki attunements. Hematocrit values were analyzed using absolute numbers to determine the net change without reflecting directionality. Two blood samples were taken 24 hours apart. Those who received Reiki attunements experienced significant changes ($p > .01$) in in-vivo hemoglobin and hematocrit values as compared to the control group. One individual who had been experiencing iron deficiency anemia experienced an approximately 20 percent increase in hemoglobin and hematocrit values. She took no medications, and her diet and fluid intake was unchanged. She continued to treat herself with Reiki, and her increase was maintained upon re-test three months after her initial Reiki attunement.

Brewitt, Vittetoe, and Hartwell (1997) studied five patients with chronic disease (two with multiple sclerosis, and one each with lupus, fibromyalgia, and thyroid goiter) to evaluate the effect of 11 one-hour Reiki sessions over a 9 week period. Outcomes were quantified by electrodermal screening at acupuncture/conductance points. Only 3 of the 40 points measured showed significant differences before and after Reiki sessions; however, these improvements were noted in points of the neuroendocrine-immune system. All patients reported increased relaxation, a sense of centeredness, a reduction in pain, and an increase in mobility after Reiki sessions.

Singg and Dressen (2000) studied the effects of Reiki on pain, mood, personality, and faith in God in a study of 120 chronically ill patients. All participants had experienced pain symptoms due to different medical conditions for at least one year. Subjects were randomly assigned to one of four groups (Reiki, progressive muscle relaxation (PMR), placebo, and control). The Reiki, PMR, and placebo groups each received 10 biweekly sessions of the therapy. Significant Reiki effects were found on pain, affective and personality measures. Reiki seemed to enhance "desirable changes in personality indicated by reduction in trait anxiety, enhancement of self-esteem, shift toward internal locus of control and toward realistic sense of personal control" (p. 75). The effect of strengthened faith in God was significantly stronger in women than in men. Importantly, Reiki gains tend to persist over time. Researchers found that after a 3-month period, there were significant reduction trends in sensory and affective qualities of pain and total pain rating index. One of the most astonishing reports came from an HIV-positive patient whose lab work following only 2 of the 10 Reiki sessions indicated a dramatic rise in CD4 cell count.

National Institutes of Health (NIH)-funded rehabilitation trials using Reiki with subacute stroke patients were conducted (Kessler, 2000), involving 30 subjects randomly assigned to either a Reiki practitioner or a sham Reiki condition. These conditions were double-blinded. Subjects received up to 10 Reiki treatments in addition to standard rehabilitation. An additional 40 patients receiving standard rehabilitation served as controls. The study used outcome measures for function and mood in an inpatient rehabilitation program. Reiki was not found to have detectable effects on these measures. Improvements that occurred were attributed to natural healing and rehabilitation.

One of the challenges of well-controlled research on Reiki outcomes is using an adequate placebo. Mansour and colleagues (1999) have successfully developed a standardized Reiki placebo control and suggest the use of their techniques in research designs to test the Reiki intervention.

Reiki and Holistic Changes

It is frequently claimed that Reiki produces holistic and life changes. However, there are few studies to test this because research design to evaluate such changes is a challenge. Some promising work in this regard is as follows.

Mansour and colleagues (1998), Canadian researchers, approached the problem of suitable research design to capture the holistic nature of Reiki with a qualitative study of five women's experience of Reiki. They chose to use a phenomenological approach because "human experiences are relational and depend on the context and meaning they have for the individual" (p. 213). The researcher's question was, "What is the essence of this phenomenon called Reiki as experienced and perceived by the patients themselves?" (pp. 213–14). Data was collected on 5 subjects, ages 38–52, by in-depth interviewing over a 5-month period, focusing on why the informants behave or develop in a particular manner.

Mansour and colleagues (1998) found that "the overriding theme in the participants' stories is that of 'experiencing existential changes.' Participants spoke about experiencing major psychospiritual and/or physical changes" (p. 215). All women initially asked for Reiki because they had exhausted conventional therapies. They all indicated that it took some time to experience substantial changes, indicating that Reiki has a cumulative effect. This study suggests that Reiki may be holistic and cumulative in nature. Mansour and colleagues recommend that "future studies include a broader spectrum of outcome measures and investigate the cumulative effects, which may be missing if post-testing is conducted after only one session, which has been the norm in quantitative studies. The cumulative effect of Reiki might be investigated by way of repeated measures" (p. 216).

Engebretson and Wardell (2002) conducted a qualitative study of the experience of a Reiki session. Findings suggest that many linear models used in researching such therapies are not complex enough to capture the experience of the recipients.

Acceptance of Reiki as an Alternative Health Care Choice by Patients

A Canadian study conducted by Kelner and Wellman (1997) compares the social and health characteristics of 300 patients being treated by five kinds of practitioners: family physician, chiropractors, acupuncturists/Traditional Chinese Medicine doctors, naturopaths, and Reiki practitioners. There were striking health and social differences between patients of family physicians, patients of alternative medicine practitioners, and groups of alternative medicine patients. Reiki patients were found to have a higher level of education and were more likely to be in managerial or professional positions than other alternative medicine patients. It should be noted that almost all alternative medicine patients also consulted a family physician.

Reiki Research in Plan and Process

Reiki biofield energy healing and other alternative therapies are being studied in the treatment of diabetes and the management of chronic pain in diabetic neuropathy at the University of Michigan (2001) which is a research center for complementary and alternative medicine (CAM) and cardiovascular disease. This 5-year research study began in 1998 and is supported by a $7 million grant, with $100,000 earmarked for the Reiki study. Patients in the study have Type II diabetes and have experienced pain in feet and legs for at least 6 months. Participants commit to a 15-week time period, with an initial physical exam at week 1, followed by 13 weeks of weekly treatments, and an assessment by a final physical exam. Quality of life and attitude measures as well as hard parameters are included in this study (Gillespie, E., June 5, 2000, personal communication), which should be completed after this book goes to press.

A $20,000 grant from the Canadian Breast Cancer Research Initiative supports a study in progress investigating the effects of Reiki on anxiety, physical problems, spiritual well-being, and complete blood counts of breast cancer patients undergoing chemotherapy (University of Saskatchewan, 1999).

Research on the use of Reiki therapy for adolescent stress and substance use and abuse (Anderson, T., June 18, 2001, personal communication) is also in process. The subjects are teenagers at risk for substance abuse who are residents of a clinical program that seeks to engage teens in activities and therapies that promote awareness of the negative consequences of substance abuse and encourage activities that increase self-esteem, relaxation, self-control, and physical and emotional well-being.

Case Studies

Total Hip Replacement

Monica is a 76-year-old female who was referred to homecare following a left total hip replacement. She experienced a significant increase in low back pain since her discharge from the hospital. Monica lives with an impaired caregiver in a two-story home. The client was referred for traditional occupational therapy (OT) intervention for strengthening and activities of daily living (ADL) training. An in-home OT assessment revealed the client had decreased strength and endurance, required minimal assist transferring out of bed, and was dependent for lower extremity (LE) bathing and dressing. The client was also unable to participate in any standing activities due to reports of significant low back pain. She was seen in the home three times a week for 4 weeks, and received about 45 minutes of OT intervention at each visit.

Monica was alert, cooperative, and oriented in all spheres. During the third session, Reiki was incorporated for pain management and relief of the lower back. This was used during each treatment, for about 15 minutes each session, for six sessions. The client reported progressive relief from pain after each Reiki session. Research supporting use of Reiki with pain includes Olson and Hanson (1997) and Singg and Dresson (2000). At the time of discharge, Monica reported minimal low back pain and was able to resume normal activities within the home, including light housecleaning and meal preparation.

Abnormal Extensor Tone in Infant

Timothy is a 6-week-old baby boy who had abnormal extensor tone when held in supine position in a caretaker's arms or in supported seated position. His family noted his preference for resting his head to the left side and his inability to track objects side to side. He would arch his back when held in one's arms, as if recreating his body pattern at the time of his delivery. Timothy was seen by a physical therapist to facilitate normal growth and development and general well-being. Therapy was provided at the personal residence of his single mother, who lived with her parents and sister. The baby was healthy and otherwise appeared to be developing normally. Timothy was evaluated and treated at 6 weeks old for two 30-minute sessions, and at 9 weeks and 16 weeks for one 30-minute session each time.

Initial assessment revealed an obvious increase of extensor tone in his body that was exaggerated in the head, neck, and torso, with restricted range of motion of his neck and shoulders. Treatment consisted of neuromuscular reeducation techniques with inhibition of extensor tone through positioning and passive proprioceptive neuromuscular facilitation (PNF) exercises. The caregivers were instructed in holding and positioning the baby and in appropriate active-assist exercise and "tracking" exercises in prone, supine, and supported sit positions.

On the second visit, the baby had a significant reduction in the extensor tone and a mild to moderate deficit of active range of motion of neck and shoulders. Treatment was again facilitation of normal range of motion for the neck and shoulders utilizing gentle neuromuscular techniques. The therapist felt intuitively guided to use cranio-sacral techniques for infants along with Reiki during this session. Within 10 minutes of intending Reiki energy, this 9-week-old infant regained full active ROM of his neck and shoulders. The deep state of relaxation that occurred allowed the baby to fall asleep.

On the third visit, this infant presented with full range of motion of head, neck, and shoulders, and had maintained normal balance and function from the previous treatment session. The family has stated that weeks following this second visit, the baby was moving his body freely at will and was now turning his head side to side without difficulty and without restriction. For them, full recovery had been noted.

There is no known research supporting the use of Reiki specifically with this kind of problem.

Hyperactivity in Deaf Child

Hugh is a 7-year-old boy enrolled in a school for the deaf. He is tactile defensive and has developmental delays in addition to being deaf. He was referred to OT because of hyperactivity, difficulties in fine motor, gross motor, perceptual motor planning, and behavioral problems. He received occupational therapy twice weekly for 45-minute sessions and was treated for 6 months by an occupational therapist certified in sensory integration who is also a Reiki master. The therapy site was an area of the school equipped with sensory integration equipment.

At the initial evaluation, Hugh was unfocused and would run around the therapy room, unable to participate in any structured activity. The therapist started to beam (send) Reiki across the room. The child would gradually come closer to where the therapist was sitting. After three sessions, he came over to the therapy mat where the therapist was able to give him Reiki and unruffle (smooth and balance) his energy field. Hugh started to actually enjoy this and would initiate these motions the next time that he came to therapy. He would lie down on the mat and show the therapist how to move her hands to smooth out his energy field. He would lie quietly as the therapist gave him Reiki as hands-on healing. He was much more cooperative, enjoyed coming to therapy sessions, and gradually became involved in the traditional goals and objectives of his IEP (Individualized Education Program). Reiki intervention outcomes were an increased ability to cooperate, increased attention to task, facilitation of the establishment of a trust relationship, and increased ability to engage in traditional OT goals (fine motor, gross motor, perceptual motor skills, and decreased sensory defensiveness). Reiki was also provided for Hugh in the classroom whenever his teacher would ask the therapist to calm him down.

There is no known research on the use of Reiki with children in this type of therapy, although clinicians report that Reiki is successfully used to balance and relax clients before treatment (Behar, 1997). The client was seen over a 6-month period. His progress was sustained; he continued to receive Reiki to maximize the full benefit of engaging in his OT program.

Chronic Pain, Fibromyalgia, and Chronic Fatigue Syndrome

Sarah, a single 38-year-old woman, came to her local Veteran's Administration Medical Center with diagnoses of longstanding chronic pain, fibromyalgia, and chronic fatigue syndrome. She reported that she was receiving disability income because she was not able to sit, stand, or do paperwork as required by many jobs. In addition, her unpredictable illness exacerbations resulted in frequent, unavoidable tardiness or absenteeism, and subsequent loss of jobs. Sarah lived with her parents and caregivers because she was often dependent on them for help with some self-care, cooking, shopping, housekeeping, and laundry. Her physicians were not able to remediate her presenting symptoms of draining fatigue and generalized severe aching pain with movement. She reported that sometimes she spent 3 to 5 days in bed, unable to get up during an exacerbation. OT was ordered to increase Sarah's functional capacity.

An initial evaluation and two 60-minute OT visits were provided. OT consisted of traditional modalities, including education regarding the disease process, explanation of ergonomic principles, pacing, energy conservation, and work-simplification strategies. Stretching exercises for fibromyalgia and stress management strategies were provided, and leisure activities were identified. Hot packs, range of motion, splints, and compression gloves were issued, and support group information was offered. The therapist suggested Reiki for relaxation and stress. Reiki was explained briefly, and the client agreed to consider this treatment option.

Two days later, Sarah scheduled an appointment for Reiki. The appointment was scheduled at noon so that the otherwise busy clinic would be quiet. The OT provided a 30-minute Reiki session during which the therapist's hands remained several inches above Sarah's body. As this was her first experience with Reiki, she briefly lifted her head during the session and opened her eyes to see what the OT was doing. She quickly settled back onto the plinth. Afterward, Sarah reported having experienced deep relaxation for the first time in months. She left the clinic appearing calm and peaceful.

Beginning research finds Reiki is effective for chronic pain and depression (Singg & Dresson, 2000), for pain (Olson & Hanson, 1997), and for relaxation effects (Wardell & Engebretson, 2001). Sarah was not scheduled for additional occupational therapy. However, she appeared in the clinic 2 weeks later, beaming, and said she was still feeling the deep relaxation she experienced in her Reiki session. In later weeks, the OT saw her occasionally in passing, and she reported sleeping more restfully, doing some cooking, having more endurance, and spending some time with friends.

Summary

The intention and use of Reiki by the practitioner in daily living becomes the true internal teacher of the power and depth of this healing modality. Reiki healing is a journey of the healer in the healing of the self. The Reiki practitioner manifests his or her own healing in a willingness to be present, to offer healing, and to be of service to others, in many ways, as life "initiates" opportunities to do this.

Reiki has merits that distinguish it from other forms of holistic medicine. It is noninvasive, can be learned easily by everyone, and has no required assessment. Reiki purports only to enhance the natural healing process of the body itself: to move towards balance in all systems. Mansour and colleagues (1998) suggest that "Reiki is one of several therapies that figure in a medical treatment model that focuses on Primary Health Care (PHC), a model defined by the World Health Organization as being essential health care that is made universally accessible to individuals and families in communities by means acceptable to them, through their full participation, and at a cost that the community and country can afford" (p. 211).

Reiki is a rapidly growing healing art that blends with ease into all circumstances. In health care, it balances the increasing technology that threatens to dominate client care with human caring presence and healing intention. It supports the Reiki healer in a self-healing and self-realization process. The Reiki technique can be "given away" to families to bolster caregiving in the home. In wellness programs, it empowers the client's clear intent to engage in healthy lifestyle change.

STUDY QUESTIONS

1. Define Reiki.
2. How can Reiki be used in rehabilitation? With what types of problems or conditions does research support using Reiki?
3. What is meant by the "way" of Reiki? How does the "way" compare with hands-on healing techniques? Does the "way" have a place in rehabilitation?
4. How does one choose a Reiki teacher or training program?
5. Describe Reiki training.

SUGGESTED READING

Barnett, L., & M. Chambers with S. Davidson. (1996). *Reiki Energy Medicine*. Rochester, VT: Healing Arts Press.

Horan, P. (1992). *Empowerment Through Reiki* (2nd ed.). Wilmot, WI: Lotus Light Publications.

Lubeck, W., F. A. Petter, & W. L. Rand. (2001). *The Spirit of Reiki*. Twin Lakes, WI: Lotus Light Publications.

Narrin, J. (1998). *One Degree Beyond: A Reiki Journey Into Energy Medicine* (2nd ed.). Seattle, WA: Little White Buffalo Publishing.

Rand, W. L. (1998). *Reiki, The Healing Touch* (Rev. ed.). Southfield, MI: Vision Publications.

Upczak, P. R. (1999). *Reiki: A Way of Life*. Nederland, CO: Synchronicity Publishing.

RESOURCES

American Holistic Nursing Association
P.O. Box 2130
Flagstaff, AZ 86003–2130
(800) 278–2462
www.ahna.org

International Center for Reiki Training
21421 Hilltop St., Unit 28
Southfield, MI 48034
www.Reiki.org

International Society for the Study of
Subtle Energies and Energy Medicine
(ISSSEEM)
11005 Ralston Rd., Suite 100D
Arvada, CO 80004
www.issseem.org

Institute of Noetic Sciences
475 Gate Five Rd., Suite 300
Sausalito, CA 94965
www.noetic.org

Reiki Pages by Light & Adonea
www.angelfire.com/az/SpiritMatters
Comprehensive Web site with links to extensive Reiki resources

REFERENCES

Alandydy, P., & K. Alandydy. (1999, Apr.). Using Reiki to support surgical patients. *Journal of Nursing Care Quality, 13*(4), 89–91.

Ai, A. L., C. Peterson, B. Gillespie, S. Bolling, M. Jessup, A. Behling, & F. Pierce. (2001). Designing clinical trials on energy healing: Ancient art encounters medical science. *Alternative Therapies in Health and Medicine, 7*(4), 83–90.

Baginski, B. J., & S. Sharamon. (1988). *Reiki Universal Life Energy*. Mendocino, CA: Life Rhythm.

Barnett, L., & M. Chambers with S. Davidson. (1996). *Reiki Energy Medicine*. Rochester, VT: Healing Arts Press.

Becker, R. O., & A. Seldon. (1985). *The Body Electric: Electromagnetism and the Foundation of Life*. New York: William Morrow.

Behar, M. (1997, Feb.). Reiki: Bridging traditional and complementary healing techniques. *OT Practice*, 22–23.

Benor, D. J. (2001). *Spiritual Healing: Scientific Validation of a Healing Revolution* (Vol. I). Southfield, MI: Vision Publications.

Brewitt, B., T. Vittetoe, & B. Hartwell. (1997). The efficacy of Reiki hands-on healing: Improvements in spleen and nervous system function as quantified by electrodermal screening. *Alternative Therapies in Health and Medicine, 3*(4), 89.

Bullock, M. (1997, Jan.–Feb.). Reiki: A complementary therapy for life. *American Journal of Hospice and Palliative Care, 14*(1), 31–33.

Byrd, R. C. (1988). Positive therapeutic effects of intercessory prayer in a coronary care unit population. *Southern Medical Journal, 81*(7), 826–829.

Dossey, L. (1999). *Reinventing Medicine: Beyond Mind-Body to a New Era of Healing*. New York: HarperCollins.

Engebretson, J., & D. Wardell. (2002). Experience of a Reiki session. *Alternative Therapies in Health and Medicine, 8*(2), 48–53.

Eos, N. (1995). *Reiki and Medicine*. Grass Lakes, MI: Nancy Eos.

Gerber, R. (2001). *Vibrational Medicine: The #1 Handbook of Subtle-Energy Therapies* (3rd ed.). Rochester, VT: Bear and Company.

Gleisner, E. (1992). *Reiki in Everyday Living*. Laytonville, CA: White Feather Press.

Hebner, S. I. (2000). Use of Reiki during childbearing: A descriptive study of Reiki practitioner perspective on uses, benefits, and risks. Unpublished master's thesis. Yale University School of Nursing, New Haven, Conn.

Horan, P. (1992). *Empowerment Through Reiki* (2nd ed.). Wilmot, WI: Lotus Light Publications.

ICRT (International Center for Reiki Training). (1990–2001). Reiki News Article Archive. Includes personal accounts of Reiki healings of many conditions. [online]. Available www.reiki.org.

Kahne, L. (1998). Applied Reiki: The use of Reiki for police and emergency services. Reiki Peace Network. [online]. Available http://www.reikipeacenetwork.com/magazine/emergency.html.

Kelner, M., & B. Wellman. (1997). Who seeks alternative health care? A profile of the users of five modes of treatment. *Journal of Alternative Complementary Medicine, 3*(2), 127–140.

Kessler Medical Rehabilitation Research & Education Corporation. (2000, Feb.). Effect of energy healing treatments on post-stroke rehabilitation patients. [online]. Available www.kmrrec.org.

Lubeck, W., F. A. Petter, & W. L. Rand. (2001). *The Spirit of Reiki*. Twin Lakes, WI: Lotus Light Publications.

Mansour, A. A., G. Laing, A. Leis, J. Nurse, & A. Denilkewich. (1998). The experience of Reiki. *Alternative & Complementary Therapies, 4*(3), 211–217.

Mansour, A. A., M. Beuche, G. Laing, A. Leis, & J. Nurse. (1999, June). A study to test the effectiveness of placebo Reiki standardization procedures developed for a planned Reiki efficacy study. *Journal of Alternative & Complementary Medicine, 5*(3), 221–222.

Narrin, J. (1998). *One Degree Beyond: A Reiki Journey Into Energy Medicine*. Seattle, WA: Little White Buffalo Publishing.

Nield-Anderson, L., & A. Ameling. (2001, Apr.). Reiki: A complementary therapy for nursing practice. *Journal of Psychosocial Nursing, 39*(4), 42–49.

Olson, K., & J. Hanson. (1997, June). Using Reiki to manage pain: A preliminary report. *Cancer Prevention Control, 1*(2), 108–113.

Pert, C. (1997). *Molecules of Emotion*. New York: Scribner.

Petter, F. A. (1999). *Reiki: The Legacy of Dr. Usui* (2nd ed.). Twin Lakes, WI: Lotus Light Publications.

Petter, F. A. (1997). *Reiki Fire*. Twin Lakes, WI: Lotus Light Publications.

Rand, W. L. (1998). *Reiki, The Healing Touch* (Rev. ed.). Southfield, MI: Vision Publications.

Rivera, C. (1999, Feb./Mar.). Reiki therapy: A tool for wellness. *Imprint, 46*(2), 31–33, 56.

Rowland, A. Z. (1998). *Traditional Reiki for Our Times: Practical Methods for Personal and Planetary Healing*. Rochester, VT: Healing Arts Press.

Rubik, B. (1995). Energy medicine and the unifying concept of information. *Alternative Therapies, 1*, 34–39.

Severino, E. (1995). *Reiki: The Healer's Touch*. Cherry Hill, NJ: The Healing Connection Books.

Singg, S., & L. Dressen. (2000). Effect of Reiki on pain and selected affective and personality variables in chronically ill patients. *Subtle Energies & Energy Medicine, 9*(1), 51–82.

Stanley, L. M. (1999). Reiki in prisons. *The Reiki Spiral Network Newsletter*, Golden, CO.

Stevens, W. (2001, June). Reiki and HIV. Presentation at 4th Annual Adjunctive Management in HIV/AIDS Complementary Therapies sponsored by University of Medicine and Dentistry of NJ, NJ AIDS Education and Training Center and Association of Nurses in AIDs Care, Newark, NJ.

University of Michigan. (2001). Complementary and Alternative Medicine Research Center for Cardiovascular Diseases, Ann Arbor, MI. Reiki Study: A study of Reiki to control pain in diabetic patients. [online]. Available www.med.umich.edu/camrc/research_reiki.html (updated 8/09/01).

University of Saskatchewan. (1999, Apr.). Office of Communications, College of Nursing. Nursing research receives funding or unconventional breast cancer therapy. [online]. Available www.usask.ca/communications/ocn/Apr24/news8html.

Upczak, P. R. (1999). *Reiki: A Way of Life*. Nederland, CO: Synchronicity Publishing.

Wardell, D. W., & J. Engebretson. (2001, Feb.). Biological correlates of Reiki touch[sm] healing. *Journal of Advanced Nursing, 33*(4), 439–445.

Wetzel, W. (1989). Reiki healing: A physiologic perspective. *Journal of Holisitic Nursing, 7*(1), 47–54.

Wirth, D. P., & J. R. Cram. (1994). The psychophysiology of nontraditional prayer. *International Journal of Psychosomatics, 41*(1–4), 68–75.

Wirth, D. P., R. J. Chang, W. S. Eidelman, & E. Paxton. (1996). Hematological indicators of complementary healing intervention. *Complementary Therapies in Medicine, 4*, 14–20.

Wirth, D. P., J. T. Richardson, & W. S. Eidelman. (1996). Wound healing and complementary therapies: A review. *Journal of Alternative & Complementary Medicine, 2*(4), 493–502.

Wirth, D. P., D. R. Brenlan, R. J. Levine, & C. M. Rodriguez. (1993). The effect of complementary healing therapy on postoperative pain after surgical removal of impacted third molar teeth. *Complementary Therapies in Medicine, 1*(3), 133–138.

ACKNOWLEDGMENTS

Special thanks to Sandra Cram, OTR; Karen M. Frame, PT, ESMT; Margaret Behar, OTR; and Joanne E. Farrar, MSC, OTR, for contributing Reiki case studies, and to Phoebe Darlington, artist, for the hand-painted design of Japanese Bamboo with Reiki Lessons (Figure 19–1).

20

Relaxation, Meditation, and Breath

Judith A. Parker

CHAPTER OBJECTIVES

- Define relaxation and its components.
- Identify the methods of relaxation.
- Articulate the two basic types of meditation.
- Outline four different methods for meditation.
- Identify the components of breathing.
- Explain the difference between mouth and nasal breathing.
- Identify the advantages and disadvantages of chest and diaphragmatic breathing.
- Discuss how the methods of relaxation outlined in this chapter are relevant to therapy practice.
- Instruct a client in at least one form of meditation, breathing, and relaxation exercise.
- Identify the contraindications of using specific methods with different clients.

A small child sits on the bank of a river on a warm, sunny afternoon, watching the never-ending ebb and flow of the river as it makes its way to the great unknown. The wind rustles the leaves softly, and the heavenly smell of newly mown grass fills the air. The child heaves a sigh of utter contentment. The child exists in the present and is in the "here and now."

How many people can say that this is how they live their lives? In Western society there is often a constant rush to get places and to accomplish things. People often live in the past with regrets about what might have been, or in the future, focused on what could be, or both past and future. This constant shift from the past to the future, as opposed to living in the present, results in an undercurrent of stress.

All people cope with stress on an ongoing basis. When a life challenge such as a physical or emotional illness, aging, or the death of a loved one occurs, this compounds the stressors people live with and can weaken the individual (e.g., increasing fatigue, decreasing immune response). Such stress (both ongoing and episodic stress) is especially relevant for therapists, since it directly impacts on therapy. If an individual is very stressed, his or her focus is on the

Therapists often work with clients in very stressful situations. Clients come to therapy as a result of emotional or physical challenges (or both) and are already faced with a wide range of stressors. As a result, although they may be invested in therapy, they are fearful and can have difficulty focusing. Their autonomic nervous system is firing, and their bodies and minds are working to survive the situation by either "fighting" or "fleeing." The muscles in their bodies are often tight, more easily damaged, and can fatigue more easily. Decreased oxygen going to their brains also results in difficulty focusing. They are often less mentally flexible and adaptable during therapy. They may also be more irritable and less willing to follow directions. Once therapists help them relax, they are much better equipped to face the challenges of therapy and to integrate what they experience in therapy in their daily lives.

The methods outlined in this chapter have several advantages. They

- are very portable.
- are easily learned.
- can be practiced in nonstressful situations and then used under stressful circumstances.
- do not require outside equipment.
- can be practiced unobtrusively and in a wide range of situations.
- can be easily integrated into a person's lifestyle.
- allow the client autonomy and can be used at his or her discretion.

One of the most important factors in teaching clients to use these methods is that they help clients develop autonomy and a sense of control in situations that usually cause clients to feel out of control and fearful. These techniques can also increase immune response, concentration, and attention to self and task performance.

stress. Overstressed clients are less likely to hear or understand instructions given to them. The therapist may observe this when clients tend to ask the same questions over and over again. This is not because the clients are being difficult, but rather, because of the stress, they are having problems understanding and remembering the directions. By learning and using the techniques outlined in this chapter, the therapist can help clients calm down, relax, and focus on what they have to do to heal.

The key to counteracting stress is to use opposite bodily responses, or relaxation (Benson, 1975; Ornish, 1990). The focus of this chapter is to examine what can be done to alleviate stress by using meditation, breath, and relaxation.

The Stress Response

Under stress, the body is put into a flight or fight mode (Selye, 1975). In this response there is an increase in heart rate and blood pressure, a constriction of the blood vessels to the major organs, and the brain is put on "red alert." Hormones are secreted, which keep the body ready to fight or flee. Although initially adaptive, when this response goes on for long periods of time, there is a breakdown in function. Such disease states as diabetes, cardiac conditions, hypertension, headaches, susceptibility to illnesses, and allergies have been linked to these responses (Bartrop, Lazarus, & Luckhurst, 1977; Cohen, Tyrell, & Smythe, 1991; Rasmussen, 1969; Solomon, 1990). Emotional challenges such as depression, anxiety disorders, and anger have also been linked to ongoing stress. Thus it is important to counteract stress and the ultimate detrimental effects.

As part of human existence, a certain amount of stress is normal. However, prolonged stressful experiences can deplete the system and lead to illness or exhaustion. Stress is costing the American economy billions of dollars in lost productivity, wages, and doctor's visits. To counteract this, many employers are instituting stress-reduction programs for their employees. In fact, it is estimated that 40 percent of all U.S. worksites will offer stress-reduction programs in the near future (Buhler, 1999). These stress-reduction programs are taking many forms, but the techniques most often used are meditation, relaxation, and yoga (Luthar, 1999), along with T'ai Chi and visualization. The key to all of these methods is the focus on helping the body, mind, and spirit relax.

The Relaxation Response

The term *relaxation response* was first coined by Dr. Herbert Benson, a cardiologist at Harvard Medical School, in 1975 when he began to work with people with cardiac conditions and to use meditation to effect change in blood pressure. He was initially exposed to meditation by a group of practitioners of transcendental meditation (TM), who asked him to study their physiological responses. Dr. Benson, collaborating with Dr. Robert Wallace, found that TM practitioners showed a drop in heart rate, metabolic rate, and breathing rate. Additionally, they had lower than normal blood pressure. This led to the current definition of the relaxation response, which is a reduction in heart rate, metabolic rate, blood pressure, and breath rate (Benson, 1975). This state of quietude also offered an essential survival mechanism, because in this relaxed state the body and mind is able to heal and rejuvenate. Thus, the relaxation response provides individuals with the ultimate stress survival tool.

To induce the relaxation response, Dr. Benson stated that it is important that an individual have a mental device to focus on, such as a phrase or mantra, and a passive attitude. A passive attitude refers to self-acceptance: putting aside distractions and simply focusing on being in the present. Initially, he indicated that two other factors played a role: a quiet environment and a comfortable position. However, he discovered that the relaxation response can be evoked while walking, running, or performing activities of daily living.

Jon Kabat-Zinn (1990) approaches response to stress in another way, saying that it is important to *respond* to stress rather than *react* to it. By looking at the stressors and actively choosing a response meaningful for the individual, a person can lower stress levels, and in so doing, allow the body and mind to relax. Dr. Kabat-Zinn also advocates meditation, or as he refers to it, *mindful meditation,* and working with the breath. Key to all models of working with stress is meditation and breath.

Although the methods outlined in this chapter seem to be relatively safe and usable with all clients, it is important to remember that each person is an individual and one method may increase fear or the feeling of being out of control for him or her.

For example, a person with asthma may have difficulty with deep breathing exercises initially because of fear that he or she won't be able to breath. It might be more effective to begin by using a relaxation method that focuses on relaxing the body before employing a breathing exercise.

Another type of challenge may be with a client who has faced great emotional trauma and has suppressed it, as occurs with posttraumatic stress disorder. These individuals may have great difficulty with meditation because when they begin to clear their minds from chatter, they begin to experience that which they fear. These individuals may benefit from psychological therapy and counseling before working on such things as body awareness, meditation, and breath work. Other clients are able to learn meditation and participate in counseling simultaneously.

Always use the client as a gauge for what is most successful for them. Do not judge for them ahead of time.

Meditation

Meditation has been practiced for centuries. Initially, it was a part of religious practices. Buddhist monks have practiced meditation as a part of their daily lives for centuries. Judaic practices include mindful meditation with the scriptures on a daily basis. Christians in the 14th century practiced a chanting of a daily prayer to Jesus Christ. Although some researchers (Benson, 1979) advocate this spiritual base for meditation, it does not need to be a part of the meditative practice. This depends on the framework or beliefs of the client. However, it is helpful if the individual has a belief in a greater power that will support his or her development and growth (Benson, 1979; Kabat-Zinn, 1990; Leyden-Rubenstein, 1998). A belief in a greater power allows the meditation practitioner to believe that there is always hope in any situation and that problems can be worked out. Thus, the practice of mindfulness or contemplative acts creates a safe place for the practitioner and allows him or her to heal.

There are many types and practices of meditation, and they all have one element in common: They all work to help eliminate the distracting thought, or "chatter," in the mind. In day to day existence, the mind is constantly working (e.g., planning, learning, remembering). The more stress an individual is under, the more chatter occurs. As the chatter is reduced through meditation, the body and the mind can relax and achieve peace and quiet. In this relaxed state the body can begin to heal itself and work towards health and balance.

All meditation techniques work by focusing the mind on one particular object or centering device. Some of the more traditional objects are breath, exercises, images, thought, and mantras.

Approaches to Meditation

There are two basic approaches to meditation: concentrative meditation and mindfulness meditation. In concentrative meditation the practitioner focuses on a specific object, such as breath, an image, or a sound, to help calm down the mind and allow for clarity and relaxation.

Mindfulness approaches meditation another way. In mindfulness meditation the practitioner simply opens her or his attention to be aware of what is going on internally and externally. In observing themselves, they are a witness to their own process. Through this process the practitioner becomes calmer, clearer, and less reactive to life's stresses. Although there are basically two types of meditation practices, there are many versions of these types.

Transcendental meditation was made popular in the 1960s by the Beatles. It has grown in popularity with the work of Deepak Chopra, who has practiced and encouraged others to practice this technique for over 20 years (Benson, 1979).

TM is a very simple technique. An instructor chooses a mantra such as *ohm* or a set of sounds specific for each person, based on their unique characteristics. Once the client is given a mantra or set of sounds, he or she sits in a comfortable position and repeats the mantra over and over again. This process allows the client to let go of distracting thoughts and to disregard any extraneous ideas. This practice is to be done for 20 minutes, twice daily.

One challenge for many people is that they rarely experience their bodies—people often exist in their bodies, but is it rare that people truly experience who they are in the context of their own physical form. *Muscle tension relaxation* helps people to increase body awareness. When using the muscle tension relaxation approach, the practitioner focuses on each muscle group, tensing and then relaxing each. This is done in a systematic way to allow all muscle groups to be addressed and relaxed. One of the beliefs of this practice is that it is important to experience the tensed state to know what a relaxed state feels like. This practice can be used not only to increase body awareness but also to facilitate centering (i.e., a calm, very focused state). It may be viewed as a form of meditation because it allows the practitioner to meditate on the body and how it feels without focusing on the distractions.

Autogenic relaxation is a form of muscle tension relaxation; however, the mind simply asks the body to relax. The practitioner focuses her or his attention on a body part, becomes aware of how much tension she or he feels in it, and then simply asks the body part to relax. This process allows the practitioner to experience the body in its present existence and in a more relaxed state. In *breath meditation* the centering device is the breath itself and the breathing process. The focus is on the movement of air in and out of the lungs. Through this focusing the practitioner develops an awareness of the body and the interaction of the breathing process with the body.

In *mantra meditation* the practitioner simply chooses a word or phrase that is personally meaningful (e.g., love or hope), as opposed to TM in which the mantra is given to the client, and then keeps repeating it. When the client's mind wanders to other areas, the client observes where the mind wandered to and then refocuses on the mantra. This single focus allows the thoughts to quiet down and creates a calm place without extraneous chatter.

Affirmation meditation is similar to mantra meditation, except a positive statement is chosen, such as "I am relaxed" or "I am in control of my life and my body." The phrase is repeated over and over again, allowing the individual to not only create a calming effect, but also to effect a change in self-perception and attitude. In the form of meditation called *letting go of thoughts,* the client simply watches what is going on in his or her mind. As the thoughts go by, they are watched as if they were clouds floating in the sky. The client appreciates the thoughts and simply lets them go by.

In *present moment* meditation the focus is on the moment—what a person is doing, experiencing, smelling, tasting, and thinking. The purpose of this type is to fully be in the present. One of the challenges of many people's current lifestyle, as discussed in the introduction, is that they live in the past and/or the future with little attention to the present. It is only through living in the present that life can be fully experienced.

Guided meditation is meditation while listening to sounds, viewing images, or both. Guided meditation can use natural sounds, such as ocean waves or falling rain, but more often utilizes spoken instructions to help clients attain specific mind states. Facilitated either by a live therapist or via audio/video tape, sound offers outside support in reaching a meditative state.

Some people are concerned that they do not know if they are "doing" meditation correctly. Others might be preoccupied and find that instructions increase their ability to focus. Guided meditation can be used to overcome such issues either initially (to "learn" to meditate) or on an ongoing basis. It is critical that the images used are relevant to the client to induce the desired state of meditation and relaxation. For example, if a person is afraid of the water, ocean imagery may not be a good choice to induce relaxation. Ultimately, the therapist can offer suggestions, but the final choice must rest with the client. There are many audio and video tapes available that provide this type of support through the meditative process.

There are many other forms of meditation developed as a part of religious or healing practices. Some examples are *insight meditation,* or *Vipassana,* which is central to Theravada Buddhism, *superconscious meditation, integrative meditation* and *Harsha meditation.* All of these practices share common beliefs, and many have been practiced for thousands of years (Burton Goldberg Group, 1995).

Breath

One important component of all healing practices is breath. All people take an average of 6 to 12 breaths per minute. Through breath, all of the cells in the body are supplied with oxygen, and waste products are eliminated. If a person goes without breathing or oxygen for more than 6 minutes, there is damage to the body and brain, and ultimately death. Breath is one of the autonomic bodily functions that an individual can consciously experience and monitor as well as affect the process.

The two basic components of breath are inhalation and exhalation. During the inhalation process, air is brought into the lungs through either the nose or the mouth. In the exhalation process, the air is pushed out of the lungs to eliminate waste products and to make room for a new breath.

Breath is affected by both physical and psychological factors. When an individual is very stressed, his or her breathing may become shallow and irregular. An individual may breath too fast or even hold his or her breath.

Breathing is an extremely portable therapeutic tool. Nearly every contemplative tradition makes use of breath and allows the person to connect to her or his body (Burack, 1999). Breath is also linked to meditative practices for many self-help methods. The Hindus focused on breathing and repeating a phrase of the scriptures on the out breath. Early Judaism, Christianity, Islam, Shinto, Taoism, and Confucianism all focused on the breath, especially on the exhalation. Breath is also linked to many meditative practices for self-help.

Chest Versus Diaphragmatic Breathing

Chest breathing is a common method of breathing for many individuals. During chest breathing, a person is shallow-breathing with only about 500 cubic centimeters of oxygen moving through the lungs, and there is minimal movement of the rib cage or diaphragm. As a result of this shallow method of breathing, there is also minimal exchange of oxygen or elimination of waste and toxic materials. Continuous chest breathing results in fatigue and susceptibility to illness, since there is always a large residual volume of air in the lungs with each breath. This large residual volume of air contains waste products, such as carbon dioxide, moisture, and particles of substances. Additionally, since the air is relatively static, mucus cannot be removed from these areas. This causes the individual to be more susceptible to respiratory infections, such as pneumonias.

Diaphragmatic breathing uses the diaphragm as well as rib cage expansion. This is a much deeper form of breathing, with 4,000 to 5,000 cubic centimeters of air being moved with each breath. This method of breathing allows the body to eliminate large amounts of waste and toxins with each breath.

Exercise: Diaphragmatic Breathing

To experience diaphragmatic breathing, gently place your hands on your abdomen. Exhale slowly through your mouth until you feel as if all the air has slowly and gently left your body. Now slowly breath in, first filling the lungs so that your hands over your abdomen begin to move up. Once this area is filled continue to breathe until your rib cage is fully expanded. At this point your diaphragm has been used to fully fill your lungs with air. Complete this process for several breaths. You will probably notice that you feel lighter and more energized.

Diaphragmatic breathing also decreases heart rate, metabolic rate, blood sugar levels, pulmonary stress, muscle tension and fatigue, and the perception of pain (Leyden-Rubenstein, 1998). Many methods of relaxation, meditation, yoga, visualization, and exercise methods use diaphragmatic breathing.

Nose Versus Mouth Breathing

Inspiration and expiration can occur through either the mouth or the nose. Many methods of breath work encourage inspiration through the nose and expiration through the mouth. According to Werntz, Bickford, and Shannohoff-Khaalsa (1987), nose or nasal breathing affects the higher cortical centers of the brain, such as the hypothalamus and the pituitary gland, as well as the endocrine and immune systems. This affects mental awareness, levels of consciousness, meditative states and internal states of awareness. Mouth breathing, on the other hand, affects the brain stem centers of respiration, which in turn affects physical awareness, bodily responses, kinesthetic sense or emotions, and awareness of the environment.

With nose breathing, the air brought into the body through the nose is filtered through the nasal hairs, and many impurities are removed. Additionally, the air is warmed before it enters the lungs. Nose breathing is generally a slower process of bringing air into the lungs and allows the air to gently move from the environment to the lungs and then back out to the environment. This method is frequently used in meditation, relaxation, yoga and many breath work methods.

When a person breathes in through the mouth, the air is not cleaned by the nasal hair and nasal passages, nor is it warmed. Mouth breathing tends to be more rapid and is usually associated with activity that is stressful on the body, such as exercise or emotional stressors. The advantage of mouth breathing is that air can be brought into the lungs more quickly, but the quality is less conditioned. In this way, the focus is on quantity of air rather than quality.

During rapid mouth breathing or hyperventilation, an imbalance between the oxygen and carbon dioxide levels develops, resulting in rapid uncontrolled breathing. The major problem during this challenge is the decrease in carbon dioxide levels in the lungs and then in the blood. To ameliorate this situation, it is helpful to have the person breath into their hands or into a paper bag to better balance these levels.

Expiration of air through the mouth or pursed lips is frequently used in breathing exercises. Expiration in this way allows for forcing more air out of the lungs to make space for more air in during inspiration. This promotes better exchange of oxygen, carbon dioxide, and waste materials.

Ways of Using Breath

Many methods of meditation have the client focus on the movement of air in and out of the lungs. The object of these methods is to simply watch the air move in and out—to act as a voyeur. It is as if the client is watching the waves on a beach, or a stream flowing by. The mindfulness of breath also allows the client to gently watch the breath slow down, and in so doing, slow down the mind and the body (Kabat-Zinn, 1990). This is one of the key factors in allowing the body to experience relaxation.

A basic principle of yoga is the connection between the breath and the mind. It is believed that if the flow of breath is jerky or uneven, the body will be in a state of unrest or a person will experience an uneven flow of thoughts. When the mind is calm, then the body will also be calm, and vice versa. *Pranayama* is the process whereby the practitioner focuses on regulating breath by creating a rhythmic breathing pattern. The key is the rhythmic flow of air in and out, which helps the mind and body relax. Pranayama is frequently used in preparation for meditation.

Nadi shodhana (purification of the channels) is a method of *alternating nostril breathing*, also known as *cleansing breath*, commonly used in yoga and other relaxation practices. The exercise begins with the practitioner sitting upright and comfortable and breathing in and out slowly and evenly three times. Then the right nostril is closed with the thumb of the right hand, and the practitioner exhales fully through the left nostril. When the exhalation is complete, the practitioner then closes the left nostril with the index finger and inhales through the right nostril. This cycle of exhalation and inhalation is repeated two more times. It is important that the inhalation and exhalation are equal.

At the end of these three cycles, the process is repeated with the exhalation through the right nostril and the inhalation through the left nostril. This is repeated three times, which completes another cycle. This method should be practiced twice a day. The focus of this method is to increase the length of the inspiration and the expiration and to keep each of them equal. This type of breath helps people relax and allows greater focus on tasks.

Breath Play was developed by former Olympic bicycle trainer Ian Jackson. The focus of this method is the full expiration of air through pursed lips, using the diaphragm, and then a relaxation of the system so that inspiration is a passive activity. This method allows for an increase of energy and endurance (Thomason, 1998). Breath Play can be used during exercise and during relaxation. Energy conservation occurs during the inspiration phase. An added benefit of this method is a relaxation of the mind and body, allowing for fuller enjoyment of activities. Athletes, individuals with respiratory challenges such as chronic obstructive pulmonary disease (COPD), and individuals with anxiety challenges have utilized this method (Thomason, 1998).

Methods to Increase Alertness

When an individual becomes tired or stressed, feelings of fatigue can affect performance and alertness. One note of importance is that when the body is moved, as with walking, running, or using the arms, there is an increase in arousal levels simply for survival—that is, when a person is moving, the mind increases levels of alertness to be awake and avoid injury. Methods to increase alertness combine breath and body work.

Exercises: Combining Breath and Body Work

The use of breath can be combined with arm movements. The practitioner begins by standing with knees slightly bent and feet shoulder width apart. The arms are straight ahead at shoulder height. The practitioner breathes out in three short exhalations through pursed lips with the final expiration a long one, as if blowing a feather across a room. As the person is exhaling, the arms are brought down to the sides. Then a slow inspiration begins, with the arms moving up to their starting position. This method is repeated three to four times. The advantage of this method is that there is an increase in oxygen in the lungs relatively quickly.

In another method the focus is on a full expiration of breath through pursed lips, followed by three rapid inspirations.

Case Study

Preparation for Surgery

Brad was born with transposition of the great vessels of his heart. At age 5 months, open heart surgery was attempted to increase oxygen supply to his body. During the operation, he stopped breathing a number of times. This resulted in permanent brain damage. He had multiple physical issues, including digestive problems, an irregular heart beat that necessitated a pacemaker, and hormonal and growth problems. Functionally, he has severe dyspraxia and minimal speech. At age 18, his pacemaker needed to be replaced. The challenge for this operation was that Brad had limited lung capacity and additionally was terrified of further surgery. He had had a range of procedures performed on him since the original heart operation. His mother asked for help so that this procedure would not frighten him.

The challenges with Brad were that his dyspraxia made it difficult for him to follow physical or verbal directions, so the tasks had to be broken down and taught in segments; he was afraid of anything being placed over his face; and because of his limited lung capacity, he had difficulty with anything strenuous: Most activities that were stressful resulted in an erratic rapid heart rate.

The initial phase of treatment involved simply learning how to blow out a complete breath through pursed lips. This was accomplished with the use of a variety of activities, such as blowing a feather and using a Blowpen™. Once this was accomplished, the next focus was to become comfortable with a mask over his face. A mask similar to the one used in surgery was used for approximately 5 minutes per session, twice a week for 1 month. At the end of this time, he was comfortable with the mask over his face. The next challenge was to help Brad relax during the procedure and feel safe. The procedure was reviewed with him and he was asked to think of it as a new adventure. Approximately 10 minutes per session, twice a week for approximately 1 month, focused on the process of relaxation using a gentle in and out breath pattern while imagining the procedure.

At the end of the month, Brad underwent the replacement of his pacemaker. His mother reported that he did not fight the face mask, smiled before the procedure, and did not have any problems with the anesthesia. He was allowed to go home 3 hours after the procedure. Brad's mother was extremely pleased with the results, and Brad did not have any problems with the procedure. This was a marked contrast to a procedure performed approximately 1 year earlier, during which he fought the face mask, needed to be hospitalized overnight, and had been ill for a few days afterwards. Brad's mother credits the difference to the use of breath and relaxation training prior to the procedure.

Summary

In this chapter different approaches to meditation, relaxation, and breath were explored. As outlined in each of these sections, there are several key components for each practice. The key to all of them is to allow the body to relax so it can heal itself and become rejuvenated. The body cannot do this if it is in a state of stress. In a relaxed state a person is able to fully experience his or her life, respond to the environment in a positive way, be flexible, and learn from what he or she experiences. These are the keys to each person's living his or her life to the fullest.

Imagine a day without stress, like the child by the stream, living in the moment. What a wonderful way to experience existence. Therapists have the opportunity to help clients on a daily basis let go of some of the stress they face, gain some autonomy, and live, even if just for the briefest of times, in the moment.

STUDY QUESTIONS

1. Imagine you are working with a 25-year-old man with an L5 spinal cord injury who is wheelchair-bound and is having shortness of breath when manually driving his chair. What method would you use with him, and how would you instruct him in its practice?

2. You are working with five 6-year-old students who are having difficulty focusing on classroom material. What method would you use to help them out and how would you teach them?

3. The nursing home that you are working in has several agitated clients who complain of difficulty in sleeping at night. What method would you consider using with them?

4. A 17-year-old rape victim, who suffered a broken elbow and recently had the cast removed, receives a prescription for therapy three times a week. Every time you get close to her she begins to sweat and hyperventilate. What method would you use, and why?

RESOURCES

Jon Kabat-Zinn's Mindfulness Meditation
    Tapes (audio)
Stress Reduction Tapes
PO Box 547
Lexington, MA 02173

REFERENCES

Bartrop, R., L. Lazarus, & E. Luckhurst. (1977). Depressed lymphocyte function after breavement. *Lancet, 1,* 834–839.

Benson, H. (1975). *The Relaxation Response.* New York: New American Library.

Benson, H. (1979). *The Mind/Body Effect.* New York: Simon & Schuster.

Buhler, P. (1999). Stress: A concern for everyone. *Supervision, 64*(12), 14–16.

Burack, C. (1999). Returning meditation to education. *Tikkun, 14*(5), 41–48.

Burton Goldberg Group. (1995). *Alternative Medicine: The Definitive Guide.* Fife, WA: Future Medicine Publishing.

Cohen, D., D. A. Tyrell, & A. P. Smythe. (1991, Aug.). Psychological stress and susceptibility to the common cold. *New England Journal of Medicine, 325,* 606–612.

Kabat-Zinn, J. (1990). *Full Catastrophe Living.* New York: Delacorte Press.

Leyden-Rubenstein, L. (1998). *The Stress Management Handbook.* New Canaan, CT: Keats Publishing.

Luthar, H. (1999). Learning the tao of meditation training. *Workforce, 78*(2), 10–11.

Ornish, D. (1990). *Reversing Heart Disease.* New York: Ballantine Books.

Rasmussen, A. F. (1969). Emotions and immunity. *Annals of New York Academy of Science, 164*(2), 458–462.

Selye, H. (1975). *Stress Without Distress.* New York: New American Library.

Solomon, T. (1990). Cope in office. *British Medical Journal, 310*(6742), 32–33.

Thomason, B. (1998, July 13). In quick-fix world there's a need to return to basics. *Advance for Respiratory Care Practitioners,* 24–25.

Werntz, D. A., R. G. Bickford, & D. Shannohoff-Khaalsa. (1987). Selective hemispheric stimulation by unilateral forced nostril breathing. *Human Neurobiology, 6*(3), 165–171.

21

Shiatsu

Scott Gold

CHAPTER OBJECTIVES

- ◆ Understand the basic principles of Shiatsu.
- ◆ Understand how Shiatsu may be integrated into a rehabilitation session.
- ◆ Understand current trends and research regarding Shiatsu as a tool for rehabilitation.
- ◆ Identify several sources of further education and resources.

Shiatsu is the Japanese word for a manual treatment also known as acupressure. There are two views on the purpose of Shiatsu. The Eastern-oriented view is that Shiatsu is used to manipulate chi, considered in Eastern thought to be the essence of life and to improve the balance of yin and yang. Shiatsu manipulates chi through the pressing of acupoints that are found on energy channels called meridians. These meridians are located along specific routes that have been defined through centuries of observation in the Far East. This view is espoused by Wataru Ohashi and Shizuro Masunaga. The Western-oriented view, espoused by Turo Namikoshi, is that Shiatsu should be used to manipulate nerves, muscles, and sweat glands: the physical being.

Sources indicate that Shiatsu predates 2000 BC. Documented use of bodywork with acupoints is dated around 200 BC (Dubitsky, 1997). In the 1950s, Japanese practitioners began opening Shiatsu clinics in America. Practitioners such as Namikoshi, Ohashi, and Masunaga applied a standard to Shiatsu practice, and the Japanese government formally recognized it as a healing practice and officially licensed it in 1957 (Namikoshi, 1981).

Although Shiatsu is a physical bodywork modality and is defined within a massage framework in state licensing, in the Eastern framework it is not a massage in the strict sense of the word. Massage works on the physical essence of the body, including the joints, muscles, lymphatic system, and fascia. Shiatsu, from an Eastern framework, works on the energetic plane of the body. Shiatsu can be introduced into the therapy session, depending on state licensure requirements, as a massage modality or as a manual/energy therapy. Benefits will be

243

described in different terms (e. g., back or hip release in the Western orientation and centering or calming in the Eastern tradition) according to therapy goals and the orientation of the practitioner.

Mechanism of Action

Eastern and Western medical frameworks each have their own theories on how Shiatsu affects the body. The Eastern perspective embraces the idea of wholeness/oneness of being, which stresses that all aspects of existence are intertwined with and affect each other. Therefore, pressing acupoints affects the body's spiritual and physical essence as a whole. The Western perspective focuses on specific symptoms rather than on a pattern of influences, with the pressing of acupoints focusing on alleviating particular physical symptoms. A combination of the two views is increasingly being espoused by many practitioners.

Shiatsu and the Eastern Paradigm: The Human as an Extension of the Universe

Fundamental to Traditional Chinese Medicine (TCM), from which Shiatsu evolves, is the idea that people exist within the universe and as part of the universe. Health or sickness are defined relatively, since nothing in the universe is absolute (Beinfield & Korngold, 1991). A person's state of health is considered relative to his or her state of illness. A person can have a high degree of health, as there may be a small degree of illness, and vice versa. A person may also be said to have a degree of health relative to those around him or her. In TCM, as with the universe, a healthy organism or state of being depends on the circulation of chi, the balance of yin and yang, and the balance of the five elements.

Therapy Focus

Shiatsu is classified as a manual therapy. It can be used as a manual/energetic intervention (focusing on the manipulation of chi and balancing of yin and yang) to manipulate the physical body or alleviate symptoms. The integration of Shiatsu in the traditional rehabilitation setting must be compatible within the overall nature of the session and must fit within the client's plans and clinical goals and objectives. To accomplish this, the therapist must have a sound working knowledge of what Shiatsu can be used for, what goals it will address, and how to individualize the approach. One must check state license laws regarding the use of this modality, because Shiatsu is defined within the massage and bodywork framework. It is also imperative that the therapist receive proper training and certification.

Shiatsu works by opening up meridians (energy channels) to enable circulation of chi. These meridians receive and provide chi to and from organs. When meridians are open, and chi is flowing, it may be directed to or away from various parts of the body. Shiatsu is used to direct the flow of chi by way of acupoints within a meridian. These acupoints act like irrigation systems to direct the flow of energy within a body. They can be used to either fill up with chi or empty out excess chi. The points may also influence energies regarding the five elements. When flowing evenly, chi will act to balance and regulate the organs as well as their energetic influences on the mind and body (Maciocia, 1989). Shiatsu on the correct points on a meridian of an effected organ can serve to restore balance. There may be instances where pressure on a point, or pressure in general, may be contraindicated (for example, in cases of skin rash or a low tolerance of pressure). In this case, an individual may stretch out a meridian by stretching out the defined limb or body part. There is a series of exercises and stretches, called *Makka-Ho,* that stretch out all major meridians.

The Western Medical Paradigm

Whereas in Eastern terms the body works as one unit, which is manifested by chi, the Western outlook takes a more reductionistic approach. The Western medical framework looks to specific systems and individual body parts to find dysfunction causality, and Shiatsu from a Western perspective targets these systems and body parts to alleviate problems.

The Effects of Shiatsu: A Comparison of Eastern and Western Perspectives

Muscular System

West: Overly contracted muscles can be painful, develop fatigue, and build up toxic waste materials, such as lactic acid. The location of some acupoints are at muscles. Compression of muscles via Shiatsu can decrease contraction, alleviating strain and fatigue. It also activates the lymphatic system to drain waste materials. Transportation of oxygen and other nutrients via blood vessels can also become more efficient.

East: Muscle tone is tonified ("tonify" refers to normalizing muscle tone or organ function) by the redirection of chi flow, which the therapist seeks to increase or decrease. Specific points along the meridians may be used for this purpose (Masunaga and Ohashi, 1977).

Central Nervous System (CNS)

West: When pressure such as Shiatsu is used on the body, especially deep pressure along muscle regions, endorphins are released. These endorphins act as pain inhibitors and stress relievers, which can put the receiver in a state of relaxation. This state of relaxation can allow the body to rest, decreasing stress on all other systems, such as muscles, nerves, and lungs.

The CNS is dependent on cerebrospinal fluids to transport waste toxins out. Pressure along the spinal grooves facilitates cerebrospinal transportation of waste and allows fresh fluids and blood in.

East: The CNS is affected by many aspects of living, such as exercise, diet, environment, and air quality. Shiatsu is a valued tool to circulate chi to vitalize the nervous system. Also, because nerves spread to every part of the body, the effect of the stretching and compression used in Shiatsu is spread throughout the body.

Autonomic Nervous System

West: A Shiatsu session to specific points activates the peripheral nervous system (PNS), which acts to reduce and conserve energy by putting the body in a state of rest, softening muscle tone and relaxing respiration, as well as improving digestive processes. Stress is a state that hinders the immune system and hampers the rehabilitation process. By activating the PNS to balance out the sympathetic nervous system, Shiatsu can enhance the body's healing process (Dubitsky, 1997).

East: The Eastern perspective views appropriate levels of stress as an important source of motivation and goal-directed behavior. Too much stress, however, is a sign of imbalance. Clients must be assessed to determine where the imbalance lies, and Shiatsu on specific acupoints would be used to address imbalance. TCM notes that stress also affects the kidney (Ohashi, 2001), so both treatment and preventive care must be given or prescribed to control stress through bodywork, diet, meditation, and exercise.

Other Systems

- The cardiovascular system is able to more efficiently circulate blood when muscles are less tense. From a Western perspective, acupressure can lower muscle tone so that the heart pumps blood with less work. This puts the client in a more relaxed state, which can improve performance during the rehabilitation session. In Eastern practice, the heart has its own meridian. The heart can be tonified through acupoints on the heart meridian.
- The respiratory system is at peak efficiency when the chest is able to expand at a greater intensity and the lungs can fill with more air. A variety of factors, including improper positioning when standing or seated, or a stressed state, can restrict chest expansion and therefore limit air intake. A Shiatsu session, from a Western perspective, can improve respiratory efficiency by relaxing chest muscles, improving posture, and consequently improving air intake. In Eastern practice, the lung also has its own meridian and can be tonified through work on acupoints along this meridian. Work at these points, for example, can help to clear coughs, expel phlegm, decongest, and promote air circulation in the lungs (Maciocia, 1989).
- Histological considerations. Individual cells become nonfunctional and die if too many toxins build up in them. This may occur when capillaries are unable to circulate fresh oxygenated blood, and when the lymphatic system is unable to adequately access the cell area. From the Eastern perspective, TCM values the importance of circulation to maintain vitality and Shiatsu is used to clear out toxic build-up. From a Western perspective, the manual compression of Shiatsu, which stretches passive muscles and opens up blood vessels, enables greater transport of waste and clean fluids to affected cells (Namikoshi, 1981).

◆ Intestinal functions. The intestines absorb nutrients from food and facilitate elimination of wastes. From a Western perspective, Shiatsu therapy can assist in helping intestines to more efficiently regulate these functions if an irregularity caused by inefficient absorption or excess ingestion of poorly digested foods should occur (Namikoshi, 1981). From an Eastern perspective, there are meridians for both large and small intestines in TCM. Shiatsu to these meridians enhances the function of the intestines.

Pediatrics

Children come with unique conditions that make them especially vulnerable to imbalance and illnesses. Their young and developing bodies are assailable to a variety of conditions that are defined within the TCM framework. TCM treatment in pediatrics, as in adults, focuses on the overall process of recommending dietary changes, as well as chi flow clearing through meridians and balancing of yin and yang. Modern Chinese approaches with children focus on two areas—treating the insult and strengthening the body (Scott, 1986). In other words, if a child suffers an insult such as a birth injury or brain injury, the process focuses on treating the injured area as well as strengthening chi flow. Shiatsu can be used, then, to address both the injured area or dysfunctional system and chi flow.

Mental Health

In TCM, an emotion becomes an issue only when it is expressed for too long or too severely. The emotion is seen as a result of imbalance. When one treats the imbalance, one then treats the emotion. Anger, depression, and anxiety are all natural consequences of human existence. It is when they interfere with normal daily routine that they must be treated.

Emotional imbalance may either cause or be caused by body disharmony. TCM acknowledges seven basic emotional states: anger, joy, worry, pensiveness, sadness, fear, and shock (Maciocia, 1989). Each has a connection to an organ and overall chi flow. There is no mental

Indications

- ◆ Emotional stress or anxiety
- ◆ A need for the least possible invasive process to normalize muscle tone
- ◆ A need to reinforce normal body mechanics or image in children with neurological or neurodevelopmental delays
- ◆ A need to increase range of motion in a particular joint while minimizing discomfort during movement
- ◆ A need or desire for a modality that will simultaneously help clients improve physical function while maintaining a steady emotional balance—for example, for clients with cerebral palsy, brain trauma, multiple sclerosis, stroke, or other neurological disorders

Contraindications

- ◆ A recent orthopedic insult
- ◆ An acute condition such as an infection, gastrointestinal upset, hemorrhage, shock, asthma attack, or recent cerebral vascular accident (CVA) (not stabilized)
- ◆ A very significant or recent heart condition
- ◆ Skin infection
- ◆ General poor condition such as dehydration, malnutrition, advanced organ disease, circulatory dysfunction
- ◆ Advanced stage of pregnancy (six months or over)
- ◆ Recent gastrointestinal bleeding (ulcers)

The general rule of thumb is summarized in one simple statement: If you have any concerns, don't perform the treatment.

illness per se in TCM; rather, the symptoms of mental illness are seen simply as manifestations of the organ's imbalances.

Shiatsu for emotional conditions will work to restore circulation and balance to reduce emotional disorder. The inclusion of Shiatsu in any form, be it applied by a therapist or by clients themselves, can work to alleviate emotional "baggage" that may hinder a client's functioning or performance. Other common procedures to balance the body would be to perform body (meridian) stretches and to perform the mind-calming exercises described later.

Typical Treatment Session

The first session of a Shiatsu bodywork massage begins with an interview about specific complaints, a medical history, and habits such as sleeping, eating, and working. The practitioner assesses the client by taking pulses and observing the tongue, eyes, and facial color. Acupoints are assessed both during the evaluation and during treatment sessions.

Preparation

Like most bodywork interventions, prior to a Shiatsu session, the therapist must be focused within himself or herself. Otherwise, the energies given off by the therapist may disrupt any benefit the massage might offer. The therapist can utilize the following exercises to enhance centering:

1. The therapist can access the *Hara* (the center of chi storage in the body) by standing or sitting still and placing his or her hands gently on the abdomen, inhaling deeply through the nose while concentrating on breathing air into the abdomen slowly and with a relaxed mood. Slow exhalation through the mouth is repeated three times. Attention should be paid to how the air is directed to the abdomen; it should rise with each inhale and fall with each exhale. Following this breathing regimen, some slow stretching for increasing flexibility as well as chi flow is recommended. Occasionally, a slow deep intake and exhale at the chest may be done to stretch chest cavity.
2. The therapist should perform a brief relaxing meditation if feeling stressed or distracted.
3. Brief deep massage to hands is helpful in circulating chi.

The client is usually clothed in a loose-fitting, comfortable shirt and pants, and socks are optional; the only time bare skin is needed is if moxa sticks[1] are used. The therapist begins at the back, proceeding down to the feet, providing stretches and pressure along points and meridians. The therapist works medial to peripheral, down to the feet, and then upward to hands. When finished in the prone position, the client turns over, and the process repeats in supine, beginning with abdominal "massage." Hand pressure depends on the client's tolerance, and the length of time spent at each acupoint depends on meridian's chi flow. Approaches within Shiatsu may be adapted to suit individual needs. For example, those who are intolerant of touch, and those who are sensitive to pressure on their skin can be provided with either different levels of touch or stretches to open the meridians to improve chi flow.

Shiatsu may be provided during a session, either by the therapist pressing on acupoints or by clients pressing on their own points. (The latter practice is called *do-in*. Stickers can be placed at acupoints in children to facilitate learning.) The client may need to lie still beneath a blanket following the massage because the chi has been circulated and the client may feel chilly due to the effects of the sudden circulation of energy. He or she may want the energies to settle a bit prior to getting up. Follow-up sessions spend a brief period on diagnosis and interview, with more time on the treatment process.

---

[1]Moxa Sticks are herbs compressed into a stick form. They are held above acupoints at the skin and burned as a form of heat therapy to stimulate deep chi flow. Moxa cones may be used on the surface of the skin.

Training is required for a therapist who wishes to seriously consider adding Shiatsu to his or her skills. A weekend course is offered to learn fundamentals of pressure technique, and the full course consists of 500 hours of training. This includes training in Shiatsu technique, meridians, acupoints, pulse assessment, general assessment skills, yoga, meditation, macrobiotic cooking , practice in clinical observation, anatomy and physiology, business skills, training in other types of Chinese massage, and pediatric massage. Schools are listed in a variety of sources, such as holistic health magazines, the Yellow Pages, and on the Internet. To check if the school's instructors are fully certified, the American Oriental Bodywork and Therapy Association (AOBTA) may be contacted.

The National Certification Commission for Acupuncture and Oriental Medicine (NCCAOM) is an agency that oversees credentialing of Asian bodywork therapies such as the AOBTA. The AOBTA is a national nonprofit association of TCM practitioners. Its credentialing process requires documentation of formal training by a certified instructor. The AOBTA provides insurance and continuing education. As of this writing, there is no license for Shiatsu practitioners.

Once a therapist is trained, the individual must determine how to best integrate Shiatsu into occupational or physical therapy practice. A therapist may include Shiatsu in the session or may decide to go into private practice as a "holistic practitioner." In each case, one must check with local license laws regarding such scenarios.

Research

There is a fair amount of research on Shiatsu outcomes, but unfortunately, some of the best controlled studies have little relevance to rehabilitation populations. A sizable portion of the research on Shiatsu has focused on its benefits in treatment of nausea. For example, Dibble and colleagues (2000) researched Shiatsu to treat nausea resulting from chemotherapy for breast cancer. Results indicated that Shiatsu helped reduce this type of nausea. Belluomini and colleagues (1994) evaluated the effectiveness of Shiatsu to reduce nausea and vomiting associated with pregnancy. This randomized, double-blind study showed that Shiatsu on a specific point (pericardium 6, also known as P6) significantly decreased nausea in the treatment group as compared with the control group. Other researchers have confirmed the positive effects of stimulating P6 on decreasing nausea and vomiting (Steele et al., 2001).

Researchers have investigated the effect of Shiatsu on a variety of factors, such as quality of sleep, cardiovascular system health, and hemiplegia. Chen and colleagues (1999) found that Shiatsu improved sleep quality in institutionalized elderly residents. Improved quality of sleep would be of great benefit to many clients receiving therapy sessions. Felhendler and Lisander (1999) studied the effects of Shiatsu on the cardiovascular system. The study showed that skin blood flow, arterial pressure, and heart rate were all significantly affected with improved circulation by the Shiatsu treatment. Finally, Chen (1997) studied the effectiveness of what he terms *digital acupoint pressure (DAP)* in treating apoplectic hemiplegia.

Results showed a 90.5 percent effectiveness in treating this condition, with results ranging from being "cured" to marked improvement.

There are also studies that show that Shiatsu is a useful adjunct treatment. Garvey, Marks, and Wiesel (1989) compared the effects of Shiatsu with lidocaine, lidocaine with a steroid, and a vapocoolant spray on lower back pain. Results indicated that Shiatsu paired with lidocaine was as effective as lidocaine with a steroid. Clients seeking to minimize use of pharmaceuticals or avoid steroid side effects might benefit from a similar approach.

As therapists and reimbursement sources continue to embrace evidence-based practice, clearly the use of Shiatsu as an adjunct to therapy practice will need to be researched further.

Case Studies

Closed Head Injury

Mark, a 20-year-old male, was 15 years old when he was in a car accident resulting in a closed head injury. He had no significant medical history prior to the accident. As a result of the accident, he was unable to verbally communicate, muscle tone increased significantly (impairing range of motion in all extremities), and he became nonambulatory. He also became dependent in all areas of activities of daily living (ADLs), but appeared within normal range of awareness and cognition. The client lives at home with his family and has a full-time registered nurse. The client was referred to physical therapy for muscle tone management and gait training, and to occupational therapy for upper extremity (UE) control and adaptive ADLs.

During the course of treatment, the OT, a Shiatsu practitioner, was able to increase active range of motion (AROM) of the client's shoulders by pressing along acupoints in shoulder, scapular, and neck area, as well as in the upper back. When this area was released, the client's muscle tone decreased and he was able to access switch controls. The client preferred Shiatsu because he found it less invasive than massage, vestibular stimulation, and myofascial release. The following demonstrates how Shiatsu was documented in OT progress notes using the SOAP note (subjective, objective, assessment, plan) format:

S: Client in wheelchair ready for session. High tone is noted in upper back and arms.
O: Continued to work on switch access, which is impaired by high tone in shoulders and elbows, limiting extension and preventing client from reaching switch. Placed client on tablemat and pressed on acupoints in shoulders, arms, and upper back. After 10 minutes, client returned to wheelchair and continued to work on switches for EC (environmental control).
A: Prior to acupressure, shoulder flexion passive range of motion (PROM) was 85 degrees; post-acupressure was 110. Elbow extension was previously 20 degrees, and post-acupressure extension was 50, which enabled pressing a switch 7 out of 10 times with minimal delays. Client was able to turn radio on and off and switch stations. Nurse requested to learn acupoint sequence to release upper extremities.
P: Continue with EC activation.

(The session involved other activities that have no bearing on Shiatsu).

Shiatsu was performed for approximately 10 minutes of the session and resulted in marked improved performance.

Physical therapy goals focused on improving hip mobility and postural stability. This was typically accomplished through traditional stretching techniques. The PT was taught to stretch the area while pressing along acupoints to decrease the amount of time spent on stretching from 30 to 60 minutes to 10 minutes per session. The PT documented the intervention as follows:

Goal: Erect sitting posture with head erect and arms relaxed to allow use of upper extremities and/or head for switch access.

Problem: Tightness of quadratus lumborum muscle, causing left lateral flexion and hip hiking, resulting in falling to the left side in static sitting posture. The implantation of a backlafen pump on client's right side has increased this tightness.

Results: Generally, with 30 to 60 minutes of relaxation, stretching, and facial release techniques, the client has been able to obtain erect sitting posture.

With application of 10 minutes of OT-demonstrated acupressure treatment to left hip, foot, and lower extremity, the client was able to maintain an erect posture, independently sitting in an upright position for 2 minutes longer than previous session without accupressure, and 5 minutes longer with back support, with improved head control for switch access noted.

Down's Syndrome and Cerebral Palsy

Tara is a 5-year-old girl with Down's syndrome and mild cerebral palsy. She presented with high impulsivity and poor postural stability, which impaired body mechanics during tablework and accuracy in visual motor activities. She is unable to hop or stand on one leg. Therapy goals include being able to kick a soccer ball to target, cut along a curved line, and maintain proper seating position when engaged in tablework. These skills support school objectives for class and gym participation.

The client generally arrived to therapy hyperactive and highly distracted. Both the OT and PT initiated sessions with deep breathing and stretching Shiatsu meridians, which would facilitate concentration. The breathing and stretching helped focus and center the client to a calmer, more relaxed state of being. The therapists noted that, when focused, the quality of the client's work improved. The client did not tolerate touch well, so she was taught to perform meridian stretches independently. This enabled work on balance, trunk stability, and body image. Also, stretches were performed slowly to reinforce motor planning skills. A combination of stretches and graded breathing, which take approximately 10 minutes of the half hour session, are used to reduce impulsivity. The teacher was taught to carry over these techniques into the class routine. Preparatory work was followed by more traditional OT modalities, which included but were not limited to use of a rocker board, physioball, balance beam, writing skills practice sheets, and cutting sheets. After several weeks of treatment (once a week each for OT and PT) the client

1. Neck work: The base of the neck holds several important points related to mental and emotional processes. These points may be pressed by the therapist or by the client. GB20, located below the occipital bone, is an acupoint that benefits concentration and inhibits fright. B10, located approximately three fingers below the lateral aspect of the occipital node by the trapezius muscle, inhibits stress, tension, and overexertion.
2. Shoulder work: The shoulder and upper back also have several points for balancing emotional states and reducing anxiety and tension. TW15, located on top of scapular angle, reduces tension and stress. GB21 (located between C7 and T1, approximately three fingers from spinal groove on either side) reduces nervousness and irritability. The meridian at this point is the channel regulating decisions, so this point will also help reduce indecision.

Press fingers gently into these points with firm but not hard or gouging pressure. Hold for three to four breaths and release.

(Source: Reed-Gach, 1980.)

was able to relax and prepare herself independently prior to treatment sessions. This enabled the therapists to concentrate the entire 30 minutes of treatment on standard therapy goals. Effective communication with the teacher focused on several issues: that the preparatory activities were not time consuming or invasive, and that the focus was on enabling improved function within the classroom environment, and that the purpose was not to make a "Zen master" out of the child.

Cerebrovascular Accident

Eve is a 72-year-old female with recent right cerebrovascular accident (CVA). She was ambulatory with a quad cane and had right upper extremity flexor synergy. She was very concerned about being dependent on her family for ADLs and was referred for home care OT for UE exercises and ADL treatment.

Eve reported that she is "excitable to begin with." When asked to relax to allow PROM exercises, she became agitated, causing increases in flexor synergy. Range of motion did not improve for several sessions. The OT decided to use Shiatsu, gentle self-stretching, and breathing exercises to address agitation. These interventions, with Shiatsu on the back of Eve's neck and shoulder points, helped Eve to relax. She was then able to extend her elbow and grossly grasp objects. Once Eve was able to overcome her initial anxiety, sessions proceeded with arm stretches and hand rehabilitation. Self-range of motion exercises were provided. Eve's family was able to see how the relaxation process directly affected her ability to improve her clinical performance. In fact, her husband, who has a heart condition, atrial fibulation, and hypertension, also tried and benefited from the relaxation procedure. (Clients with long-term cardiac conditions such as atrial fibulation or a stenosis may receive some Shiatsu bodywork by a more experienced practitioner.)

In each case, Shiatsu was utilized locally to balance tone in affected areas and to improve chi flow to enhance functional outcomes.

Summary

Shiatsu is a manual intervention that stems from Traditional Chinese Medicine. It can be used to balance the flow of chi, to address the physical body alone, or both, depending on which paradigm the practitioner espouses. Therapists must check with state licensing boards before determining how Shiatsu can be integrated into therapy practice.

STUDY QUESTIONS

1. Explain how the following terms relate to each other: chi, meridians, and acupoints.
2. A client with a CVA displays a spastic elbow with limited extension. As a Shiatsu trained therapist, you note that release to points along the shoulder and wrist will improve elbow ROM. Explain to your puzzled coworkers how manipulation of acupoints can affect symptoms at a different site.
3. A client is very apprehensive about standing after a hip surgery, and this anxiety is preventing full compliance. This has been ongoing for days and the "usual methods of engagement" are not working. You ask if you can press along certain points along the neck and shoulders. When asked why, you explain you know of certain points that, when pressed, could help calm the client. Explain to the client and coworkers, from both an Eastern and Western framework, how this may occur.
4. A child with cerebral palsy displays spasticity in the lower extremities and may require a release to decrease the tone. The child, however, is hypersensitive to touch and refuses to let the therapist provide pressure on points. Name two other methods by which Shiatsu could be performed.
5. Name at least five conditions in which Shiatsu would be contraindicated.
6. You wish to add Shiatsu as a therapeutic modality to your practice, but are hesitant to describe it in an Eastern framework, being concerned that terms such as chi, yin, yang, and so on would not be within your clients' understanding. Pick three systems of the body (e.g., muscular, nervous) and explain how Shiatsu would benefit these systems. Put explanations in "layman" terms.
7. You are late for an appointment and are somewhat stressed out, having hurried to be there. There are still concerns in your mind, but you feel able to provide full attention to your client. The client wants some more of that "nice delightful shoulder relaxation work" you did last time. Explain to your client why, then, you must take some more time before you can actually work on her.
8. Describe a technique to prepare the practitioner prior to performing Shiatsu.

RESOURCES

American Oriental Bodywork and Therapy
   Association (AOTBA)
1010 Haddonfield-Berlin Rd., Suite 408
Vorhees, NJ 08043
(856) 782-1616
AOBTA@prodigy.net

National Certification and Commission for
   Acupuncture and Oriental Medicine
11 Canal Center Plaza, Suite 300
Alexandria, VA 22314
(703) 548-9004

REFERENCES

Beinfield H., & E. Korngold. (1991). *Between Heaven and Earth: A Guide to Chinese Medicine*. New York: Random House.

Belluomini, J., R. C. Litt, K. A. Lee, & M. Katy. (1994). Acupressure for nausea and vomiting of pregnancy: A randomized, blinded study. *Obstetrics and Gynecology, 84*(2), 245–248.

Chen, M. L., L. C. Lin, S. C. Wu, & J. G. Lin. (1999, Aug.). The effectiveness of acupressure in improving the quality of sleep of institutionalized residents. *Journal of Gerontology, 54a*(8), M389–394.

Chen, R. (1997, Sept.). Treatment of apoplectic hemiplegia by digital acupoint pressure—A report of 42 cases. *Journal of Traditional Chinese Medicine, 17*(3), 198–202.

Coseo, M. (1992). *Acupressure Warm-up*. Brookline, MA: Paradigm.

Dibble, S. L., J. Chapman, K. A. Mack, & A. S. Shih. (2000). Acupressure for nausea: Results of a pilot study. *Oncology Nurse Forum, 27*(1), 41–47.

Dubitsky, C. (1997). *Bodywork Shiatsu*. Rochester, VT: Healing Arts Press.

Felhendler, D., & B. Lisander. (1999, Dec.). Effects of noninvasive stimulation of acupoints on the cardiovascular system. *Complementary Therapies in Medicine, 7*(4), 231–234.

Fugh-Berman, A. (1999, Jan.). Acupressure for nausea and vomiting of pregnancy. *Alternative Therapies in Women's Health, 13*(9), 9–11.

Garvey, T. A., M. R. Marks, & S. W. Wiesel. (1989, Sept.). A prospective, randomized, double-blind evaluation of trigger point injection therapy for low back pain. *Spine, 14*(9), 962.

Liechti, E. (1998). *The Complete Illustrated Guide to Shiatsu*. Boston: Element Books.

Maciocia, G. (1989). *The Foundations of Chinese Medicine*. Singapore: Longman Singapore.

Masunaga, S., & W. Ohashi. (1997). *Zen Shiatsu—How to Harmonize Yin and Yang for Better Health*. Tokyo: Japan Publishing.

Namikoshi, T. (1981). *The Complete Book of Shiatsu Therapy*. Tokyo: Japan Publishing.

Ohashi, W. (2001). *Do It Yourself Shiatsu—How to Perform the Ancient Art of Acupuncture Without Needles*. New York: E. P. Dutton.

Reed-Gach, M. (1980). *Acupressure's Potent Points*. New York: Bantam Books.

Reed-Gach, M., & C. Marco. (1981). *AcuYoga*. Tokyo: Japan Publishing.

Scott, J. (1986). *Acupuncture in the Treatment of Children*. Seattle, WA: Eastland Press.

Steele, N. M., J. French, J. Gatherer-Boyles, S. Newman, & S. LeClaire. (2001). Effect of acupressure by Sea-Bands on nausea and vomiting of pregnancy. *Journal of Obstetrical Gynecological Nursing, 30*(1), 61–70.

Travell, J., D. Simons, & B. Cummings. (1991). *Myofascial Pain and Dysfunction: The Trigger Point Manual*. Baltimore, MD: Lippincott, Williams and Wilkins.

Zhao-Pu, W. (1991). *Acupressure Therapy: Potent Point Percussion of Cerebral Birth Injury and Stroke*. Singapore: Longman Singapore.

22

Structural Integration (Rolfing)

Judith Deutsch, Patricia Judd, and Irene DeMasi

CHAPTER OBJECTIVES

- ◆ Understand the goals and assumptions of structural integration.
- ◆ Describe the focus of a complete structural integration series.
- ◆ Discuss research on structural integration.
- ◆ Describe training in structural integration.

Rolfing was developed by Dr. Ida Rolf and is described in the book *Rolfing: The Integration of Human Structures* (1977). Dr. Rolf was born in 1896 in New York. She graduated Barnard College in 1916, and received her Ph.D. in biological chemistry from the College of Physicians and Surgeons of Columbia University in 1920 (Rolf Institute for Structural Integration, 2001).

Rolf was interested in complementary therapies such as yoga, chiropractic, and Awareness through Movement (a Feldenkrais Method concept). She combined her training as a scientist, her interest in complementary therapies as well as her own experiences with physical trauma to develop Rolfing. Initially she trained health care practitioners but then expanded her audience. At the time of her death there were 200 certified Rolfers (Rolf Institute for Structural Integration, 2001).

Background

The primary goal of SI is to restore the alignment of the body with respect to gravity in order to improve mobility and well-being. This is achieved by remodeling the structure of the body, specifically the fascia. Dr. Rolf believed that a body that was aligned with respect to gravity functions more efficiently. Proper alignment allows muscles to function at their optimal length-tension relationship. She writes, "In a structurally integrated body the flexors flex and the extensors extend" (Rolf, 1977, p. 35).

Optimal alignment requires that the blocks, which represent the different segments of the body, be centered on the pelvis and aligned in all three planes. A body becomes malaligned or disorganized with respect to gravity as a result of trauma or the cumulative effects of poor posture. Segments of the body can be malaligned in all three planes, producing asymmetries and torsions. In Rolf's view, "the body is a plastic medium that succumbs to the unequal torque in everyday life" (Rolf, 1977, p. 30).

One of the main assumptions of SI is that the fascia acts as an organ to connect the entire body. Superficial fascia, which encases muscles and separates compartments, is very flexible. When damaged, this tissue becomes shortened and denser, creating the effect that a snag might have on a sweater. Therefore, damage in one part of the body can have an effect on the alignment and structure of the entire body. The damage to the tissue also changes the tone in the tissue.

The intervention is also based on the assumption that the tissue can be remodeled using manual pressure and the body's alignment restored with respect to gravity. Rolf postulated that the addition of pressures add energy to the tissue colloids. The application of this energy is believed to turn colloid gel into solution (Rolf, 1977). Therefore, the intervention reverses the disorganization or malalignment of the body.

SI consists of 10 sessions of soft-tissue mobilization and movement reeducation. Client posture and selected movements are evaluated at each session. Postural assessments are performed in standing from anterior, posterior, and both lateral views. The body is viewed as a series of blocks that should be aligned in all planes. The pelvis is considered the central and pivotal block. The absence of this alignment indicates that structure is not integrated (Rolf, 1977). The treatment is aimed at restoring this alignment.

Evaluating and Treating

Evaluation and treatment are combined in a session, using the evaluation to direct the treatment. The evaluation and treatment process have general principles for every session and specific elements that are related to the objectives of each session. The practitioner may

Indications

- Normalize soft tissue mobility
- Release muscle spasms
- Decrease pain
- Improve musculoskeletal alignment
- Increase movement efficiency

Contraindications

- An acute exacerbation of arthritis
- Advanced osteoporosis
- Advanced diabetes
- An increase in symptoms with prior soft tissue mobilization

Precautions

Avoid areas being treated for:

- malignancy
- inflammation
- fracture
- hemorrhage
- obstructive edema
- infection
- aneurysm
- osteomyelitis
- deep vein thrombosis

(Adapted with permission from Edmonds, 2001)

reevaluate often within a session, asking the client to stand or perform a movement. Documentation of the evaluation can be in a narrative form and is often supplemented with photographs. A single session will typically last 1 hour. The sessions are spaced 1 week apart. This interval allows the body to adapt to the changes in alignment between each session.

Each of the 10 sessions of a complete SI series has a specific purpose and focuses on a different part of the body. The emphasis of the sessions alternates from a focus on the upper body (sessions 1, 3, and 5) to the lower body (sessions 2, 4, and 6). In session 7 the head is the focus. Sessions 8 and 9 address either the upper or the lower body, depending what is required. The final session emphasizes large fascial planes and integration across the body. The goals, depth of the work, and key myofascial structures are summarized in Table 22–1.

The evaluation consists of observing a client's posture in standing from anterior, posterior and lateral views. The practitioner uses the pelvis as the central block and visualizes additional blocks above and below the pelvis, observing their alignment with respect to the line of gravity. There may also be an observation of movement, attending to whether

Table 22–1 Session Goals of Structural Integration

Session	Goals	Depth	Key Myofascial Structures
1	• Establish rapport with the patient • Increase movement with each breath of the thorax and ribs • Horizontalize the pelvis	Superficial	Rib cage and costal arch
2	• Restore alignment between the calcaneus and the ischial tuberosities • Restore balanced movement between the hip, knee, and ankles • Direct attention to the relationship of the feet to the ground	Superficial	Peri-articular ankle retinaculum, plantar fascia, and lateral arch
3	• Lengthen the lateral line • Increase the space between the pelvis and the 12th rib • Release the shoulder and pelvic girdles	Superficial	Quadratus lumborum, 12th rib
4	• Reduce excessive rotation of the lower limb • Align the pelvis in all planes • Align the foot with respect to the spine	Deep	Medial retinaculum of the ankle, attachments of the adductors and hamstrings to the pubic ramus
5	• Lengthen the anterior thorax • Align the clavicles in all planes • Facilitate movement of the arm with proper scapular alignment • Facilitate movements of hip flexion	Deep	Psoas, pectoralis minor, rectus abdominus, and diaphragm
6	• Vertically align the lower limb • Align the pelvis, sacrum, and spine	Deep	Hip rotators, sacrotuberous ligament, thoracolumbar fascia
7	• Align the head • Separate the fascia of the head and arms	Superficial to deep	Sternocleidomastoid, scalenes, masseter, occipital atlantic ligaments, deep cervical muscles, and cranial fascia

(continued)

the "sleeve" (i.e., arms and legs) moves freely over the "core" (i.e., the spine, pelvis, and clavicle).

A global examination of posture precedes a more focuses observation that is dictated by the goals of the session. In the third session, for example, the focus is the lateral line of the

Table 22–1 *Continued*

Session	Goals	Depth	Key Myofascial Structures
8 and 9	◆ Focus on either the upper or lower body ◆ Balance and relate the girdles to the dorsal lumbar hinge ◆ Relate the limbs to the spine	Varied	Mobility of fascial planes
10	◆ Integrate a functional whole ◆ Maximize movement strategies and efficiency	Varied	Fascial planes across joints

trunk. This is a line that extends from the greater trochanter to the head of the humerus. Key structures in this session are the quadratus lumborum and the 12th rib. The therapist observes the alignment from the ear to the lateral malleolus, notes if the length of the 12th rib and the iliac crest is symmetrical between both sides, and whether the lateral lower chest expands during breathing.

The treatment consists of soft-tissue mobilization and movement awareness cues. The soft tissue work is performed with the client in supine, sidelying, sitting, and prone positions. The hands and elbows are used to impart the force on the tissues. The depth of the soft-tissue work varies with the session. In sessions 1 to 3 the work is more superficial, at the skin-fascia interface. During sessions 4 to 6 the work is deeper, at the fascia-bone interface. Sessions 7 to 10 are considered integrative in nature, and the work is done along large fascial planes.

There is some general tissue work that occurs at each session, with an emphasis placed on the structures that are the focus of the session. In session 3, for example, with the client positioned in sidelying, work is done at iliac crest, thoracolumbar fascia, 12th rib, quadratus lumborum, greater trochanter and iliacus (to separate the ileotibial band from the vastus or biceps femoris), the tensor fascia latae, gluteals, and quadratus femoris, down to the fibular head. The shoulder girdle is released from the rib cage by working on the teres major, subscapularis, serratus anterior, latissumus dorsi, pectoralis major, deltoids, and intercostal spaces. The fascia between the trapezius, levator, splenius, sternocleidomastoid, and scalenes is differentiated. Movement awareness cues focus on rib expansion. Movement education is performed in sidelying, having the client reach or extend extremities in an effort to lengthen the lateral line.

Research

Research about the outcomes of SI interventions has been conducted on individuals who are healthy as well as on those who have a disease. Cottingham and his colleagues (Cottingham, Porges, & Lyon, 1988; Cottingham, Porges, & Richmond, 1988) researched the effects of

There are two organizations in the United States that certify practitioners and support the development of Rolfing: the Guild for Structural Integration and the Rolfing Association. Each organization has a useful Web page that lists practitioners as well as resources such as books and videotapes. Both offer courses that lead to certification and advanced training.

The Rolf Institute for Structural Integration was founded in 1971 by Dr. Ida Rolf. Its mission is to train Rolfing practitioners and Rolf movement practitioners, support research, and promote Rolfing to the public. According to the Rolfing Association, there are over 1,000 certified Rolfers in 27 countries.

Only people trained and certified by the Rolf Institute are licensed to use the Rolfing service mark. To receive the basic certification takes approximately 2 years. The process is composed of three units interspersed with clinical practice: Unit 1 (214 hours), Foundations of Somatic Practice, teaches background on anatomy, physiology, and kinesiology, Unit 2 (244 hours), Embodiment of Rolfing and Rolf Movement Integration, and Unit 3 (269 hours), Clinical Application of Rolfing Theory, with a focus on theory and clinical application of the techniques. The institute also offers advanced certification. It publishes *Rolf Lines*, which is available to practitioners.

The Guild for Structural Integration is a private, nonprofit vocational school that was founded in 1972. It is a teaching and research service organization that promotes SI as a method and philosophy of personal growth and integrity. To become certified as a structural integration practitioner through the Guild, one must complete a three-part course series, which consists of a prerequisite class in anatomy, kinesiology, and biomechanics; an auditing class (264 hours in evaluation training), and a practicing class. An interview is required before progressing to the practicing phase (264 hours), in which individuals practice the manual skills on models and each other. Advanced training and continuing education courses are also offered. The Guild publishes the *Guild News*, which is available for practitioners.

SI on healthy subjects. They studied the effects of a single Rolfing maneuver, the pelvic lift, on parasympathetic tone. In both studies they found an increase in parasympathetic tone after the application of the maneuver. This work provides some quasi-experimental evidence for a role of the autonomic nervous system in explaining the mechanism of SI.

Studies about the efficacy of SI with different patient populations consist of case studies (Cottingham & Maitland, 1997; Deutsch, Judd, & DeMasi, 1997) and correlational studies (Deutsch et al., 2000; Talty, DeMasi, & Deutsch, 1998). These studies were conducted with different patient populations, such as those with chronic pain (Deutsch et al., 2000) low back pain (Cottingham & Maitland, 1997), cerebral palsy (Perry et al., 1981), and traumatic brain injury (Deutsch, Judd, & DeMasi, 1997). The outcomes of these studies are in general supportive of the efficacy of SI, but the research was conducted with small samples and designs that were not rigorous. They can be interpreted as preliminary support for the approach and enough positive findings to justify further study.

Importantly, in all the research that has been conducted on SI there have been no adverse effects reported. This suggests that in the populations in which SI was studied (i.e., the healthy and individuals with chronic musculoskeletal and neurologic diagnoses) there is some merit in the approach. The primary outcomes have been reductions in pain, increases in flexibility, improvements in posture, improvements in function, and reports of well-being. With the exception of the brain injury case study (Deutsch, Judd, & DeMasi, 1997), none of the studies looked at long-term effects of SI.

Case Study

Multiple Sclerosis with Special Seating Needs

A 52-year-old female with a 14-year history of progressive MS punctuated with exacerbations and subtotal remissions lived at home with her husband. She used a walker for household ambulation. Early in 1993 she experienced a deterioration in her mobility and cognitive status, which was attributed to the progressive nature of the disease. In August 1993 she underwent a sacretomy and partial ischietomy with flap repair to manage sacral and right ischial infected decubiti. She also experienced loss of bowel and bladder control.

This client was admitted to a rehabilitation center 10 days after her surgery. She received physical therapy 5 times a week for 90 minutes per session. Her documented physical therapy goals were to improve bed mobility and increase lower extremity (LE) range of motion (ROM). Her posture was not assessed, since she was unable to sit due to postsurgical precautions. Wheelchair seating prescription was delayed, although it was considered a goal. The client required contact guarding to minimal assistance for rolling and was unable to perform other mobility skills due to precautions from the sacral flap repair. Her movements were described as having severe hip and knee flexor and hip adductor posturing, and she exhibited moderate ROM limitations in both lower extremities.

Cognitively, the client was oriented to person and place, but not to time. She was able to follow one- and two-step commands but not more complex directions. Also, her memory was impaired—she was unable to recall events from a week ago or describe her past medical history.

Twenty days after admission, a sitting tolerance program was initiated. The client tolerated 30 minutes of sitting without any skin complications. By 24 days, tolerance for sitting increased to three 30-minute sessions. At 27 days after admit, she sat for two 2-hour sessions a day. In sitting she required moderate assistance and verbal cues to maintain a symmetrical position; her posture was described as windswept to the right.

Pharmacological intervention, aimed primarily at management of spasticity, began 2 weeks after admission with an increase in her baclofen dose to 10 mg t.i.d. Six weeks after admission, baclofen was increased and prozac was added. Baclofen dose was increased again 2 months after admission, and lioresal was prescribed 10 days before discharge.

The client was referred for an SI program almost a month after admission to acute rehabilitation to supplement physical therapy. She was not responding to stretching techniques used by her treating therapist, and her poor sitting posture precluded wheelchair prescription.

The goals for this client, to be achieved with the SI program, were to increase vital capacity, improve postural alignment for carryover to wheelchair seating, and promote healing with increased scar tissue mobility of the sacral ischial flap. In her assessment of the client, the SI therapist documented an average vital capacity (three trials) of 1,000 ml and used photographs to describe the client's sitting posture in and out of the wheelchair. Sitting posture was described as kyphoscoliotic, with excessive lumbar flexion, sacral sitting, left lateral trunk flexion with LEs windswept to the right, and a forward head. Seating in the wheelchair required the addition of an abduction wedge to separate her LEs, a Styrofoam pad to prevent excessive knee flexion, and a belt across the thighs to prevent excessive hip flexion. The client's primary therapist continued to treat and document on her progress.

The therapist modified some of the SI sessions due to positioning and endurance constraints. These modifications are described in detail to explain the physical therapist's thought process and skill at adapting the SI approach for this particular client. Only the sessions that required modification are mentioned. In general, the therapist had to work slowly and in smaller arcs of motion to prevent eliciting reflexive tonal responses of the LEs.

The emphasis of the second session was on the foot contacting the ground. Typically, the client is asked to walk "through the foot." Movement reeducation includes standing and walking, which the client was unable to do. In sitting, however, the client was cued to bear weight through her heels. This was done to improve her sitting balance by increasing her base of support and reducing the effect of the LE's tonal influence on balance. The movement reeducation component focused on directing her to "feel" the weight of her foot contact the ground while she adjusted her trunk in a seated position.

Minor modifications were required in the third session to attain the sidelying position and direct the client to attend to her breathing. The session is typically performed in sidelying with a focus on lengthening the lateral trunk. Given the client's lower trunk restrictions, the therapist focused on the attachments to the sacrum, greater trochanter and head of the femur, and the quadratus lumburom. The movement education component for this session focuses on having the client attend to breathing and to note how the breath influences the thorax. The therapist added positioning and reaching activities to encourage the client to maintain the newly acquired ROM of the trunk.

Modifications to the fourth session were required to accommodate the client's decreased active isolated LE movement and strong hip and knee flexor and hip adductor posturing of both LEs. The fourth session focuses on the inner line, requiring work on the adductor surface of both LEs. The treatment was performed in sidelying, and positioning was achieved by using firm Styrofoam rollers to abduct the lower extremities.

During session four, the therapist applied deep pressure in order to reduce the activity of the adductor muscles. She applied this pressure longer than she might with a client with an intact neurologic system. She had to avoid light contact on the inner thigh, which she found stimulated the adductor posturing. Care was taken not to trigger any tonal responses by proceeding with the work in a slow and sustained manner.

The movement reeducation component for lesson four is typically performed supine, requiring active flexion and extension of the LEs, which the client was unable to perform. The therapist modified the session to include work in sitting to weight bearing on the ischial tuberosities. enhancing the client's ability to move from the pelvis. This session was much longer than a typical hour. Parts that are performed in standing, where the client is asked to reference the calcaneus to the pelvis, were omitted.

Session five, performed in supine, focuses on the anterior thorax and "front of the back" (iliopsoas and the structures anterior to the spine). Positioning was modified from supine to supine with flexed knees over a firm bolster and a wedge to abduct the lower extremities. Generally, movement reeducation consists of selectively activating the psoas to flex the hip in the supine position. The client was unable to isolate this movement. Instead, the movement was performed in sitting, using pelvic rotation over the femur while maintaining the spine extended. Attention was given to positioning her feet so that they were in contact with the ground.

Positioning and movement reeducation were modified for session six, where a major focus is to increase the length of the tissues in the lumbar spine area. Typically performed in prone, the client required a modified prone position to accommodate her extreme LE flexion. The therapist was able to work from the heels to the thoracolumbar junction, lengthening the deep tissues, derotating the femur, and integrating the sacrum and coccyx as part of the spine by working on the attachments to sacrum. Movement reeducation of fine movements of the leg was not possible due to the client's decreased motor control. The client was not fully able to direct her attention to the "breathing pelvis" or to movement of the core. There were no modifications noted for sessions 7 through 10.

Interpretations about the outcome of the intervention are speculative. Factors that may have enhanced or detracted from the client's progress that were not controlled for are the changes in her medications, the timing of her clearance to sit, concurrent physical therapy sessions, and the chronic disease process, which manifested itself in an impaired cognitive status. The client demonstrated both transient and sustained changes at the impairment level and sustained improvements at the ability level. Specifically, the therapist measured changes in LE ROM, which were concomitant with the SI but did not persist once SI was completed. However, functionally, especially with rolling, wheelchair management, and mobility, she improved from minimal assist to a supervised level. Her alignment in sitting and ability to sit improved progressively; she required moderate assistance for sitting at the beginning of SI and improved to requiring supervision by the end of SI. Improvements in sitting posture after receiving the third session included a partial correction of her left lateral trunk flexion and improved alignment of her thorax and head with respect to her lower trunk. Sitting alignment improved after the eighth session. Compared with the beginning of the third session, the client exhibited a decrease in kyphoscoliosis, decrease in excessive posterior tilt and lumbar flexion, and greater symmetry in weight bearing. She no longer required assistance to sit.

The authors speculate that important ROM increases in the pelvic and lumbar areas, not specifically measured but observed, were instrumental in improving the client's mobility for rolling, supine to sit, and wheelchair propulsion. An increase in pelvic and lumbar spine PROM allowed the client to superimpose active mobility. In addition, the improved upper trunk alignment reduced the need for extensive wheelchair modifications.

The client was discharged to a nursing home and maintained her mobility status for a year after discharge. It was reported that attendant costs at the nursing home were decreased by her improved mobility status. After 1 year of living in the nursing home, her cognitive and motoric status deteriorated, and she was no longer able to manage low-level mobility.

Summary

Structural integration, or Rolfing, is a manual therapy with movement reeducation components. It is a systematic, holistic approach, the goal of which is to restore structural alignment with respect to gravity in order to enhance function. There is some evidence to support the application of SI for people with musculoskeletal complaints that can be from a neurologic or musculoskeletal etiology. Becoming a practitioner requires approximately 2 years of training. Two organizations that offer training are the Guild for Structural Integration and the Rolf Institute for Structural Integration.

STUDY QUESTIONS

1. What is the role of gravity in SI?
2. Based on literature to support SI, would you apply the technique to a client with poor posture? Justify your response.
3. How does NCCAM classify structural integration?
4. What is the most important structure in SI?
5. Describe in general how an SI evaluation is conducted.
6. Describe in general the types of treatment used in SI.
7. What is the difference between the Guild for Structural Integration and the Rolf Institute for Structural Integration?

SUGGESTED READING

Feitas, R. *Ida Rolf Talks.* (1978). New York: Harper & Row.

Guild for Structural Integration. (2001, August 1). [Online]. Available: http://rolfguild.org.

Kotzsch, E. (1993). Restructure the body with Rolfing: Deep massage that realigns the human form. *East West Natural Health*, 35.

Mixter, J. (1983). In C. Lowe & J. Nechas (Eds.), *Whole Body Healing*. Philadelphia: Rodale Press.

Rolf, I. P. (1973). Structural integration: A contribution to the understanding of stress. *Confina Psychiatrica, 973*(16), 69–79.

Urbanczik, A. (1994). A tour of the first three sessions. *Guild News, 4,* 32–35.

Urbanczik, A. (1995). A tour of the basic series—Sessions 4, 5, and 6. *Guild News, 5,* 21–23.

RESOURCES

The Guild for Structural Integration
PO Box 1559
Boulder, CO 80306
(800) 447-0150

Rolf Institute for Structural Integration
205 Canyon Blvd.
Boulder, CO 80302
(800) 530-8875

REFERENCES

Cottingham, J. T., & J. Maitland. (1997). A three-paradigm treatment model using soft-tissue mobilization and guided movement awareness techniques for a patient with chronic low back pain: A case study. *Journal of Orthopedic and Sports Physical Therapy, 26,* 155–167.

Cottingham, J. T., S. W. Porges, & T. Lyon. (1988). Effects of soft tissue mobilization (Rolfing pelvic lift) on parasympathetic tone in two age groups. *Physical Therapy, 68,* 352–356.

Cottingham, J. T., S. W. Porges, & K. Richmond. (1988). Shifts in pelvic inclination angle and parasympathetic tone produced by Rolfing soft tissue manipulation. *Physical Therapy, 68,* 1364–1370.

Deutsch, J. E., L. Derr, P. Judd, & B. Reuven. (2000, Sept.). Structural integration applied to patients with chronic pain. *Physical Therapy Clinics of North America, 9*(3), 411–427.

Deutsch, J. E., P. Judd, & I. DeMasi. (1997). Structural integration applied to patients with a primary neurologic diagnosis: Two case studies. *Neurology Report, 21*(5), 161–162.

Edmunds, S. (2001). Musculoskeletal course. University of Medicine and Dentistry of New Jersey, Doctor of Physical Therapy Program.

Perry J., M. Jones, & L. Thomas. (1981). Functional evaluation of Rolfing in cerebral palsy. *Developmental Medicine and Child Neurology, 23,* 717–729.

Rolf, I. P. (1977). *Rolfing. The Integration of Human Structures*. New York: Harper & Row.

Talty, C., I. DeMasi, & J. E. Deutsch. (1998). Structural integration applied to patients with chronic fatigue syndrome: A retrospective chart review. *Journal of Sports Physical Therapy, 27*(1), 83.

The Rolf Institute for Structural Integration. (2001, August 1). [Online]. Available: http://www.rolf.org.

23

T'ai Chi

Sandy Matsuda

CHAPTER OBJECTIVES

◆ Describe the evolution of T'ai Chi into a movement therapy.
◆ State ways T'ai Chi can be used therapeutically by rehabilitation professionals.
◆ Describe health benefits of T'ai Chi.
◆ Choose resources to help learn T'ai Chi and incorporate it into one's work.

T'ai Chi is a slow-moving exercise originally practiced as a martial art in China but now practiced around the world for its health benefits. T'ai Chi became a way of life based on Taoist philosophy and was practiced by the Chinese for centuries as an exercise to balance mind and body. T'ai Chi masters passed the teachings on to chosen students or descendents for many generations. Health professionals today increasingly use T'ai Chi as a safe and gentle form of exercise with physical and psychological benefits for people of all ages, especially older adults. Health improvements are attributed to the combination of movement, meditation, and breathing patterns practiced in T'ai Chi. Recent research suggests that regular practice of T'ai Chi has a positive effect on balance, flexibility, circulation, blood pressure, cardiopulmonary function, general fitness, and fall reduction in the elderly (Lan et al., 1996; Wolf et al., 1997; Young et al., 1999). Anecdotal reports claim people improved from a variety of disabling conditions, such as arthritis, chronic pain, and fatigue, with regular practice (Shaller, 1998).

T'ai Chi is firmly rooted in principles and philosophy developed in the East that differ from the foundation of exercises developed in the West. T'ai Chi practice emphasizes relaxation, proper breathing, and soft, graceful, slow movements done with a meditative focus. Practitioners of T'ai Chi seek to integrate body, mind, and spirit in order to "function in harmony with the external world" (Harlowe & Yu, 1997, p. 9). People may initially question the principles and benefits claimed for such a slow and gentle form of exercise when they compare T'ai Chi to more familiar exercise or sports whose benefits are explained by Western

T'ai Chi is a slow and gentle form of exercise that is useful when a more strenuous form of exercise is not appropriate. Younger clients who need a low impact form of exercise, for example, may find it a viable alternative as they heal from injuries. It is particularly suitable for the elderly, for people with progressive neuromuscular diseases, and for clients in hospice care or coping with cancer and chronic illness and pain. T'ai Chi is also useful in increasing postural control, dynamic balance, active range of motion, strength, coordination, and respiratory function. Although T'ai Chi is done at a slow and steady pace, studies have shown it to have a positive effect of improving VO2 uptake compared to an age-matched control group of sedentary elders (Lai et al., 1995).

Some people use T'ai Chi as part of their personal wellness program and find that it reduces stress and tension while increasing their general well-being. It has been used with senior housing residents in California to improve socialization and health (Clark et al., 1997) and in senior centers throughout the country. Home health therapists also incorporate the principles and movements of T'ai Chi in home exercise programs for clients. Therapists are frequently in a position to recommend and encourage physical activity and exercise for clients, and T'ai Chi is a safe and enjoyable form of activity to recommend when studied with a qualified teacher.

scientific principles. The principles of Chinese medicine and health underlying T'ai Chi are equally valid and rigorous but may differ dramatically from those in the West (Williams, 1999). Western-trained therapists who want to use T'ai Chi therapeutically would benefit from becoming acquainted with the historical, philosophical, and theoretical roots of this ancient practice, for as an alternative therapeutic approach, it can enhance and expand one's practice (Bottomley, 1997).

History

T'ai Chi is rooted in ancient Chinese culture and Taoist philosophy. The term is usually translated as *the supreme ultimate* or *the way* (Man-Ch'ing & Smith, 1983). The term *T'ai Chi Chuan* loosely translates *as supreme ultimate boxing or fist* and is associated with the martial art forms of T'ai Chi. Hence, the word Chuan is often dropped when referring to the meditative form of the exercise. No real historic evidence exists on T'ai Chi's exact origin, but some claim that it began approximately 1,700 years ago as a way of life based on the theory of mutually dependent opposites represented by the yin and yang energies observed in the natural world (Liao, 1990).

Lao Tzu, an early pioneer in the philosophy of Taoism, stressed that the soft will overcome the hard (Liao, 1990). Like water meeting a stone, the soft and yielding motion of T'ai Chi deflects the aggressive energy of a forceful opponent back onto himself and throws him off balance. Later masters of Taoism stressed the importance of exercise coordinated with breathing.

The efficient movements of T'ai Chi coordinated with the in and out breath focuses energy. Today's T'ai Chi exercises are based on the idea that movement provides the foundation of efficient body function and health (Bottomley, 1997). Meditation complements or balances the energy of movement, contributing to the power of T'ai Chi. T'ai Chi remains grounded in the Taoist philosophy of seeking balance and harmony by performing healing exercises that emphasize relaxation, breathing, and inner calm rather than strength and force.

T'ai Chi is believed to have evolved into a soft martial art around the 13th century. Legends report that a Taoist monk created a set of postures that were connected into movement patterns based on the monk's observation of a crane and snake engaged in a fight. Hence, many of the moves imitate and describe nature such as "snake creeps down," "monkey retreats," or "white crane spreads its wings." Ancient T'ai Chi martial art forms often bear the family name of masters who taught them. While T'ai Chi can be learned for self-defense and as a martial art, the T'ai Chi done publicly today in China and in the West is done slowly, gently, and evenly, and appears more like a dance than a martial art (Bottomley, 1997).

T'ai Chi Forms

Several forms, or styles, of T'ai Chi have been developed, with numerous offshoots that are suitable for therapeutic use. The length of forms varies from as few as nine to as many as 108 moves. The most common form practiced in the United States is probably the 24 form, which is short and easy to learn. Yang style short form has 37 moves and is also popular among serious practitioners. All movements are performed in a continuous, flowing, and mindful manner that helps increase awareness of the body-mind connection. The ultimate goal of T'ai Chi is to do all the moves as if they were one move. Practitioners hope to "gain the pliability of a child, the health of a lumberjack, and the peace of mind of a sage" (Man-Ch'ing & Smith, 1983, p. 1).

One of the more recent offshoots of T'ai Chi is a set of non-martial movements, called T'ai Chi Chih. It was originated by Justin Stone, a T'ai Chi Chuan master, now in his mid 80s, after discovering that many people could not master the more complex moves of ancient forms (Shaller, 1998; Stone, 1994). These movements are easier to learn than traditional forms and accessible to a range of people, including some with physical or functional limitations. While not considered a T'ai Chi form, they are based on the same principles and offer some of the same benefits to practitioners.

A rather new development are classes in which T'ai Chi is done in water. For people who cannot tolerate sustained weight bearing on one leg, indoor water T'ai Chi could be a viable alternative if it becomes more widely available.

Another program that has been developed over the last 20 years is the ROM (range of motion) dance, based on the movement principles of T'ai Chi Chuan. The ROM dance is an exercise and relaxation program developed by Diane Harlowe, MA, OTR/FAOTA, and Tricia Yu, MA (Harlowe & Yu, 1997). They have created moonlight variations for people with Lupus, seated versions for those who cannot stand. More recently, Tricia Yu and Jill Johnson, a physical therapist, have developed a training and certification program called T'ai Chi Fundamentals for Health Care Practitioners (McKean, 2000). This program teaches how to use a simplified version of T'ai Chi movement patterns and forms suitable for people with some physical limitations.

Several movement patterns or derivations of T'ai Chi forms have been adapted for the elderly and those with balance disorders. Xu (2000) developed nine movements to help seniors improve their balance. These are the same movements used in a National Institutes of Health study that demonstrated that regular practice of T'ai Chi could successfully reduce falling and injury among the elderly (Xu, 2000). The movements were combined with warm-up exercises and many repetitions to make it easier for seniors to learn and practice safely.

Another simplified set of T'ai Chi movements centers around the heart and is called the Phoenix style. In Traditional Chinese Medicine the heart is believed to be the meeting place of heaven and earth. Developed by Ni Hua-Chiang, a T'ai Chi master, this style is particularly suited to women. The moves revolve around the energy center of the heart, a yang center, to balance the practitioner's female energy and lower center of gravity. In contrast, older forms, originally practiced only by men, balanced male energy and a higher center of gravity around a yin center of energy, the solar plexus (Cis Hager, personal communication, 2000).

Principles

Central principles are often taught as the foundation for a T'ai Chi form or movements. These principles originate from metaphysical, Taoist concepts. Variations exist in how the principles are stated, but the five principles given here are central to many forms. One essential principle is *separation of yin and yang*. Yin and yang energies are opposites, one passive, the other active, one yielding, the other advancing. Practicing this principle requires both mental and physical flexibility. This principle is evident in practicing what is called *separation of weight* or *empty stepping*. In essence, T'ai Chi is shifting weight from one foot to the other in an incredibly mindful way.

In practicing the T'ai Chi walk, for example, one constantly shifts weight from one foot to the other or between opposites of empty (yin) and full (yang) legs. One advances by stabilizing body weight over the yang leg while the advancing leg makes contact with the ground and then assumes weight. Initially, it takes great concentration and restraint not to rush forward onto the advancing leg, but with practice, one's walk becomes more stable, smooth, and effortless. One's body weight sinks down over the center of gravity, giving the feeling that one is anchored to the ground like a tree with a deep root. Moving gracefully between yin and yang helps one attain equilibrium and harmony. It improves balance while strengthening the lower extremities (Chung, 1998).

A second principle is *keeping the body upright*. The body is always grounded with the center of gravity either within one foot or between both feet. One maintains good postural alignment by looking forward and keeping the head and spine straight, as if one's spine were a string of pearls gently suspended from above. One avoids leaning forward or back and keeps the arms and legs slightly bent at the knees and elbows during the exercises. Good posture and natural, deep breathing work together to allow the *chi*, or energy, to flow freely throughout the body. The flow of chi is important for health and inner strength.

A third principle is that *the waist is the commander*. This means that movements are initiated from the energy center located in the region just below the navel in the hip and waist area of the body. Practitioners draw the chi up from the earth through the bubbling well on the bottom of the foot, and the waist directs the flow of energy out the extremities like water flowing through a garden hose. When properly rooted and focused, a practitioner can deflect the force of a powerful opponent back into himself by using only the weight of a fly landing on the surface of the opponent's body. The practitioner's body is always grounded and unmovable as one part of the body's movement is counterbalanced by the rest of the body.

A fourth principle is that *the body is relaxed and movement is flowing and yielding*. This principle emphasizes relaxation and proper breathing. One learns to relax the mind as well as the body. By calming the mind, relaxing every muscle, and breathing naturally through the nose, one can eliminate stiffness and avoid tense or forced movements. Focus is achieved by centering, maintaining equilibrium, and moving from the center of gravity. Eventually, one moves from the center of gravity in all daily activities without thinking about it. Flowing means that movements should not be abrupt and that when one part of the body moves, it should be accompanied by movement in the rest of the body. Muscles not directly used for a particular move are soft, yielding, and fully relaxed.

A fifth principle is *attention to present*. T'ai Chi is considered a form of meditation in which complete focus needs to be on the experience of moving and responding to the present circumstance. The mind and body stay grounded as one attends to the here and now. T'ai Chi is sometimes called a moving meditation or Chinese moving yoga because it integrates and coordinates the mind and body into a single whole.

Indications and Contraindications

Indications

T'ai Chi may be beneficial as therapeutic exercise for people

- who are socially isolated or prefer exercising in a group.
- who are in long-term care facilities and can imitate and learn movements through repetition.
- who are well elderly living in the community.
- with arthritis or chronic pain.
- with breathing problems.
- with mild balance difficulties.
- with activity restrictions that eliminate other forms of more vigorous exercise.
- with ambulation devices who can still move lower extremities.

Contraindications

T'ai Chi may not be appropriate for people with

- severe balance disorders or vertigo.
- significant health problems for which mild activity would be inadvisable.
- debilitating stages of diseases, such as Alzheimer's or Parkinsons.
- severe arthritis.
- cerebellar dysfunction or cerebral palsy causing ataxia.

Typical Practice

People of all ages practice T'ai Chi. It offers a safe form of exercise for people who have suffered an injury in sports, high-impact aerobics, or the hard-style martial arts. It is often taught to senior adults as a therapeutic program of wellness, for prevention of falls, or to improve concentration, balance, and relaxation. The success of serious practitioners suggests that it is a movement therapy well suited for older people who wish to continue improving as they age. T'ai Chi can be done by people with arthritis or other mobility-limiting diseases. People who want to improve balance, cardiorespiratory function, or flexibility also find it useful. And it can benefit those in palliative care and those being treated for cancer or chronic pain who may need help with relaxation and pain management (LeFort, 2000). Although T'ai Chi is typically done from a standing position, exercises based on the principles of T'ai Chi have been developed that can be performed while seated or holding onto a stable surface. The breathing, relaxation, and meditative features of T'ai Chi, for example, can be practiced under a variety of circumstances, including from a chair (Harlowe & Yu, 1997).

T'ai Chi is not typically a substitute for therapy or medical care but rather is used as a complementary or adjunct approach to improve or maintain balance, flexibility, range of motion, and general health and fitness. Movement is essential in preventing disability and promoting health and well-being. The basic movement patterns of T'ai Chi can be applied in many ways to therapeutic and functional activities. Whyte (1997) describes the similarities of body mechanics used in T'ai Chi and energy conservation and suggests ways to grade T'ai Chi movements for beginners in cardiac rehabilitation who are learning energy conservation techniques for activities of daily living. In a traditional practice setting, T'ai Chi movements may be incorporated into therapeutic activities for strength, active range of motion, balance, pain and stress reduction, and improving cardiorespiratory status. In home health and community settings T'ai Chi movements can be taught as a way of enhancing the way people move while performing functional activities of daily living. For example, incorporating T'ai Chi movements in standing, sitting, walking, and reaching activities improves dynamic balance and gives clients a greater freedom from fear of falling. This increased confidence and sense of well-being can lead to a richer quality of life. Some therapists integrate T'ai Chi into their repertoire of skills, teach classes in community centers or YMCAs, or recommend that their clients take instruction in community classes.

Numerous tapes and books are now available but are not recommended as the only source of instruction. Therapists new to T'ai Chi may want to study with a qualified T'ai Chi teacher, take a course in the fundamentals of T'ai Chi for health care practitioners, or invite practitioners to provide an in-service or seminar for staff at their facility (McKean, 2000; Yu & Johnson, 1999).

In a typical T'ai Chi class, one begins with 15 to 30 minutes of warm-up exercises. These focus on proper breathing, relaxation, and gentle turning of the waist while shifting weight from one foot to the other. Other warm-ups might include doing the T'ai Chi walk, which involves empty stepping before shifting weight into the advancing foot. Another warm-up is holding the opening posture of *wu chi*, where weight is equally distributed in both feet, and the arms form a circle as if holding a ball in front of the body at waist level. Warm-ups are followed by practice of the form in which one or two moves are learned and practiced for a week or more before adding new moves. The yang form, for example, can be learned in as short as 3 months of daily practice, but usually takes 1 to 2 years to learn well, and a lifetime to perfect. Because changes and benefits appear slowly and with consistent practice, some older people become discouraged with classes that are taught by teachers who are "purist" in their approach or are accustomed to teaching younger learners. It may be better for many people to seek a beginner's class that is taught by someone who explains the moves and gives both feedback and encouragement. Teachers and therapists need to be sympathetic to participants who cannot practice rigorously each day but who attend sessions faithfully.

Each person's body is unique, and T'ai Chi should be tailored to avoid injury to weakened or compromised joints and muscles. Clients performing T'ai Chi can experience sprains or strains. The risk of injury can be reduced by proper warm-ups and by performing the movements slowly (*Nurses Handbook*, 1998). Likewise, a level surface, good lighting, appropriate nonskid footwear, and a stable surface such as a table or grab bar to use during one-footed postures should reduce the risk of falling. If someone should fall and is not able to get up without help, the person should be assessed on the ground and able to move extremities before being helped to a chair. The incident should be documented and the person's doctor notified as appropriate (*Nurses Handbook*, 1998). Some people report that T'ai Chi has stressed their lower back and knees. While moves are usually done in a low stance position with knees bent, a more upright posture should be recommended for those with back or knee pain. Moves that require complete separation of weight may need to be modified for individuals due to pain, balance, strength, or range of motion limitations. For example, some persons with hip or knee replacements may need to restrict standing on one leg or the degree of internal rotation normally practiced in some of the moves.

Usually, discharge from therapy services is indicated when goals are achieved or when disabling conditions make continuing an exercise program contraindicated. T'ai Chi is less a treatment and more a lifestyle change related to goals of preventing falls, maintaining wellness and movement, and improving balance and postural stability. These goals can continue throughout a person's life. Many people, for example, report taking a 6- or 8-week T'ai Chi class over and over again because they want to continue to practice and learn. If T'ai Chi is offered outside of a third-party payer system, continuing practice should be encouraged for as long as the person feels it is beneficial.

Therapeutic Goals

Therapists can introduce T'ai Chi movements and incorporate these principles into broadly defined goals that fit most exercise groups. Some examples of broad goals stated for a T'ai Chi movement group designed for senior adults might be the following:

◆ Participate in daily exercise routine with increased benefit and enjoyment.
◆ Increase ability to cope with stress and pain through relaxation and pain management techniques.
◆ Facilitate social interaction.
◆ Increase awareness of health, body awareness, and well-being.

More specific physical goals for individuals might be to improve respiration status, decrease pain, develop trunk control, as well as to improve balance, flexibility, strength, and range of motion (Bottomley, 1997).

Many schools, forms, and styles of T'ai Chi exist and are taught through YMCAs, health clubs, community centers, and martial arts studios. To choose a class for yourself or your clients, consider the following:

1. *Teachers.* The teacher should have at least 5 or more years of experience and should be willing to spend time with beginners, explaining the moves. "The most famous instructors are not necessarily the most qualified, and a qualified master may not be in a position to teach his skills to others" (Liao, 1990, p. viii).

2. *Purpose of class.* If the class is taught in a martial arts studio, one should be cautious of high-pressure tactics, clothing requirements, and T'ai Chi being last on a long list of martial arts taught. Health clubs, YMCAs, adult education programs, and senior centers generally have more affordable classes and may be geared to older participants interested in the health aspects rather than martial art applications of T'ai Chi.

3. *Size and requirements of class.* One should ask to visit a class and talk with other students as well as the instructor. Choose a small class that gives individual attention and does not require special clothing or equipment or a large financial investment. T'ai Chi can be done in casual, loose clothing or exercise-wear.

4. *Client's acceptance.* Consider a client's past exposure to, or interest in, T'ai Chi when recommending classes. A client's level of participation and follow-through may be determined by how that person and his or her social and cultural group view exercise, relaxation and meditation activities (Whyte, 1997).

No single organization oversees training or certification of teachers. Therapists with little or no T'ai Chi experience can receive training in using the ROM dance, a simple set of exercises based on T'ai Chi principles, suitable for many older adults. They can also begin with a workshop or video that provides T'ai Chi Fundamentals for Health Care Professionals (described in the resource list) and become certified in using this method. A therapist can learn these exercises and integrate them into his or her practice with individuals or groups in long-term care, rehabilitation, or community-based wellness programs. For more advanced training, therapists should study with a qualified teacher before teaching T'ai Chi to clients. However, a knowledgeable therapist, working in collaboration with a qualified teacher, can develop therapeutic T'ai Chi classes for clients. Providing leadership is an emerging role for therapists in planning and promoting community, population-based services designed for wellness and health promotion (Clark et al., 1997; Moyers, 1999). Some resources are listed at the end of this chapter that may be helpful in designing programs for seniors, people with disabilities, and rehabilitation clients.

Research

There has been a steady increase in Western research documenting the benefits of T'ai Chi. Several studies have substantiated the value of T'ai Chi in decreasing blood pressure (Young et al., 1999), improving postural stability and balance (Tse & Bailey, 1992; Wolf et al., 1997), and as a means of reducing the risk of falls (Hain et al., 1999; Wolf et al., 1996). Likewise, studies have shown that cardiovascular functioning, strength, and flexibility improve in regular practitioners (Lan et al., 1996).

A study by Wolf demonstrated that T'ai Chi practice can decrease blood pressure and the risk of falling. Wolf, a physical therapist, and his colleagues (1996) coordinated a major study among the elderly called the Atlanta FICSIT Group studies (Frailty and Injuries: Cooperative Studies of Intervention Techniques). They tested T'ai Chi movements because the movements were believed to "dynamically tax balance mechanisms while facilitating concentration of body position" (p. 490). T'ai Chi showed the most significant difference among various programs that focused on endurance, flexibility, use of balance platforms, education, functional activities, and behavioral and medication changes as they affected falls (Province et al., 1995; Shaller, 1998; Wolf et al., 1996).

Tse and Bailey (1992) studied Chinese-Americans retrospectively, comparing nine T'ai Chi practitioners with nine nonpractitioners, and found a significant difference in postural stability on three tests of balance with eyes open. Schaller (1996) studied two groups of volunteers and found a significant improvement in balance for the T'ai Chi group compared to a control group, but no significant difference in measurements of mood, flexibility, health status, and blood pressure. Hain and colleagues (1999) studied the effects of T'ai Chi on balance and concluded that it could be a useful modality for balance rehabilitation and reduce the risk of falls.

Lan and colleagues (1996), in a 15-week study of 76 community-dwelling elderly in two groups, found that the T'ai Chi group showed higher trunk flexibility and an increase in cardiorespiratory function (measured by oxygen uptake). A later study of 38 community-dwellers in two groups over 12 months substantiated the significant increase in trunk flexibility and in torque muscle strength in the T'ai Chi group compared to controls (Lan et al., 1998).

Other studies examined the safety and potential use of T'ai Chi for clients with arthritis and found less joint tenderness and swelling and greater grip strength in T'ai Chi practitioners than in controls (Kirstein, Dietz, & Hwang, 1998; Lumsden, Baccala, & Martire, 1998). A pilot study was done on the ROM dance program, which uses T'ai Chi principles, to determine if it provided an enjoyable alternative to traditional daily exercise programs recommended to people with rheumatoid arthritis. Participants found it an enjoyable and sustainable alternative, which seemed to improve their ability to cope with pain (Harlowe & Yu, 1997). An ongoing study using the ROM dance with adults with chronic pain has preliminary results indicating that the exercise was effective in reducing and controlling pain (LeFort, 2000).

Case Studies

Because T'ai Chi is often done in groups, these case studies are of people who have participated in T'ai Chi classes with a therapist or other qualified teacher. While the case studies do not follow the usual format of this text, they illustrate the wide range of applications and benefits of using T'ai Chi as a movement therapy. The case studies describe the changes in the participants as well as changes in the teachers. The teachers were a massage therapist, a college teacher, and an occupational therapist, who have 14 to 20 years experience in practicing T'ai Chi. The clients ranged in age from 52 to 98 years old.

T'ai Chi as Transformational Learning

Learning T'ai Chi can be a kind of transformational learning that results in being able to integrate new perspectives. Research within the medical model often focuses on physical benefits and instrumental learning. Learning T'ai Chi can be much more than instrumental learning of an exercise routine, however. T'ai Chi can have a transformational or emancipatory effect on the lives of some participants. Cedar, a T'ai Chi teacher from Seattle, who was asked to reflect on the benefits experienced by seniors in her classes, reported the following:

"I think the most significant stories I have gotten from my classes with seniors fit into three categories:

1. The physical improvements, including mobility and safety experiences;
2. The mental/emotional changes, including decreased depression and overall more open appreciation of living;
3. The developing understanding of [T'ai Chi] principles and being able to feel and follow the energy of the body."

In addition to the "expected physical improvements in leg strength and balance," the most important and pervasive effects she witnessed in seniors occurred in their "emotional body and outlook on life." For example, she reports having seniors who "move out of depression from loss of their husbands, wives, children; heal from chronic fatigue syndrome; become less 'bitchy' to friends and family . . . , [and move] to dealing with family crisis better and making necessary boundary decisions more easily." She reflects that the "increased vitality and mental clarity" they experienced from doing T'ai Chi seems to grant seniors a chance to function more like they may want to in daily life, "with a calm mind and heart." While noting that seniors may not learn movements as quickly, she found a slower pace does not prevent seniors from gaining deeper understanding from T'ai Chi. Rather, the "personal transformation is definitely present, as is the personal development of understanding principles of the art itself. The alchemy happens over time, just as it does with any student consistently and mindfully practicing."

Finally, there was a transformation for Cedar, the practitioner/teacher, as well. She shifted her own perspective of what seniors could learn and accomplish through practicing T'ai Chi. "Working with seniors has taught me patience and gradually the realization that they can do what anyone else can do with T'ai Chi—understand the depth of practice of an energy art" (Personal communication, 2000).

Norma, now a teacher and a long-time practitioner of T'ai Chi, chose to pursue T'ai Chi over yoga because she tended to hurt herself doing yoga but not doing T'ai Chi. She describes her practice of T'ai Chi as a journey of "becoming or embodying the physical and metaphysical principles of T'ai Chi" in her life. Like many Eastern mind-body movement arts, T'ai Chi is always presented as having spiritual or philosophical components or roots. The "yielding and moving out of harm's way" practiced in T'ai Chi is in contrast to more aggressive moves in Western approaches to building strength and endurance through exercise and sport. Norma reports that T'ai Chi has allowed her "to be still, to be centered, to be rooted, and to learn how to move through space in a way that is the least harmful, the softest way. T'ai Chi is about learning to live, be, exist, and move through space in a much more conscious way" (Personal communication, 2000).

Two of Norma's students, women in their 70s, have been doing T'ai Chi twice a week for 3 years and 1 year respectively. Both walked and exercised to stay physically active but had experienced falls resulting in a broken ankle for one and a broken shoulder for the other. T'ai Chi was important in their recovery of mobility and balance after their falls. When asked about the health benefits they had experienced, surprisingly, both students spoke of a shift in attitude, a new awareness of their bodies and a sense of well-being in addition to physical benefits. In their own words,

Judy: In the beginning I was thinking of exercise. It is somewhat strenuous and I do it for balance, which I think it definitely helps with. But I discovered there is much more to T'ai Chi than that, a mind, body spirit combination at work there. I get a lot of that out of it. There is an attitude. You are certainly more aware of your body, but there is also a rejuvenation of the spirit with these exercises; it's a slowing down, focusing on your body and where it fits in the universe, and the energy aspects of it, and we do reading (about T'ai Chi). I feel it is a sort of three-pronged approach. I just have the feeling, the general feeling, of well-being when I do it, and I miss it very much when I can't make the class. . . . I definitely feel I am in better shape, and I am much more aware of my body.

Marilyn: In the fall, I broke my ankle, not serious but incapacitating. I found that once I could go back to T'ai Chi, I felt a lift in my spirit. I had felt restrained in the cast and I felt that I gained mobility in my ankle. I took it because I heard it was good for balance and I don't have very good balance. It has helped some in balance. I just find it a very good thing to do and I feel better, more in touch with my body. [It is] more than the physical exercise— to be aware and in the present—and my general well-being improved.

The author's experience as a therapist, practitioner, and teacher has been that the longer forms of T'ai Chi are often hard for some people to learn. Among those who seek out a class because of health problems may be people who have not exercised or not been successful in doing other forms of exercise. These people may need to start with a class based on T'ai Chi principles but modified for beginners with health problems. The following experience of one 75-year-old is not unusual among seniors who do T'ai Chi.

I was always interested in it because I heard it was a meditative thing. But my husband had Parkinsons and I wanted something active we could do together. After he died, I continued to seek out classes and have been in several other classes of T'ai Chi Chuan. But they were often too difficult for me! By some strange coincidence, the Y started offering this easier, simpler form of T'ai Chi Chih. That made a lot of sense to me, and it's doable. The other was too difficult for me. But this [T'ai Chi Chih], because there are separate movements, one can learn one or two or three moves and practice them.

Benefits in my life don't come easily and don't come quickly, but I find it totally relaxing, totally wonderful, and I'm totally concentrating on the movements. It's that doable! Afterwards, I was energized. Encourage people to look into that [T'ai Chi Chih] rather than the longer forms, which [we older people are] thinking we'll never learn!

It is never too late to start doing T'ai Chi if the desire is present. The author's oldest student, Grace, began attending a weekly class at age 97. She lived in a retirement hotel and was almost completely blind. She began by sitting in a wheelchair immediately to the right of the therapist, because she has some peripheral vision on that side. The therapist both described the moves and formed Grace's body into the various postures as the class progressed. Grace wore a 3-inch lift on one shoe and held onto her walker as she stood. After about 6 weeks, she was able to release her hold on the walker and perform the hand movements while standing in her walker but without holding it. She progressed to holding onto a sturdy chair back placed in front of her while moving her feet and practicing single-foot stances. She reports that she practices her postures each time she rides up and down the elevator. She begins by standing in the corner of the elevator and holds the grab bars at the back and side of the elevator as she practices single-leg stances. Grace's posture and balance have improved, and she is ambulating around the facility using a walker.

Grace leads the class in a warm-up exercise some days by singing and demonstrating a Chinese children's game. Seated in a chair, she directs the class to begin moving one foot, then the other, progressively adding the movement of a new body part with each verse of the song until the legs, arms, and head are all moving. While not strictly a T'ai Chi exercise, this routine evolved from discussing the history and principles of T'ai Chi from Chinese culture. The class calls the routine "Moving with Grace."

Another woman in her mid-50s started doing T'ai Chi shortly before she was diagnosed with terminal cancer. During the last months of her life, she found doing T'ai Chi with a friend a way to calm her anxiety, reduce her pain, and help her focus on something other than the difficult tasks of coping with medical problems and putting her affairs in order. She came to associate doing T'ai Chi with a meditative state of relaxation that brought her relief and comfort.

Summary

As a meditative movement therapy, T'ai Chi helps to balance the mind and body. It is based on principles of Chinese medicine and philosophy that emphasize relaxation, mindfulness, and proper breathing. Conscious weight shifting, an upright posture, and flowing movements are practiced. People of all ages can gain physical and psychological health benefits by doing this safe and gentle form of exercise over a long period of time. Therapists can learn the movements and principles from a qualified teacher of T'ai Chi. When these principles are integrated into treatment, clients learn better balance and postural stability, energy conservation, and relaxation techniques. T'ai Chi also fits nicely into a wellness, education, or fall-prevention program.

STUDY QUESTIONS

1. What do researchers see as the benefits of T'ai Chi?
2. What do participants see as the benefits of T'ai Chi?
3. What are the principles upon which T'ai Chi is based?
4. What precautions and contraindications are important when using T'ai Chi as a movement therapy?
5. What recommendations would you make to clients seeking a class in T'ai Chi?
6. How can therapists use T'ai Chi principles in traditional practice settings?
7. How can therapists use complementary therapies like T'ai Chi in expanding practice areas?

RESOURCES

Harlowe, D., & P. Yu. (1997). *The ROM dance: A Range of Motion Exercise and Relaxation Program,* Madison, WI: Uncharted Country Publishing. (Instruction book and videos). Diana Harlowe, MS, OTR, FAOTA, and Tricia Yu, MA, developed a 7-minute exercise and relaxation routine based on T'ai Chi principles under an Arthritis Foundation Grant, which sponsored research on its effectiveness (Harlowe & Yu, 1997). Tricia Yu and Jill Johnson, a physical therapist, developed a version of Tai Chi movement patterns and a simplified Tai Chi form that can be used by rehabilitation professionals and those that want to teach beginners who may have some physical limitations. They offer workshops and certification for instructors, as well as a book and a video called *T'ai Chi Fundamentals for Health Care Professionals.* Tricia Yu has also developed teaching videos based on the Cheng Man Ch'ing short form of T'ai Chi practice. For more information on certification and workshops contact

The ROM Dance Network and T'ai Chi
  Center
408 S. Baldwin St.
Madison, WI 53703-4805
(608) 242-9133
email: ucp@taichihealth.com
www.taichihealth.com and
  www.romdance.com

Stone, J. (1996). *T'ai Chi Chih/Joy Thru Movement: A Photo Textbook,* Fort Yates, ND: Good Karma Publishing, and (2000) *T'ai Chi Chih/Joy Thru Movement,* the video, include both instruction and practice in this form. Good Karma Publishing can be contacted for a list of accredited teachers in your area who teach T'ai Chi Chih. These 19 easy-to-learn movements, done in one pose, are based on principles of balancing and circulating internal energy (chi). Proponents claim they can produce benefits in weeks instead of years (Schaller, 1996). Contact

(701) 854-7459 or (888) 540-7459
www.taichichih.org

T'ai Chi: A Gift of Balance by Tingsen Xu is a video of nine movements taught in a large National Institute of Health study that successfully reduced falls and injury in seniors. It is available along with other videos and books on T'ai Chi and Qi Gong and Eastern Philosophy from

Wayfarer Publications
PO Box 39938
Los Angeles, CA 90039
(323) 665-7773
taichi@tai-chi.com

Whyte, N. (1997, Oct.). T'ai Chi for clients in cardiac rehabilitation. *OT Practice, 2*(10), 38–41. Describes the similarities of body mechanics used in T'ai Chi and energy conservation and suggests ways to grade T'ai Chi movements for beginners in cardiac rehabilitation.

For a lengthy listing of research abstracts on T'ai Chi done at institutions in the East as well as the West, the World T'ai Chi & Qigong Association provides a Medical and Scientific Research Fact Sheet through its Web site: *www.worldtaichiqigongassn.org.*

Many popular videos, books, and magazines are available for learning traditional forms of T'ai Chi. Local libraries and bookstores as well as the Internet are good sources of information. A comprehensive listing of resources can be found on the Internet at *www.tai-chi.com.* This site contains information about *T'ai Chi Magazine* as well as other publications, products, and workshops.

References

Beling, J. (1999). 12-month T'ai Chi training in the elderly: Its effect on health fitness [review of study]. *Physical Therapy, 79*(2), 208.

Bottomley, J. (1997). T'ai Chi: Choreography of body & mind. In C. Davis (Ed.), *Complementary Therapies in Rehabilitation: Holistic Approaches for Prevention & Wellness.* Thorofare, NJ: Slack.

Burd, A. (1998). The Effects of T'ai Chi on geriatric perceived quality of life: An occupational therapy perspective. Unpublished master's thesis, Rush University, Chicago.

Chung, L. (1998, October 1). Complementary care corner: T'ai Chi—Shall we dance? *OT Week, 12*(40), 15.

Clark, F., S. Azen, R. Zemke, J. Jackson, M. Carlson, D. Mandel, J. Hay, K. Josephson, B. Cherry, C. Hessel, J. Palmer, & L. Lipson. (1997). Occupational therapy for independent-living older adults: A randomized controlled trial. *Journal of the American Medical Association, 278,* 1321–1326.

Hain, T. C., L. Fuller, L. Weil, & J. Kotsia. (1999). Effects of T'ai Chi on balance. *Archives of Otolaryngology—Head & Neck Surgery, 125*(11), 1191–1195.

Harlowe, D., & P. Yu. (1997). *The ROM DANCE: A Range of Motion Exercise and Relaxation Program.* Madison, WI: Uncharted Country Publishing.

Kirstein, A., F. Dietz, & S. M. Hwang. (1991). Evaluating the safety and potential use of a weight-bearing exercise, T'ai Chi Chuan, for rheumatoid arthritis patients. *American Journal of Physical Medicine and Rehabilitation, 70,* 136–141.

Lai, J., C. Lan, M. Wong, & S. Teng. (1995). Two-year trends in cardiorespiratory function among older Tai Chi Chuan practitioners and sedentary subjects. *Journal of the American Geriatrics Society, 43*(11), 1222–1227.

Lan, C., J. Lai, S. Chen, & M. Wong. (1998). 12 Month T'ai Chi training in the elderly: Its effect on health fitness. *Medicine and Science in Sports and Exercise, 30*(3), 345–351.

Lan, C., J. Lai, M. Wong, & M. Yu. (1996). Cardiorespiratory function, flexibility, and body composition among geriatric T'ai Chi Chuan practitioners. *Archives of Physical Medicine and Rehabilitation, 77,* 612–616.

LeFort, S. M. (2000). A test of Braden's self-help model in adults with chronic pain. *Journal of Nursing Scholarship, 32*(2), 153–160.

LeFort, S. M. (1998). ROM Dance in Canadian chronic pain self-management program and research. *Pain, 74,* 297–306.

Liao, W. (1990). *T'ai Chi Classics.* Boston: Shambhala.

Lumsden, D. B., A. Baccala, & J. Martire. (1998). T'ai Chi for osteoarthritis: An introduction for primary care physicians. *Geriatrics, 53*(2), 84, 87–88.

Man-Ch'ing, D., & R. W. Smith. (1983). *T'ai-chi: The "Supreme Ultimate" Exercise for Health, Sport, and Self-defense.* Rutland, VT: Tuttle.

McKean, L. (2000, Spring/Summer). From the editor: New instructional resources. *Uncharted Country Newsletter, 2*(1), 3.

Morris, K. (1999, March 13). T'ai Chi gently reduces blood pressure in elderly. *The Lancet, 353*(9156), 904.

Moyers, P. (1999). The guide to occupational therapy practice. *American Journal of Occupational Therapy, 53,* 3.

Nurses Handbook of Alternative & Complementary Therapies. (1998). Springhouse, PA: Springhouse Corp.

Province, M. A., C. D. Mulrow, & S. L. Wolf. (1995). The effects of exercise on falls in elderly patients: A preplanned meta-analysis of the FICSIT trials. *Journal of the American Medical Association, 273*(17), 1341–1347.

Schaller, K. J. (1996). T'ai chi Chih: An exercise option for older adults. *Journal of Gerontological Nursing, 22*(10), 12–17.

Shaller, K. J. (1998). T'ai Chi/movement therapy. In M. Synder & R. Lindquist (Eds.), *Complementary/Alternative Therapies in Nursing* (3rd ed.). New York: Springer.

Stone, J. F. (1994). *T'ai Chi Chih: Joy Thru Movement.* Fort Yates, ND: Good Karma Publishing, Inc.

Tse, S., & D. M. Bailey. (1992). T'ai Chi and postural control in the well elderly. *American Journal of Occupational Therapy, 46*(4), 295–300.

Whyte, N. (1997). T'ai Chi for clients in cardiac rehabilitation. *OT Practice, 2*(10), 38–41.

Williams, T. (1999). *The Complete Illustrated Guide to Chinese Medicine: A Comprehensive System for Health and Fitness.* Boston: Element Books.

Wolf, S. L., H. X. Barnhart, G. L. Ellison, C. E. Coogler, & F. B. Horak. (1997). The effects of T'ai Chi Quan and computerized balance training on postural stability in older subjects. *Physical Therapy, 77*(4), 371–385.

Wolf, S. L., H. X. Barnhart, N. G. Kutner, E. McNeeley, C. Coogler, & T. Xu. (1996). Reducing frailty and falls in older persons: An investigation of T'ai Chi and computerized balance training Atlanta FICSIT Group. Frailty and injuries: Cooperative studies of intervention techniques. *Journal of the American Geriatric Society, 44*(5), 489–497.

Xu, T. (2000, Winter/Spring). Tai Chi: A gift of balance [review of the video]. In *Wayfarer Publications Catalog.* Los Angeles, CA: Wayfarer Publications.

Young, D. R., L. J. Appel, J. SunHa, & E. R. Miller III. (1999). The effects of aerobic exercise and T'ai Chi on blood pressure in older people: Results of a randomized trial. *Journal of the American Geriatrics Society, 47*(3), 277–284.

Yu, T., & J. Johnson. (1999). *T'ai Chi Fundamentals for Health Care Practitioners and Instructors* (video). Madison, WI: Uncharted Country Publishing.

24

Yoga

Stacey Austin and Susan Laeng

CHAPTER OBJECTIVES

- Understand the history of yoga.
- Describe the benefits of yoga.
- Describe the current state of knowledge about yoga research.
- Describe how yoga can be incorporated into a therapy program.

Yoga is a vast body of knowledge from ancient India that offers the opportunity to deepen awareness and understanding of life on many levels. To present, in one chapter, what yoga really is, would be impossible. It takes years, perhaps a lifetime, of practice and study to just scratch the surface of this profound science, art, and philosophy.

This chapter will discuss one type of yoga, hatha yoga, and show how it can be used therapeutically in the Western health care system. There are a variety of resources with which to explore yoga today, but the most effective method is to take regular classes with a qualified instructor. The intention is that, with regular practice, one can learn how to relax the mind in order to let the body provide the answers from within.

History

Yoga has a broad meaning. The Sanskrit word yoga means "to yoke" or "union." Most broadly, yoga is union with the Divine, with Truth. T. K. S. Desikachar (1995), a world re-knowned yogi, stated "anything that brings us closer to the understanding that there is a power higher and greater than ourselves is yoga" (p. 6). The sage Patanjali, considered to be the father of yoga, documented his yoga sutras in India some 2,500 years ago (Iyengar, 1996). These sutras include 196 aphorisms of life and are the philosophical foundation of yoga as we know it today.

There are a multitude of styles and practices related to yoga. Hatha yoga integrates a system of physical postures (*asanas*) and breathing techniques (*pranayama*). *Ha* means sun, and *tha* means moon, referring to the integration of these two polarities within body, mind, and spirit (Iyengar, 1988). This 5,000-year-old practice is not by any means outdated and holds significant therapeutic value for the modern world.

The Eight Limbs of Yoga

Patanjali divided the philosophy of yoga into eight ashtangas, or limbs, which are named yama, niyama, asana, pranayama, pratyahara, dharana, dhyana, and samadhi (Iyengar, 1979). The principles of *yama* and *niyama* are ethical disciplines, with yama focused on social practice while niyama deals more with individual, inner codes of conduct. *Asana* and *pranayama* are the limbs used primarily in hatha yoga, in which asana relates to physical postures and pranayama to the regulation of breath or prana, the body's vital energy. Internalizing one's senses towards their source within is called *pratyahara*. *Dharana* is the act of concentration or steadying the mind, while *dhyana* is a more narrow focus of the mind, as in deep meditation. The final limb, *samadhi*, is the end stage of yoga, a much more profound meditation that cannot be practiced; instead, it happens, a result of the other seven practices. All of these eight limbs are equally important in the yogic body of knowledge and indicate the reasoning behind NCCAM classification of yoga as a mind-body therapy. This chapter focuses on asana, or the physical postures that can be incorporated therapeutically into our health care system. A discussion of breath work and meditation can be found in Chapter 20.

Yoga in the United States

Yoga was first introduced to the United States in 1893 by Swami Vivekananda at the World Parliament of Religions in Chicago (Feuerstein & Bodian, 1993). Since then, its focus has changed from a philosophical base to a more physical form. In the past century there has been a large ex-

Therapy Focus

Yoga, classified as a mind-body therapy by NCCAM, incorporates breath work, meditation, and strong body-based components to promote health. Yoga has been functioning as a form of therapy in other cultures for thousands of years. While therapy is not the only function of yoga, it is a very valuable rehabilitative tool that is finding a niche in our modern healthcare system.

One of the advantages in utilizing yoga in therapy is that it is relatively simple to apply, requiring minimal use of props. No expensive machines or large amounts of space are needed. The therapist applies kinesthetic principles and proper biomechanical alignment of the poses to address a wide variety of conditions. Many poses simultaneously address strength, flexibility, balance, and coordination as well as produce a relaxation effect.

Styles of Hatha Yoga in the United States

- Iyengar
- Ashtanga
- Power Yoga
- Jivamukti
- Kali Ray Triyoga
- White Lotus
- Integrative
- Viniyoga
- Svaroopa
- Bikram
- Phoenix Rising
- Sivananda
- Integral
- Ananda
- Ishta
- Kripalu
- Anusara

change between the East and West on the practice of yoga, as many yogis have come to America to promote yoga in all its forms. In 1920 Paramahansa Yogananda came from India to the United States as an emissary of Kriya yoga. His famous book, *Autobiography of a Yogi,* published in 1946, has since become a classic in its genre and has been translated into 18 languages. B. K. S. Iyengar developed his own style of hatha yoga and has authored many books on yoga philosophy and practice. He has done much to promote yoga as a form of health care throughout the world. His book, *Light on Yoga,* published in 1966, describes hundreds of yoga postures and pranayama techniques in detailed narratives, with photographs of himself in every pose. This classic book is considered by many to be the modern "bible" of yoga.

In the United States today, yoga is experiencing renewed popularity, primarily as a form of fitness and relaxation. There are now approximately 12 million people estimated to be practicing yoga in the United States, which is double the number of practitioners from just 5 years ago (Arnold, 1999). Yoga studios are thriving, and a multitude of videotapes and books are flooding the market. Medical doctors and other health care professionals are practicing, researching, promoting, and publishing the benefits of yoga as a form of preventative and curative medicine.

Therapeutic Yoga

Yoga works on so many levels simultaneously, in such subtle ways, that it is sometimes difficult to objectify it for therapeutic purposes. Also, the multitude of yoga styles generally do not have set standards, making it even more difficult to mainstream yoga into health care.

Yoga is a very dynamic system that can be greatly altered to accommodate individual differences and needs. Among the various forms of hatha yoga, all practitioners use most of the classic postures: standing, forward bend, seated, balancing, twists, backbend, inversion, and relaxation pose. Many postures are a combination of several of these categories. Standing poses are generally the starting point for beginners to introduce the principles of proper alignment, postural awareness, and general strengthening. Forward bends involve flexing the trunk over the lower extremities, with the flexion taking place in the hips, not the spine. This can be done seated, standing, supine, twisting, balancing, or inverted. Seated poses are generally more calming for the body and the nerves. Balancing postures develop poise, coordination, and strength. The spine, abdominal organs, and muscles are all activated and toned with twists. Backbends stretch most of the body's flexor muscles and strengthen the extensor muscles while stimulating the nervous system and creating an invigorating effect on the entire body. Inversions reverse the effects of gravity on each system in the body. More difficult inversions, such as headstand and handstand, are introduced after strength, confidence, and balance are attained in other poses. Each yoga session ideally ends with a relaxation pose in order to allow all the systems of the body to integrate the effects of the asanas.

Although there are many styles of hatha yoga, this chapter focuses on the style developed by Iyengar, well known for its therapeutic applications. Iyengar has spent decades applying his methods of hatha yoga to various medical conditions. One of his numerous contributions to modern yoga, and perhaps the hallmark of his method, is the use of props in order to adapt postures to any individual or condition. Examples of some props include mats, chairs, belts, blocks, bolsters, blankets, slings, and ropes. Props permit the exploration of various poses while maintaining the integrity and alignment of the body.

In the context of therapy, the goal is not to master a yoga pose. As a complementary approach, yoga should be incorporated with other therapy modalities that best address the client's condition and needs and facilitate functional improvement. While there are no contraindications for yoga, special adaptations are needed for certain conditions. Table 24–1 reviews indications and conditions requiring adaptations. When utilizing yoga integrated with therapy, discharge follows similar guidelines: when clients have achieved their functional goals or when maximum potential has been attained and adjustments in the treatment plan do not improve status. If a client has responded well to yoga and is highly functional, he or she can be referred to a community-based instructor for private sessions or classes after discharge.

Benefits of Yoga

Yoga benefits the whole system in gross as well as extremely subtle ways. Physically, yoga addresses flexibility, strength, coordination, balance, and circulation. Emotionally and mentally, yoga calms, builds self-esteem, clears the mind, and increases self-awareness and confidence. Iyengar (1988) states that yoga is the science of the mind. Western medicine and research are now starting to validate the connection between mind and body and its role in health with emerging fields such as psychoneuroimmunology. If the mind and thought patterns can be responsible for physical disease, then addressing the mind through asana and breathing practices can be a very powerful tool for health. A clear and peaceful mind, which is one possible by-product of yoga, provides a firm foundation for strength and vigor in the physical body.

Table 24–1 Indications and Conditions Requiring Adaptations

Indications:
- scoliosis/musculoskeletal conditions
- cardiovascular disorders
- respiratory diseases
- neurological conditions
- women's health issues, including pregnancy
- depression and anxiety
- thyroid conditions
- arthritis
- congenital disorders
- attention deficit disorder

Special Adaptations are Needed for the Following:
- pregnancy
- unstable blood pressure
- glaucoma
- postsurgical care
- acute fractures or medical conditions
- spondylolysis/spondylolisthesis
- arthritic flare-ups

Even if one's physical constitution is weak, mental fortitude and clarity are effective coping mechanisms for handling stress and disease.

The most obvious physical benefit of yoga is its effect on the musculoskeletal system. The flexibility and stability of the spine is often the key focus in poses. The Iyengar system incorporates meticulous attention to the biomechanical principles of alignment and kinesiology. In most asanas, attention begins with the foundation of the pose and is then directed up and out to every part of the body. The majority of musculoskeletal problems are simply a result of an imbalance among the opposing muscle groups that stabilize specific joints, creating either instability or immobility. This in turn sets up a series of reactions with neighboring areas and joints to try to either create more mobility or stability as needed until the original imbalance is corrected. Most yoga poses will simultaneously strengthen and increase flexibility where needed. A trained yoga instructor can choose specific postures based on individual needs and address a variety of conditions. For example, Uttihita Trikonasana, also called Triangle pose, incorporates a great degree of lateral trunk flexion combined with lumbosacral and pelvic stabilization, and can be effectively used to address scoliosis or other spinal conditions, using props as indicated. Numerous poses involve weight bearing not only through the lower extremities but also the upper ones and are an excellent exercise for those at risk for osteoporosis.

Effects of yoga on the nervous system are equally profound. Twists and forward bends tend to have a calming effect on the nervous system, while backbends can be extremely invigorating (Iyengar, 1979, 1990; Yoshikawa, 2000). Poses can be sequenced to induce a variety

Training and Certification

Training and certification is probably the most controversial issue in yoga today. The majority of the 17 styles listed earlier have their own standards for certifying instructors. One should contact each individual association for its specific training requirements. There is presently a Yoga Alliance Registry that has established a minimum set of criteria for inclusion in its national registry of yoga teachers, which is applicable to all the styles. This affiliation is perhaps the closest to a national standard that currently exists. Today opportunities abound to take numerous teacher-training courses all over the world. These range from weekend workshops to 6-month residentials. Yoga instructors are constantly updating their skills through regular teaching in a class and one-on-one situations. Also, teachers usually continue ongoing education from the more advanced instructors of their preferred style. Senior teachers of all traditions travel to various locations around the world to perform teacher training and workshops.

When choosing a yoga teacher, sample all the styles you are interested in. Ask questions and make your individual needs known. Choose a teacher that matches your goals, is inspiring, and has the knowledge and experience to help you to develop your own yoga practice. Perhaps the most invaluable quality a yoga instructor can possess is a strong and regular personal practice of his or her own. If referring your clients to a yoga instructor, become well acquainted with that teacher. Take the classes and make sure you are confident in his or her abilities and knowledge of body mechanics, alignment principles, and therapeutic applications. Yoga, like any physical activity, can cause injuries if not performed properly; therefore, choosing a skilled and well-trained teacher is extremely important for safety and therapeutic issues.

of effects, such as to ground, soothe, stimulate, or revitalize one's energy level. Properly performed inversions can tonify the nervous system and be very beneficial in treating insomnia (Iyengar, 1979, 1990; Yoshikawa, 2000). In a variety of neurological conditions where abnormal muscle tone is present, certain yoga postures can be utilized and adapted in order to help normalize the muscle tone.

Many cardiac rehabilitation programs utilize yoga to improve circulation, endurance, and strength of cardiac patients (Lipson, 1999). Inverted poses strengthen the venous system while draining and flushing the lymphatic system. Standing poses increase cardiac strength and endurance (Iyengar, 1990). Forward bends relax the sympathetic nervous system, which can be beneficial to the reduction of high blood pressure. Backbends tend to open up and expand the chest, stretching the cardiac vessels, which increases blood flow and acts as a preventive measure to arterial blockage or stenosis (Raman, 1998). Twisting poses squeeze and massage most major organs, which cleanses them, allowing the organs to work at peak efficiency, and decreases the demand for cardiac output to assist in their functioning (Raman, 1998).

The respiratory system is addressed in yoga primarily through pranayama technique and asanas that open the chest, shoulders, and rib cage. Pranayama cleanses the lungs, improves vital capacity, and increases one's sense of breath awareness and control (Iyengar, 1979, 1990; Raman, 1998). Backbends are especially beneficial for opening and expanding the chest and rib cage. Postures such as forward bends and twists, done properly, will also promote chest expansion. Movement into many of the postures is usually coordinated with the breath. Postures that flex the body are generally performed on an exhalation, while those that involve extension are coordinated with an inhalation (Feuerstein & Bodian, 1993).

In general, yoga postures prompt a lengthening of the spine, causing expansion of the abdominal cavity by a lifting of the ribs up off of the diaphragm and the underlying digestive organs, resulting in their improved overall functioning. Twisting postures most specifically benefit the gastrointestinal system. The abdominal organs are massaged, therefore increasing their blood flow and improving digestion and elimination. Backbends stretch the vagus nerve, of which one effect is the reduction of excessive gastric acids responsible for ulcers (Raman, 1998).

Reproductive health can also be improved with the practice of certain yoga postures (Iyengar, 1979, 1990; Raman, 1998; Yoshikawa, 2000). The Iyengar system has specific sequences of poses that address menstrual disorders, menopause, and pregnancy. For instance, the general focus of yoga application in the treatment of menstrual irregularities is to perform poses that energetically and physically open up the pelvic area. Such poses aid in the elimination of any congestion and sluggishness from the organs of reproduction. Yoga can be performed throughout pregnancy to prepare the body for the birthing process. Men's issues, such as prostate problems, can be addressed with hatha yoga as well, using poses that open up and increase the circulation in the pelvic area.

Inversions are specifically used to address the glandular and metabolic systems. Headstands are especially beneficial to stimulate the pituitary gland, as the head is inverted and the cranial cavity is perfused with excess blood volume and circulation. Shoulder stand regulates the highly vascular thyroid gland by compressing and massaging it by the movement of the sternum to the chin (Iyengar, 1990; Yoshikawa, 2000).

Psychological and emotional benefits are derived in many ways from yoga asanas and pranayama techniques. Poses that expand the chest and armpit areas, such as inversions and backbends, are reportedly extremely effective in treating depression. Very often in depression there is a shallow breathing pattern, which can be addressed by using pranayama techniques to deepen the breath and balance the inhalation to the exhalation time. This tends to have an immediate effect on mood. Balancing poses can help develop psychoemotional poise and strength necessary to manage the stressors of modern life. Yoga offers a great opportunity for insight, self-awareness, and growth through observation of thoughts, feelings, and experiences.

Research

There are many difficulties with yoga related research. Yoga works on many levels simultaneously and often in subtle ways that are difficult to quantify. Another challenge in objectifying yoga is that it is not a standardized practice—there are many styles of yoga with numerous inconsistencies among them. Research showing significant changes using one type of yoga may not relate to the benefits of other types of yoga.

Much of the research on yoga is being done in India and published in Indian journals such as the *Indian Journal of Medical Science*. Western research is mostly geared towards yoga's capacity to help those with specific conditions, such as heart disease, asthma, high blood pressure, and musculoskeletal problems such as low back pain, arthritis, and carpal tunnel syndrome. Yoga is also being scrutinized for its effects as a beneficial stress-reduction technique. Yoga, along with other forms of natural medicine based on stimulating the body's internal wisdom to heal, are gaining momentum rapidly. Even insurance companies are starting to recognize and pay for these modalities (Lipson, 1999).

Yoga has been researched moderately well, and the research suggests some very promising outcomes. One recent study focused on the effect of yoga in treating carpal tunnel syndrome (Garfinkel et al., 1999). This was a randomized, single-blind, controlled trial using 42 individuals diagnosed with carpal tunnel syndrome, ranging in age from 24 to 77 years. The subjects were divided into two groups, with the control group receiving traditional therapeutic treatments, including splinting. The study group received a program of Iyengar yoga consisting of a sequence of 11 asanas followed by a relaxation pose. Subjects in the yoga group showed statistically significant improvements in grip strength and Phalen sign as well as greater pain reduction versus the control group. Another study examined the effects of yoga on osteoarthritis of the hands (Garfinkel et al., 1994). This randomized, controlled clinical trial showed significant decreased hand pain and increased range of motion in osteoarthritic patients who followed a supervised yoga program.

Yoga's effects on asthma were examined in a controlled clinical study of university students. The yoga group followed a program of asanas, meditation, and pranayama practice and reported a greater sense of well-being with a more relaxing and positive attitude and better exercise tolerance. The use of beta adrenergic inhalers was also reduced after the 16-week yoga program (Vedanthan et al., 1998).

A study performed in Germany found that subjects who participated in a 3-month residential program significantly reduced cardiac risk factors, such as elevated blood pressure and cholesterol (Lipson, 1999). This program consisted of yoga, meditation, and a vegetarian diet. Perhaps the most well-known proponent of reducing cardiac risk factors and stress with yoga in the United States is Dean Ornish, M.D. Yoga is incorporated into his programs along with a low-fat vegetarian diet, group support, and moderate aerobic exercise. Ornish and his colleagues performed studies in 15 sites around the United States, demonstrating an 80 percent success rate in preventing costly and risky surgeries such as bypass and angioplasty in patients who followed this program. As a result, companies are beginning to cover the expense of Ornish's program (Lipson, 1999).

Overall, it is becoming more and more apparent that yoga will continue to grow in the United States as a therapeutic and preventative part of health care. However, additional research is clearly needed to prove yoga's legitimacy to insurance companies and the medical profession.

Case Studies

Muscular Dystrophy and Scoliosis

Michael was diagnosed with muscular dystrophy at 7 years of age. Muscular dystrophy is a hereditary and often fatal disease characterized by a progressive wasting of muscle tissue. There is no cure, and corrective surgery is used for severe scoliosis and muscle contractures. Michael came to physical therapy at 13 years of age in a school setting. He was very scared, as his older brother had recently died at age 15 from the same disease. However, he was extremely motivated and determined to keep himself strong and mobile. Michael was ambulatory but had very little pelvic and hip strength or control. He locked his knees in hyperextension to overcome quadricep weakness and had an increased lumbar lordosis to offset weak hip extensor muscles. There was a moderate right thoracic scoliosis, with resultant rib cage rotation/protusion, and a mild left lumbar scoliosis. His shoulder girdle and neck musculature were still relatively strong.

The therapist's main concern was his scoliosis and its interference with his lung capacity. The other focus was to keep Michael ambulatory. He had his brother's wheelchair and periodically was seen being wheeled around in it by his friends. In treatment Michael was started with yoga floor poses and some mild inversions with the use of ropes and other props to create length in his spine. A seated forward bend was practiced using a bolster for support of his trunk and a sandbag placed on the right posterior rib cage, which was protruding. This pose provided a good stretch for his tight hamstrings and helped him to actively lengthen and derotate his spine. Several standing poses were used with the wall and blocks for support. These poses were performed differently on each side to address the assymetry created by the scoliosis. For instance, in triangle pose, when laterally flexing the trunk to the right, towards the convexity, emphasis was on twisting to even out the spinal rotation. When laterally flexing to the left, towards the concavity, lengthening of the spine was emphasized to open up the compression on the left side of the spine and rib cage. Standing poses also worked on quadricep, pelvic, and paraspinal strengthening and hamstring, heelcord, and iliotibial band flexibility. Supported passive backbends were practiced using bolsters. Also, an active backbend was incorporated to strengthen hip and spinal extensor muscles. A standing twist using the wall and a seated twist on a chair was added with emphasis on lengthening the spine and staying longer in the twist to the left for spinal derotation. Each session was concluded with savasana, or corpse pose, for relaxation.

All of these poses were done three times a week in physical therapy sessions during the school year. Michael tried to do a little every day on his own as well. According to his friends and relatives, his follow-through was excellent. Michael continued this all through high school until he graduated at the age of 18. During his high school career, there was no progression of the scoliosis or loss of lung vital capacity, and he stopped using his wheelchair. His gait continued to be wobbly but did not stop him from being a very active member of his class and participating in extracurricular activities. He graduated high school as valedictorian of his class and showed no signs of progressing muscular weakness throughout those 4 years. He went on to college with a trunk full of yoga props. The poses not only appeared to enhance his mobility, but also seemed to soothe and calm his nervous system and mind. He grew into a poised man with good decision-making skills and strong self-confidence to deal with his disease and other obstacles in his life.

Low Back Pain

Jeanne, age 48, presented to physical therapy with severe pain and muscle spasms in her lumbosacral area bilaterally, but worse on the right, as well as radiating pain into her right hip and thigh. She had a full-time desk job and had had bouts of back pain on and off since the birth of her child 18 years ago, but never this severe. She reported "a little" pain during the week, and after a short weekend trip, which had involved a lot of driving, she woke up in severe pain. Jeanne presented with decreased lumbar lordosis and increased thoracic kyphosis. Her shoulders were rounded with tight pectoral muscles, and her head was positioned forward with tight neck flexors. Palpation revealed severe muscle guarding and spasms and tenderness at both sacroiliac (SI) joints, but more so on the right. The right SI joint was also slightly more posterior than the left. Her hamstrings, hip flexors, adductors, and external rotators were extremely tight.

The first several treatments focused mainly on patient education and treatment of her acute pain and muscle spasms with soft tissue work and electrical stimulation with heat. Gentle yoga low back and hip stretches were also introduced. Jeanne's acute pain and spasms subsided by the third treatment, but she still had some radiating pain and discomfort. A gentle supine piriformis stretch was initiated as well as mild supported backbends over a small bolster in both the thoracic and lumbosacral areas. Mild inversions using wall ropes helped her to lengthen her spine and derive a traction effect. By the third week, her radiating pain was completely gone. Her therapeutic exercise program was progressed to the more difficult standing poses, using a table for support, and some active backbends as well as gentle standing and seated twists with emphasis on creating length in the spine before rotation. By week five, Jeanne reported that her whole body felt so open and energized and that she was sleeping better than she ever had. As her hip musculature opened up, her standing poses and backbends were made more challenging by using less props, all the while stressing spinal lengthening. The poses incorporated in her exercise program not only addressed strengthening her paraspinal muscles and other stabilizers, but also increased the flexibility at her hips, shoulders, and neck. By the end of week six, she was discharged to a local yoga class with a highly qualified instructor. She continued attending classes twice a week indefinitely. She has not had any relapses since and her posture has dramatically improved.

Huntington's Chorea

Grace is a 47-year-old whose doctor ordered home health occupational therapy after a significant decline in upper extremity function with resultant decreased ability to perform activities of daily living. Grace was diagnosed with Huntington's Chorea at 42 years of age, and presently her doctor, reporting that her medications were at their maximum amounts, wanted to try occupational therapy. Upon initial evaluation, Grace required maximum assistance for ADLs. She also presented with severe apraxia, and fine and gross motor coordination was at a poor grade, with cogwheeling present.

Initially, treatment focused on passive range of motion progressing to active range of motion and coordination activities. Initial yoga techniques used were passive backbends over a bolster and gentle supine twists. Backbends aided in increasing her shoulder range of motion, and twists helped in normalizing her muscle tone. Modified forward bends were incorporated along with quadriped, standing, and twisting poses, all with the use of props. These yoga postures all worked on Grace's balance and coordination skills considerably, and increased her shoulder range of motion and normalized her muscle tone. Sessions were three times a week, and after 2 months, Grace had improved upper extremity gross and fine motor coordination skills to the fair grade that allowed her to dress herself again with minimal assistance. There was an increase in her shoulder range of motion bilaterally by about 50 percent. She was also able to safely wash dishes, including her wedding china, without breakage. She was discharged from home health services but presently continues with private yoga sessions to maintain her gross and fine motor skills at their present levels.

Cerebral Vascular Accident

Benjamin was 71 years old and suffered a right CVA, which presented as left hemiparesis with mild increased muscle tone. Home health occupational, physical, and speech therapies were ordered for Benjamin 5 weeks after the stroke, for which he received in-patient rehabilitation services. Benjamin had minimal aphasia and swallowing difficulties and progressed quite rapidly in the rehabilitation setting to moderate assist levels for mobility, transfers, and ADLs, and minimum assist self-feeding skills. He did not present with hemianopsia but had some mild discriminatory sensation deficits. Upon initial evaluation, he was beginning to show mild reflex sympathetic dystrophy (RSD) of his left arm and hand. Benjamin used a hemiwalker for ambulation. Initial home health rehabilitation goals were to increase Benjamin's function level to as independent as possible in the home. Neurodevelopmental treatment (NDT) techniques were employed, and joint PT/OT sessions were scheduled to incorporate yoga poses. Weight bearing and weight shifting of the right upper extremity in sitting, standing, and quadriped positions were used to help the RSD. Modified standing yoga poses, using the wall for support and a chair to weight bear through arms, as well as standing wall stretches were used in treatment, all addressing strengthening and flexibility where needed. Several passive backbends using bolsters were used to open the chest and improve swallowing capabilities. Most treatments were concluded with seated twists to calm Benjamin and quiet his nervous system as well as to decrease the muscle tone that was heightened slightly from his effort throughout the session. Benjamin worked hard and progressed slowly but steadily in 4 weeks, at which time he was discharged to an out-patient therapy setting. Upon discharge from home care, Benjamin was standby assist with transfers and gait using a quad cane. He was safely swallowing a regular diet and ADLs were at a supervisory level.

Summary

Since its introduction to the West, just over a 100 years ago, yoga has become an increasingly popular form of exercise, relaxation, disease prevention, and rehabilitation. Yoga addresses the mind-body-spirit connection and attempts to bring an overall sense of harmony to each and every aspect of the human system. Health care professionals throughout the country are increasingly practicing and prescribing this ancient science and integrating it into our medical and fitness systems. As Western health care continues to integrate energetic concepts and holistic views into the mainstream model of health, yoga should continue to prove itself as a valuable therapeutic resource. What seems like a simple concept of holding certain postures can actually lead, with prolonged practice, to very profound and subtle changes within the human body.

STUDY QUESTIONS

1. Define yoga.
2. Discuss the benefits Yoga practitioners have theorized yoga produces and compare these benefits with the current state of knowledge from research on yoga.
3. Choose one benefit of yoga and describe how the use of yoga can be incorporated into a therapy program to treat a problem commonly seen in rehabilitation.

SUGGESTED READING

Geeta, S. (1990). *Yoga: A Gem for Women*. Spokane, WA: Timeless Books.
Lasater, J. (1995). *Relax & Renew*. Berkeley, CA: Rodmell Press.
Mehta, S., M. Mehta, & S. Mehta. (1990). *Yoga: The Iyengar Way*. New York: Alfred A. Knopf.
Schatz, M. (1992). *Back Care Basics*. Berkeley, CA: Rodmell Press.

RESOURCES

Yoga Journal
Berkeley, CA
(800) 600-9642

Yoga International
Honesdale, PA
(800) 253-6243

Videos

Yoga Practice for Beginners with Patricia Walden
Yoga Practice for Relaxation with Patricia Walden & Rodney Yee
Yoga Remedies for Natural Healing with Rodney Yee

All available at
Living Arts
PO Box 2908, Department YJ505
Venice, CA
(800) 254-8464
www.livingarts.com

Relevant Associations

Ananda Yoga Teachers Association
14618 Tyler Foote Rd.,
Nevada City, CA 95959
(800) 346-5350.

BKS Iyengar Yoga National Association
 of the U.S.
PO Box 268
Culver City, CA 90230
(800) 899-9642

California Yoga Teachers Association
PO Box 60746
Palo Alto, CA 94306
(415) 759-7430

International Yoga Teachers Association
PO Box 13
Union Hill, NY 14563
(716) 265-2372

Kripalu Yoga Teachers Association
Box 793
Lenox, MA 01240
(413) 448-3202

Phoenix Rising Yoga Therapy
PO Box 819
Housatonic, MA 01236
(800) 288-9642

Yoga Alliance Registry
234 South 3rd Ave.
West Reading, PA 19611
(610) 376-4421

REFERENCES

Arnold, K. (1999, Winter). Retreat and rededication. *Yoga Journal,* 4.

Desikachar, T. K. S. (1995). *The Heart of Yoga.* Rochester, VT: Inner Traditions International.

Feuerstein, G., & S. Bodian. (1993). *Living Yoga.* New York: Putnam.

Garfinkel, M. S., H. R. Schumacher, A. Husain, M. Levy, & R. A. Reshetar. (1994). Evaluation of a yoga-based regimen for treatment of osteoarthritis of the hands. *Journal of Rheumatology, 21,* 2341–2343.

Garfinkel, M. S., A. Singhal, W. A. Katz, D. A. Allan, R. Rechetar, & H. R. Schumacher. (1999). Yoga-based intervention for carpal tunnel syndrome. *Journal of the American Medical Association, 18,* 1601–1603.

Iyengar, B. K. S. (1979). *Light on Yoga.* New York: Schocken.

Iyengar, B. K. S. (1988). *The Tree of Yoga.* Oxford, England: Fine Line Books.

Iyengar, B. K. S. (1996). *Light on the Yoga Sutras of Patanjali.* London: Thorsons.

Iyengar, G. S. (1990). *Yoga: A Gem for Women.* Spokane, WA: Timeless Books.

Lipson, E. (1999, Winter). Yoga works. *Yoga Journal,* 6–12.

Raman, K. (1998). *A Matter of Health.* Madras, India: Eastwest Books.

Vedanthan, P. K., L. N. Kesavalu, K. C. Murthy, K. Duvall, M. J. Hall, S. Baker, & S. Nagarathna. (1998). Clinical study of yoga techniques in university students with asthma: A controlled study. *Allergy and Asthma Proceedings, 19*(1), 3–9.

Yogananda, P. (1946). *Autobiography of a Yogi.* Los Angeles: Self-Realization Fellowship.

Yoshikawa, Y. (2000). Everybody upside-down. *Yoga Journal, 155,* 94–101, 174–177.

25

Stress Management

Franklin Stein

- Define stress and relevant terminology.
- Describe negative effects of stress.
- Describe methods of stress assessment.
- Describe common methods to treat stress.

Stress levels have risen in many demographic groups, including children, teenagers, adults and the elderly, over the last decade. Recent research (Stress, 2000) shows that 75 to 90 percent of visits to primary care physicians are for stress-related problems. Eighty-nine percent of adults describe feeling "high levels of stress" at some point in their everyday environment. Over 50 percent of adults complained of stress at least once or twice a week, and more than one in four said stress occurred on a daily basis. Most adults report that they are under much more stress now than they were in the past.

What is *stress* and its relationship to illness? Stress is a physical or psychological force that produces bodily or behavioral responses such as raised heart rate, increased anxiety, or insomnia in an individual. Stress can be conceptualized as a precipitating cause of symptoms or as an effect of an illness. As a cause, stress can be mild (driving in city traffic), moderate (applying for a job), or severe (the death of a family member). Stress can be acute or chronic. Mild stress can be a motivating force in an individual's life and create a challenge to succeed, while severe stress can be debilitating and precipitate or exacerbate symptoms of an illness.

Other examples of stressful situations are pressure to do well on an examination, the fear of being rejected by a friend, the reaction to a loss of a job, or an anxious thought about the future. When a person is able to use available resources for coping, the response to stress becomes lessened. *Eustress* is a term referring to positive stress, when an individual is challenged and puts forth his or her best efforts to succeed (Seyle, 1956). Cognitive, physical, and

Instances of stress are everyday events in a person's life that put pressure on the individual to react. While mild stress can be a motivating factor for people, moderate, severe, and prolonged stress can produce negative results. Stress seems to play an important role in determining the etiology and treatment of an illness (Larson, 1990). As much as 80 percent of the illnesses that physicians see is thought to be due to psychosocial stress (Taylor, Ureda, & Denham, 1982), and it undoubtedly effects our clients. Physically, the body reacts to prolonged stress in a variety of ways that can precipitate symptoms in an individual who is at risk or vulnerable to a disease. Therapists should be ready to address stress management with clients in order to maximize therapeutic outcomes as well as to prevent future problems.

emotional systems function efficiently in eustress, allowing the individual to perform maximally and to have the stamina to endure the demand.

Situations are referred to as *stressors* when they trigger a reaction in the individual. The body reacts to these stressors by increasing its response rate. When an individual perceives that he or she is under pressure, the body mobilizes as if it is under attack. The intensity of the stress reaction will depend on the individual's ability to cope and the resources available. An intense or prolonged stress response can lead to symptoms such as headaches, heartburn, blurring of vision, anxiety, or numerous other common problems.

Stressors are specific to the individual. There are *external stressors* that are generated by the environment, including crowds, noise, poor lighting, inadequate ventilation, and environmental pollutants. *Internal stressors* are generated by the individual and could be caused by feelings such as insecurity and fearfulness. *Social stressors* include major life changes, such as divorce, job loss, a major illness, financial problems, a car breakdown, and accidents. *Copers* are everyday activities or behavioral efforts to master, reduce, or tolerate demands created by a stressful situation. *Coping* refers to an individual's efforts to manage demands, regardless of the success of those efforts (Folkman et al., 1987). When successful, copers manage or reduce stress by bringing about a feeling of relaxation, reduced anxiety, and increased sense of well-being.

Effects of Stress

It has long been known by researchers and clinicians that psychosocial stress contributes to many illnesses and disabilities, including bronchial asthma, hypertension, headaches, rheumatoid arthritis, dermatitis, and ulcerative colitis (Goldberger & Breznitz, 1993). Walter Cannon (1939) first described the theoretical models and experimental data describing the effects of stress on the body in his classical work, *The Wisdom of the Body*. Cannon described the body's striving to maintain an internal equilibrium or homeostasis. Selye (1965) later elaborated upon Cannon's work and described the general adaptation syndrome, directly linking psychological factors with physiological responses. Since the initial research by

Cannon and Selye, scientists throughout the world have broadened the area of stress research, examining neurochemical and physiological evidence implicating stress as a contributing factor in diverse illnesses, diseases, and disabilities (Goldberger & Breznitz, 1993).

Research has presented overwhelming evidence that severe stress during prolonged periods has a detrimental effect on an individual's life (Sapolsky, 1998). Stressors can negatively impact the immune system, leading to a negative psychoneuroimmune reaction (Kemeny & Gruenewald, 1999). Studies have linked stress with several potentially life-threatening diseases, such as hypertension and coronary heart disease (Rozanski, Blumenthal, & Kaplan, 1999).

Stress can also cause changes in behavior, mental illness, and depression (Day, 1998). Stress has been linked to violence in the workplace (Antai-Otong, 2001), and work-related stress can have a secondary effect on other areas of people's lives (e.g., some individuals who are extremely angry and/or abusive to their spouses or children may also be reacting to extreme stress on their jobs).

Anger can be a self-defeating reaction to stress (Taylor, 1988). Extreme emotions of overreacting or underreacting to stress can create chronic emotional upset and attitudes of self-criticism and helplessness, and may lead to substance abuse in an effort to quiet the distress (Orioli, 1992). Also, the use of negative responses to stress, such as smoking, using illicit drugs, and abuse of alcohol, may actually increase stress and cause additional health and interpersonal problems, since they do nothing to change or manage the sources that cause the tension.

Clinical Practice

The widespread nature and detrimental effects of stress make it a particularly important issue to address. Research has shown that learning to self-regulate stress through relaxation exercises may help protect people from health problems such as heart attacks and high blood pressure (McGrady, Olson, & Kroon, 1995). Many of the individual therapies and modalities covered previously in this book address such practices. For example, from a mind-body perspective, the treatment of stress could involve imagery to assess or practice different stress responses, or meditation to elicit the relaxation response. Traditional Chinese Medicine views stress as a sign of imbalance (Barrett, 1993) and advocates chi-balancing activities such as Shiatsu. Because these topics have been covered previously, this chapter addresses more "traditional" stress assessment and management techniques, which are, however, "alternative" to most therapists' practice.

Assessment

Assessment of stress generally involves identification of an individual's stressors, response to stressors, and copers. These can be found in a number of different sources, including Davis, Eshelman, and McKay (1998).

The Stress Management Questionnaire

The Stress Management Questionnaire (SMQ) (Stein, Bentley, & Natz, 1999; Stein & Nikolic, 1989) is a 158-item paper and pencil assessment designed through pilot studies and clinical research to provide a personal stress profile for clients. Individuals identify how they respond to stress (e.g., physical, emotional, cognitive, and behavioral symptoms such as headaches, anxiety, loss of memory, insomnia), situations that cause the stress response (e.g., arguments, criticism, red tape, driving in heavy traffic), and coping responses such as exercise, listening to music, and talking to a friend.

The SMQ is a reliable (Stein, Bentley, & Natz, 1999) and valid tool that distinguishes between normal and clinical groups such as individuals with schizophrenia and depression (Stein & Nikolic, 1989; Stein & Smith, 1989). Clients who use it report satisfaction with its length, clarity, diversity of items concerning stress, and with the learning of new ways to manage stress through its administration (Stein, Bentley, & Natz, 1999).

Sorting Out Stress

Sorting Out Stress (SOS) cards are a newly devised version of the SMQ. Clients sort through three packs of cards—symptoms, stressors, and copers—identifying and then ranking the most troubling symptoms of stress, major copers, and copers that are most helpful. The client then determines whether the symptoms of stress and stressors are a major factor in performing activities such as work, self-care, and leisure.

The SOS cards can be used with a variety of clinical populations to identify activities that promote healthy adjustment, lower anxiety, and increase quality of life. The forced-choice format of the SOS cards provides an opportunity for self-monitoring of symptoms, stressors, and copers. Its game-like presentation is innovative and an appealing alternative to paper and pencil tests. Its reliability and validity are currently being assessed.

Treatment of Stress

Stress management techniques are used by a wide group of health professionals to enhance the well-being of people with a diverse group of disabilities, including spinal cord injuries and mental health issues (Courtney & Escobedo, 1990; Stein & Nikolic, 1989); traumatic brain injury (Lysaght & Bodenhamer, 1990); acute myocardial infarction (Norlan & Wielgosz, 1991); chronic pain (Strong, Cramond, & Maas, 1989; Swann; 1989); headache (Engel, Rapoff, & Pressman, 1991; King, 1992), and problems for resolving anger (Taylor, 1988). Stress management techniques for personal well-being can also be used by a normal population, such as health care professionals (Griffin, 1992); occupational therapy students (Mitchell & Kampfe, 1990); married adults (Mattlin, Wethington, & Kessler, 1990; Parkerson & Broadhead, 1995); and retired persons (Folkman & Lazarus, 1987).

Generally, three types of solutions exist for any problem. First, it can be tolerated, often leading to continued stress. Second, taking charge of the stressful situation by adapting to it can change the situation. The third solution is to escape the situation (Detherage, Johnson,

Therapists who work with clients for whom stress is a factor in their illness, such as mental health disorders or physical disorders or illnesses that are exacerbated by stress, can consider further training in stress management techniques in order to optimize their interventions. Many of the therapy approaches described in this text are geared to managing stress via manual, movement, mind-body, and energy therapies. The resources section of this chapter and others provides resources for further training.

& Mandle, 1994). Stress management involves addressing stressors, responses to stress, increasing coping activities, or a combination of these. For example, when an individual uses meditation or relaxation exercises, the body becomes calm and the sympathetic nervous system responses are reduced, making the individual's stress response calmer—addressing both stress response and coping activities.

Cognitive Strategies in Stress Management

Learning to cope more effectively with stressors is the basis for changing responses to stress (Levy, 1993). Cognitive or rational-emotive strategies (Ellis & MacLaren, 1998) are effective in reducing the effects of stress on individuals by teaching clients to self-regulate their feelings by becoming more objective in their thinking. Behaviors can be relearned by changing thought processes regarding situations that have previously been labeled stressful (Legeron, 1993). Through a cognitive approach to stress management, the client is taught to recognize, record, analyze, and modify the maladaptive behaviors that result from stressful conditions. Positive behaviors are developed through cognitive-behavioral retraining of maladaptive perceptions.

Therapists' Roles in Stress Management

A stress management program can help clients understand that by addressing everyday hassles with a healthy outlook, hardiness will be developed, and resistance to stress-related health problems will be better attained. Incorporation of daily activities that reduce tension, enhance self-esteem, and increase coping are facilitated by using a stress management program as part of a holistic approach in rehabilitation.

Stress management in therapy practice can be addressed formally (e.g., with the focused use of assessment tools and development of treatment plans), informally (e.g., providing resources that the client can use either while waiting for or during treatment, or when at home), or both. Therapists can stock their clinic or therapy site with stress management-related materials (see "Resources" in this and related chapters).

Therapists should decide whether their practice and training lends itself to formal, informal, or both types of stress management intervention. For example, therapists with training and experience in treating mental illness are particularly well suited to address stress manage-

It is important to develop strategies that can be used on an everyday basis to be better able to manage change. Flexibility in the choice of coping mechanisms also helps an individual to deal effectively with stress.

The general principles of stress management for a client include the following:

1. Incorporate the stress management technique into your everyday schedule so that it is as routine as brushing your teeth.
2. Engage in the activity at the same time each day, such as right before breakfast, for an afternoon break, or before dinner.
3. Keep a daily log of stress management activities and how it affects your mood, energy level, and productivity.
4. Be realistic in setting up a schedule that is relevant, appropriate, and attainable.
5. Do stress management techniques in increments, starting out for 5 or 10 minutes and working up to a half hour.
6. Monitor the impact of each coper in reducing anxiety and depressive feelings, and raising self-esteem.
7. Try to establish a quiet, unobtrusive environment for carrying out relaxation exercises.

ment formally under goals of cognitive retraining. Therapists without such training might opt to address stress management informally, educating clients about the physical effects of stress, encouraging clients to address the stress in their lives, or talking with clients about how to incorporate stress management techniques into his or her everyday life. The management of stress by therapists can include relaxation therapy, prescriptive exercise, creative arts, biofeedback, meditation and visualization, social skills training (Stein & Cutler, 1998) as well as manual, and movement therapies.

Laughter, relaxation, and hopefulness are examples of stress responses that increase the responses of the parasympathetic branch of the nervous system, reducing blood pressure and protecting the heart (Norlan & Wielgosz, 1991). Both physical and occupational therapists can use or advise the use of therapeutic activities that will assist in stress management, as well as use *themselves* therapeutically (e.g., with humor or empathy), facilitating the healing aspects of relationships.

The Importance of Cooperation

Client compliance and motivation are key factors in the success of any treatment. Stress, along with lack of exercise, poor diet, obesity, smoking, excessive alcohol use, and drug abuse are lifestyle risk factors that are ordinarily under the control of the individual. The elimination or reduction of these risk factors must involve the active participation of the client. For example, prescriptive exercise, individual diet, and stress management are only successful with the client's compliance and motivation. The greater the desire to change, the more willing the individual is to assume responsibility for his or her behavior. The more active the involvement in instigating change, the greater the probability that the necessary changes will occur.

Summary

Stress is a widespread health issue with far-reaching physical and emotional effects. Prolonged and excessive stress often produces negative consequences. Therapists can address stress formally and/or informally, depending on their level of training and the constraints of their practice site.

STUDY QUESTIONS

1. Define the following terms generally and provide an example of each from your life: stressors (mild, moderate, severe, external, internal, social), eustress, and copers.
2. Describe two long term effects of stress on the physical body.
3. What are the implications of behaviors such as smoking or drinking alcohol as responses to stress, and why?
4. Describe how rational-emotive strategies can be used to address stress.
5. Describe a practice area in which you are interested and two interventions you could use within it to address stress.

RESOURCES FOR IMPLEMENTING A STRESS MANAGEMENT PROGRAM

Cohen, M. (1999). *1 Amazing Way to Relax and Renew: Mike Cohen's Instant Relaxation Technique and Training Program*. Audio Educators compact disk training recording.

Davis, M., E. R. Eshelman, & M. McKay. (2000). *Relaxation & Stress Reduction Workbook*. Oakland, CA: New Harbinger.

Richardson, S. (1998). *Shakuhachi Meditation Music*. Sounds True music compact disk MM00301D.

Seligman, M. (1998). *Learned Optimism: How to Change Your Mind and Your Life*. New York: Pocket Books.

REFERENCES

Anastasi, A., & S. Urbina. (1996). *Psychological Testing* (7th ed.). Upper Saddle River, NJ: Prentice Hall.

Antai-Otong, D. (2001). Critical incident stress debriefing: A health promotion model for workplace violence. *Perspectives in Psychiatric Care, 37*(4), 125–139.

Barrett, S. (1993). Complementary self-care strategies for healthy aging. *Generations, 17,* 49–52.

Cannon, W. B. (1939). *The Wisdom of the Body*. New York: Norton.

Courtney, C., & B. Escobedo. (1990). A stress management of inpatient to outpatient. *American Journal of Occupational Therapy, 44,* 306–310.

Day, G. (1998). Stress prevention, not cure. *Director, 52,* 46.

Derogatis, L. R., & H. L. Coons. (1993). Self-report measures of stress. In L. Goldberger & S. Breznitz (Eds.), *Handbook of Stress: Theoretical and Clinical Aspects* (2nd ed.). New York: Free Press; London: Collier Macmillan.

Detherage, K. S., S. S. Johnson, C. Edelman, & C. L. Mandle. (Eds.). (1994). Stress management and crisis intervention. *Health Promotion Throughout the Lifespan*. Boston: Mosby.

Ellis, A., & C. MacLaren. (1998). *Rational-Emotive Behavior Therapy: A Therapist's Guide*. New York: Impact Publishers.

Engel, J. M., M. A. Rapoff, & A. R. Pressman. (1994). The durability of relaxation training in pediatric headache management. *Occupational Therapy Journal of Research, 14,* 183–189.

Everly, G. S., Jr., C. Harnett, R. Hendersen, E. C. Newman, M. Sherman, & R. Allen. (1986). The development of human stress in adults. In J. H. Humphrey (Ed.), *Human Stress.* New York: AMS Press.

Folkman, S., R. S. Lazarus, S. Pinely, & J. Novacek. (1987). Age differences in stress and coping processes. *Psychology and Aging, 2,* 171–184.

Goldberger, L., & S. Breznitz. (1993). *Handbook of Stress* (2nd ed.). New York: Macmillan.

Griffin, R. M. (1992). Controlling stress to attain career goals. *Occupational Therapy Practice, 3,* 39–44.

Kemeny, M. E., & T. L. Gruenewald. (1999). Psychoneuroimmunology. *Seminars in Gastrointestinal Disease, 10,* 20–29.

King, T. L. (1992). Use of electromyographic biofeedback in occupational therapy for treatment of stress-related disorders. *Occupational Therapy Practice, 3,* 50–58.

Kohn, P. M., & J. E. MacDonald. (1992). The survey of recent life experiences: A decontaminated hassles scale for adults. *Journal of Behavioral Medicine, 15,* 221–236.

Larson, K. B. (1990). Activity patterns and life changes in people with depression. *American Journal of Occupational Therapy, 44,* 902–906.

Legeron, P. (1993). Behavioral and cognitive strategies in stress management. *Encephale, 19,* 193–202.

Levy, L. L. (1993). Cognitive disability frame of reference. In H. L. Hopkins & H. D. Smith (Eds.), *Willard and Spackman's Occupational Therapy.* Philadelphia: J. B. Lippincott.

Lysaght, R., & E. Bodenhamer. (1990). The use of relaxation training to enhance the functional outcomes in adults with traumatic head injuries. *American Journal of Occupational Therapy, 44,* 797–802.

Mattlin, J. A., E. Wethington, & R. C. Kessler. (1990). Situational determinants of coping and coping effectiveness. *Journal of Health and Social Behavior, 31,* 103–119.

McGrady, A., R. P. Olson, & J. S. Kroon. (1995). Biobehavioral treatment of essential hypertension. In M. S. Schwartz and F. Andrasik (Eds.), *Biofeedback.* New York: Guilford Press.

Mitchell, M. M., & C. M. Kampfe. (1990). Coping strategies used by occupational therapy students during fieldwork: An exploratory study. *American Journal of Occupational Therapy, 44,* 543–550.

Moos, R. H., & J. A. Schaefer. (1993). Coping resources and processes: Current concepts and measures. In L. Goldberger & S. Breznitz (Eds.), *Handbook of Stress: Theoretical and Clinical Aspects* (2nd ed.). New York: Free Press; London: Collier Macmillan.

Norlan, R. P., & A. T. Wielgosz. (1991). Assessing adaptive and maladaptive coping in the early phase of acute myocardial infarction. *Journal of Behavioral Medicine, 14,* 111–124.

Orioli, E. M. (1992). Stress map. *Personnel News.* San Francisco: Essi System, Inc.

Parkerson, G. R., Jr., & W. E. Broadhead. (1995). Perceived family stress as a predictor of health-related outcomes. *Archives of Family Medicine, 4,* 253–260.

Rozanski, A., J. A. Blumenthal, & J. Kaplan. (1999). Impact of psychological factors on the pathogenesis of cardiovascular disease and implications for therapy. *Circulation, 101,* 177–178.

Sapolsky, R. M. (1998). *Why Zebras Don't Get Ulcers: An Updated Guide to Stress, Stress-related Diseases, and Coping.* New York: W. H. Freeman.

Seyle, H. (1956). *The Stress of Life.* New York: McGraw-Hill.

Stein, F. (1987). Stress and schizophrenia. *Alberta Psychology, 16,* 10–11.

Stein, F., D. Bentley, & M. Natz. (1999). Computerized assessment: The stress management questionnaire. In B. Hemphill-Pearson (Ed.), *Assessment in Occupational Therapy Mental Health: An Integrative Approach.* Thorofare, NJ: Slack.

Stein, F., & S. Cutler. (1998). *Psychosocial Occupational Therapy: A Holistic Approach.* San Diego: Singular Publishing.

Stein, F., & S. Nikolic. (1989). Teaching stress management techniques to a schizophrenic patient. *American Journal of Occupational Therapy, 43,* 162–169.

Stein, F., & J. Smith. (1989). Short-term stress management program with acutely depressed in-patients. *Canadian Journal of Occupational Therapy, 56,* 185–192.

Stress, 2000. [Online]. American Institute of Stress. Available: www.stress.org.

Strong, J., T. Cramond, & F. Mass. (1989). The effectiveness of relaxation techniques with patients who have chronic low back pain. *Occupational Therapy Journal of Research, 9,* 185–191.

Swann, C. (1989). Stress management for pain control. *Physiotherapy, 75,* 295–298.

Taylor, E. (1988). Anger intervention. *The American Journal of Occupational Therapy, 42,* 147–155.

Taylor, R. B., J. R. Ureda, & J. W. Denham. (Eds.). (1982). *Health Promotion: Principles and Clinical Applications.* Norwalk, CT: Appleton-Century-Crofts.

26

Pain Control

Guy L. McCormack

- Describe pain and the common myths that surround it.
- Contrast the conventional perception of pain with the mind-body approach.
- Describe a variety of self-help mind-body techniques that therapists can apply within their scopes of practice.

Background and History

What is pain? Pain is truly a puzzling phenomenon. Even as researchers continue to unlock its secrets, many doorways remain bolted shut.

The most widely accepted definition of pain is "an unpleasant sensory and emotional experience associated with actual or potential tissue damage or described in terms of such damage" (International Association for the Study of Pain, Subcommittee on Taxonomy Part II, 1986, p. 12). The very definition of pain suggests that it is multidimensional and subjective in nature. Like urban legends on the Internet, pain is associated with many myths. For example, the word *pain* is derived from the Greek work *poena*, which means "penalty" or "payment" (Thomas, 1993). Obviously, this definition equates pain with punishment, and there is a connotation that pain is also associated with misery. Many religious and philosophical belief systems have portrayed pain as a rightful consequence of sin or bad behavior.

Another common myth is that chronic pain can be cured. Unfortunately, a purely medical cure for some chronic pain syndromes does not exist (Corey, 1989; Sternbach, 1987) because chronic pain syndromes do not stem from one source. Chronic pain interfaces with emotional, cognitive, physical, and social parameters.

Another myth is the "quick-fix" fantasy created by advertisers and by medical breakthroughs being highly publicized in the media. The media suggest that there is a pill or a quick treatment to remedy almost every disorder. Yet chronic pain usually has taken a long time to develop and is a multifaceted problem. A single injection or a pill, such as those seen in headache advertisements, is unlikely to abolish chronic pain in one fell swoop (Corey, 1989).

Even the behavioral scientists have created myths, as can be seen in the controversial literature on the so-called "pain personality." Clinical observations have led some investigators to believe that chronic pain is correlated with a pain-prone character disorder. Again, there is very little hard evidence to support this supposition.

Another ubiquitous myth is the belief that persons complaining of chronic pain are malingerers or derive secondary gain by getting attention from others. True, some individuals fake injuries to collect insurance or worker's compensation monies. As it turns out, however, most people filing claims have suffered acute injuries, and more than 90 percent have legitimate pain syndromes (Corey, 1989; Segraves, 1989).

These myths and others surrounding chronic pain continue to exist because pain is poorly understood and often poorly managed. Pain is a phenomenon that simultaneously affects a person's mind, body, and spirit. However, the conventional wisdom of health care is inadequate to deal with such a multidimensional problem.

The conventional medical models are based on the assumption that there is a demarcation between mind and body, a philosophy known as *dualism*. This 300-year-old doctrine states that the mind and body operate as separate entities (Fields, 1987). As a result of this assumption, pain research has taken two diametric, antithetical directions: One group of investigators has followed the premise that pain is a psychosocial problem originating from unresolved emotions, aberrant behaviors, or mental disorders; a second contingent of researchers views pain as having physiological origins. This well-entrenched philosophical split has created havoc in the health care delivery system (McCormack, 1993).

It should also be noted that pain is experienced in a historical and cultural context. The health care provider's cultural mindset and technical skills determine how a person's pain is interpreted and treated. The sensation of pain is a construction—an interpretation of culturally given conceptual schemes and a product of linguistic expressions. For example, some ethnic individuals are more emotive in the expression of pain while others may tend to be restrained while expressing their pain experience.

The notion of dualism and the medical model have treated chronic pain as either a psychological response or a physical disorder arising from some organic dysfunction. The primary drawback of this traditional approach is that it fosters client dependency and a segmental interpretation of the pain experience.

One irrefutable principle of pain management is this: *The person suffering from chronic pain should be seen as a whole person, not as a disease entity.* Furthermore, pain is a personal perception of harm (hurt) that can be understood only by the individual experiencing it. The

Therapy Focus

Because pain is a factor in many problems treated by therapists, one must be familiar with approaches to treatment of pain.

ultimate standard for determining the efficacy of a pain management approach is the client's intuition about her or his everyday experiences with pain.

Methods of Managing Pain Syndromes

Pharmacologic Management of Pain

A very effective pharmacologic method of pain management is the World Health Organization's approach called the WHO Ladder, which implies a progressive stepping up approach to drug therapy. The first step in this approach is the use of nonsteroidal anti-inflammatory drugs (NSAIDs) such as acetaminophen, aspirin, and other oral analgesics. The second step is to administer an opioid such as codeine or hydrocodone for mild to moderate pain. The third step is for moderate to severe pain where more potent opioids such as morphine, hydromorphone, or methadone are prescribed on an "as needed" basis. The administration of pharmacologic management depends on the specific drug, its formulation, and the clients' individual tolerances for the drug. Analgesics can be administered orally, by rectal route, transdermally, and through transnasal routes. Other more invasive routes for the administration of analgesics are intraspinal, intraventrical, and client-controlled devices. Each analgesic has advantages and side effects. The practitioner should become familiar with the major pharmacologic agents and the potential side effects (Jacox et al., 1994).

In recent years, evidence has shown that many people with terminal illnesses, such as cancer, and other people with chronic pain syndromes have been undermedicated. Evidence-based practice has shown that few individuals become addicted to pain medications and many do not receive sufficient pain relief (Neuman, 1989).

Mindbody Interventions

Basically, there are two nonpharmacologic approaches to pain management. One involves cognitive behavioral management or central processing.

Central processing pertains to a more humoral pain abatement mechanism whereby thoughts or mind states originating in the frontal lobe of the cortex send neuronal messengers to the limbic system and the hypothalamus. Here various neuropeptides are released that act both as neuromodulators in the central nervous system and hormones in the bloodstream. The central processing level transforms negative thinking into positive thinking through visualization, guided imagery, autogenic suggestion, and positive affirmations. Central processing works on the molecular level by the transmission of ions and second messengers (McCormack, 1993).

The second nonpharmacologic approach to pain management is called peripheral processing, which involves neurogenic mechanisms. The stimuli provided by the health professional are based on counterstimulation or dermal abrasive techniques. Modalities such as heat, cold, TENS, and localized touch pressure in acupressure appear to work either through the gating mechanism in the dorsal horn of the spinal cord or through activating the cells in the periaqueductal grey of the brain stem. At the spinal cord level, pain is blocked by presynaptic inhibition. In the periaqueductal grey, the release of endogenous opioids creates a descending volley of neurotransmitter substances that blocks pain messages from reaching higher levels where pain is consciously perceived.

Therefore, it is likely that pain can be modulated or abated at the level of the skin through subcortical mechanisms and through manipulation of the mind (Raj, 1992).

Recall that chronic pain is not only an aberration of the nervous system, but of endocrine and immune systems as well. In time, pain becomes patterned into the DNA of cells and produces prolonged disturbances in cellular functions. In the nervous system, this pattern may entail alterations of neurotransmitter substances, as well as prolonged discharge caused by second messengers. By conjuring vivid, positive pictures in the mind, one can directly influence bodily processes. Furthermore, by seeing in our mind's eye how we want to be, it is indeed possible to transform behavior.

If thoughts, beliefs, attitudes, and social support systems can influence our perception of pain and immune responses to produce what has been called psychosomatic illness, why can't the same mechanisms be used to reverse the process and produce psychosomatic wellness? I do not intend to imply that some strange or mystical force is at work in this mind-over-matter approach. Thoughts are powerful medicine that tap into the natural capacity to heal. Activities that engage the mind can have a positive influence on the human body.

Visualization

Visualization, also known as *guided imagery* or *creative imagery,* is the act of conjuring up mental images. The main idea is to develop vivid pictures and sensations of places, scenes, memories, or fantasies. Like dreams, imagery contains symbolic meanings and can give the person insight into subconscious beliefs and understandings.

The brain responds to these mental images as if they were real, and they have direct effects on the body. Mental images have been known to relieve pain, reduce stress, and promote healing. Studies suggest that most people who have faithfully practiced visualization at least twice a day in order to reduce pain report favorable results within a few weeks (Weil, 1995). As consciously chosen, intentional instructions to the body, visualizations act on the subcortical components of the nervous system, especially the limbic-hypothalamus-pituitary axis.

According to Achterberg (1985), there are biochemical and neuroanatomical components to every image that have the potential to change activities at the cellular level.

Sensory Substitution

Sensory substitution is guided imagery that reinterprets the sensation of pain as a more tolerable sensation. For example, the person in pain may describe the pain as a "red-hot poker, stabbing into my lower back." The guided imagery first takes the person through a general relaxation script, then guides the person to see the pain image transform into a more benign image. For example, the hot poker might gradually change into a pointed massage vibrator providing circulating touches that dissipate the pain.

Displacement

Displacement is a visualization process that moves the pain from one area of the body to another. This type of visualization works best on well-localized pain in the limbs. The pain is seen as a spiraling form of energy that can move from one body part to another. Usually, the facilitator directs the relaxation part of the script and the image of the pain as a spiraling form of energy, but allows the person to visualize the direction and location of the movement. The advantage of this technique is that it gives the person some control over the pain and gives the site of pain some rest.

Dissociation

Another visualization strategy is to dissociate from the pain. The person is led through a visualization of "taking a mental vacation," leaving the pain in the room and journeying to another place.

End-Result Imagery/Mental Rehearsal

Korn (1990) has described a valuable central processing strategy called *end-result imagery* employed by many Olympic athletes. It involves simply mentally rehearsing an impending event and visualizing before the actual event the best possible scenario. Many athletes concur that such mental rehearsal really affects the outcome of a competitive event. One's belief system affects many physiological processes in the body as well.

Positive Event Journal

A functional activity that provides a more tangible approach to positive thinking is keeping a journal of positive events and accomplishments. Accomplishments may be physical, such as walking an extra lap, or emotional, such as feeling good about helping someone else. This journal provides an "emotional lift" during the "bad days" when pain seems unrelenting and depression sets in. Reading the positive citations and accomplishments makes it hard to dwell in the "negative zone" for long.

Meditation

The word *meditation* comes from the Sanskrit word *medha*, meaning "wisdom." Meditation is a means of tuning in, a focusing inward of attention in order to reach a purer experience of the self. Meditation can open one to transpersonal experiences; in essence, it gives one an awareness of being.

During deep meditation, the body undergoes measurable physiological changes, including increases in skin electrical resistance and the regularity and amplitude of alpha waves in the brain, and reductions in blood pressure, metabolism, heart rate, and oxygen consumption. The overall effect of slowing the body's functions to a healthier balance is called the relaxation response (Benson, 1976).

Meditation is not something one can force through some internal fusion of energy—it just happens. The meditative attitude provides a medium through which one can simply "be," not "become" or "do."

Progressive Relaxation

Progressive relaxation was developed by Jacobson in 1938. Progressive relaxation is a systematic process of voluntarily contracting and relaxing specific groups of muscles. The recipient is asked to focus on the sensations of tightness and tension and the feeling of muscle relaxation as the tension recedes. This helps the person discriminate between feelings of tension and relaxation. This technique works best with individuals who tend to be kinesthetic learners and with individuals whose primary source of pain is excess muscle tension.

Many tapes for progressive relaxation are commercially available, some with background music to enhance the script. As with all central processing approaches, the prerequisites are a quiet environment, a comfortable posture, and a receptive state of mind. The procedure consists of sequential cycles of contraction followed by relaxation with 14 separate muscle groups.

Peripheral Processing

In the peripheral processing approach the neurological mechanism involves forms of counterstimulation to alleviate pain through the gate control mechanism (Melzak & Wall, 1982). Counterstimulation appears to cause encapsulated receptors that are superficial or deep in the skin to reach action potential. Once the encapsulated receptors fire (discharge), they transmit along thick fibers to the dorsal horn of the spinal cord (substantia gelatinosa) where presynaptic inhibition takes place in the same region where thin fibers carrying pain impulses must synapse (converge). Usually, the stimuli carried by the thick fibers prevail, causing a long-lasting inhibition of thin fiber pain transmission neurons. Various dermal abrasive techniques such as coin rubbing, cupping, ice massage, and therapeutic vibration involve the gate control mechanism.

Physical Agent Modalities

Cryotherapy or cold therapy is commonly used to alleviate pain. Superficial cooling such as with ice packs is helpful for musculoskeletal and neuromuscular conditions as a source of analgesia (Bracciano, 2000). The application of cold affects nerve endings and nerve roots by providing counter irritation and by reducing metabolic activity in the tissues (Lehmann & de Lateur, 1982). Ice massage has been shown to reduce pain and decrease muscle spasms in most patients (Melzack et al., 1980). Cold can be applied by ice packs, cold/ice water immersion baths, ice towels, ice massage, or vapocoolant sprays.

Fluorimethane spray contains a fluorocarbon that is known to affect the environment, so it is not used in many settings. As with any physical agent modality, cryotherapy should be used with precautions. The practitioner should always monitor the patient's skin condition and blood pressure. Cold should not be applied over areas of impaired circulation, over wounds that are 2 to 3 weeks post injury, or for a prolonged time over superficial nerves (Bracciano, 2000).

Superficial Heat Application for Joint Pain

Superficial heat agents increase the temperature of skin and superficial subcutaneous tissues. Hot packs, contrast bath, and parafin involves physical contact and transmits thermal energy by conduction. Whirlpool bath and fluidotherapy use convection as the mechanism of heat transfer. Again, it is important that the practitioner have appropriate training in the use of physical agent modalities. Superficial heat agents have been shown to have an analgesic effect on soft tissues; heat causes vasodilation, increases metabolism, reduces byproducts of inflammatory response, and improves extensibility of connective tissues. Clients with compromised circulation or diminished sensation are not good candidates for superficial heat agents.

Additional Mindbody Techniques

Deep Breathing

Deep breathing exercises are another useful technique to acquaint the client with the relaxation response. Breathing is often forgotten as a therapeutic intervention. The object is to have the client concentrate on breathing. In doing so, the rate of breathing slows down automatically. As breathing slows, so do other physiologic mechanisms, and the mind once again is diverted from pain. To augment the effects of deep breathing, the therapist instructs the client to breath in through the nose and out through the mouth, with partly closed lips (a sighing sound may accompany the expirations). The rate of breathing can be set to a metronome so the expirations are calibrated to be twice as long as the inspirations. It is also beneficial to have the client focus on an object while breathing, with the intent of producing a concentrated gaze.

Diaphragmatic breathing is another breathing technique. The diaphragm and the muscles of the abdominal wall are extremely important to the maintenance of homeostasis. Attached to the posterior abdominal wall are the quadratus lumborum and psoas muscles, which are important for daily activities such as bending, walking, running, and adequate expulsion of air. Passing through the diaphragm from the thoracic cavity to the abdominal cavity are the aorta; the thoracic lymphatic duct; the splanchnic nerves; and the vagus, phrenic, and paravertebral ganglion chains. These important structures are the "pipelines" for nutrition, circulation, and the function of the organs in the abdominal and pelvic cavities. These structures are stimulated with deep breathing practices.

Deep breathing also benefits clients physiologically because inhalation through the nose activates parasympathetic fibers in the nasal mucosa (Guyton, 1991). Inhalation through the nose also draws oxygen into the blood, causing oxyhemoglobin levels to increase and thus promoting healing. In contrast, exhalation releases carbon dioxide and waste products. The patient in pain usually breathes in a shallow manner, using mostly the chest and intercostal muscles. Deep breathing opens up more alveoli in the lungs and oxygenates the bloodstream, allowing microcapillary beds to dilate and supply tissues (Weil, 1995).

Moxibustion

Moxibustion involves the burning of a Chinese herb called artemisia vulgaris, or commonly known as mugwort, near the skin, over acupoints, which are the sites used for needle insertion during acupuncture treatment. Moxibustion is used in conjunction with acupuncture or can be purchased as moxa rolls that look like cigars wrapped in thin paper. When one end is ignited, it burns slowly like incense. The burning roll is held about two inches away from the skin over specific acupoints and moved in a slow circular fashion. In Traditional Chinese Medicine, moxibustion is used to increase the flow of chi (qi) in the body. Moxa conveys heat by way of convection. As a heat source it is used to increase circulation and reduce fatigue, and may alleviate pain when used over distal acupoints.

Cupping

Cupping techniques involve the placement of glass cups where oxygen has been burnt out to create a vacuum or suction on the skin. The cups are usually applied over regions of the anterior trunk to assist in respiratory conditions or over the primary raimi of the posterior trunk to reduce muscle soreness from overuse or muscle strain. Both moxibustion and cupping techniques require proper training, and precautions should be followed (McCormack, 1991). For more information, contact the American Association of Oriental Medicine (see "Resources").

Reflexology

In 1917, William Fitzgerald, an American physician, observed that manual pressure to the hands and feet produced analgesic effects to larger regions of the body. He systematically identified 10 vertical reflex zones on the feet and hands.

Today reflexology is the study and science of using touch on the feet, hands, and ears to stimulate regions of the body that are believed to be topographically related. Reflexologists believe that there are both vertical and horizontal reflex zones that are somatopically related to specific areas of the body. Therefore, there are regions of the hands, feet, and outer ears that are believed to correspond to every organ, gland, and soft tissue structure of the body.

The prevailing theory for why reflexology alleviates pain comes from the concept of "eliminating blockages" and peripheral irritation of the nervous system. In theory, when a part of the body is physically overstressed, biochemical byproducts accumulate in the soft tissues surrounding nociceptive nerve endings. Massage and firm deep pressure to the hands and feet causes the biochemicals to dissipate, thereby alleviating the irritation to the nerve endings.

Reflexology has been found to relieve stress, increase circulation, remove systemic byproducts in soft tissues and restore homeostasis (see Chapter 18 for more information on reflexology).

Aromatherapy and Essential Oils

Aromatic oils have been used for over 5,000 years in China, India, Persia, and Egypt. Essential oils were found to be useful for health, as they contain antibacterial, antivirus, antifungal, and antiseptic properties. Essential oils are highly concentrated oils extracted (by cold pressing) or distilled from plants, trees, flowers, herbs, and bushes. Proportional yield from plants vary from 1 to 10 percent.

The term aromatherapy was coined in 1920 by Rene-Monrice Gattefosse, a chemist. He discovered that pure lavender facilitates the healing of burns. Lavender has high ester, a class of chemical compounds formed by bonding of an alcohol and organic acids.

Plants contain phytohormones or chemical messengers that normally protect them from infectious agents. Many people believe that phytohormones act like pharmacologic agents and have antiseptic and antimicrobial properties (Damian, 1995). Essential oils penetrate the barrier of the skin because of their small molecular size and because they are lipid (fat) soluble (water soluble molecules do not penetrate the stratum corneum because it contains keratin). Essential oils are highly volatile (evaporative). They can be diffused in the air or applied to the skin in a carrier oil. When applied to the skin, the essential oils are believed to penetrate deeply into the tissues to enter the blood stream and the lymphatic system (Lavabre, 1990).

With inhalation, diffused essential oils enter the nose and stimulate the olfactory bulbs. Impulses are transmitted to the limbic lobe and the hypothalamus. Through diverging pathways, neuronal impulses can be transmitted to the autonomic nervous system and to the pituitary gland, where hormonal effects can take place.

Essential oils are never applied full strength or directly to the skin but are mixed in a "carrier oil." Petroleum products such as mineral oils should not be used because they do not penetrate the keratin, the fibrous protein layer of the skin. Vegetable oils such as canola, sweet almond, sunflower, grape seed, or safflower are preferred carrier oils, as they do penetrate the keratin layer of skin.

Aromatherapy is commonly used in England and France in hospital settings. Diffusers are used to dispense essential oils to alleviate respiratory conditions, elicit relaxation, and elevate moods. Vaporized essential oils such as lemon, lavender, and lemongrass are known to combat airborne infectious diseases (Damian, 1995). Over all, aromatherapy is used to elicit the relaxation response.

Summary

Pain management is a multidisciplinary task. The conventional dualistic approach that views the mind and body as separate entities is limited. The distinctions between physical and psychogenic pain are illusory. New understandings derived from the field of psychoneuroimmunology have provided convincing evidence that the mind and body are one. In this chapter peripheral processing and central processing techniques were discussed to develop an understanding of how pain can be modulated. In the future, pain control methods will include more mindbody approaches, and drugs and surgery will take a less prominent role in pain management.

STUDY QUESTIONS

1. Describe four myths that are commonly associated with pain.
2. Differentiate between peripheral processing and central processing as methods of pain modulation.
3. Describe four different methods of visualization or imagery for pain management.

Resources

American Association of Oriental Medicine
433 Front St.
Catasaukua, PA 18032

References

Achterberg, J. (1985). *Imagery & Healing*. Boulder, CO: New Science Library, Random House.

Benson, H. (1976). *The Relaxation Response*. New York: Avon Books.

Bracciano, A. G. (2000). *Physical Agent Modalities: Theory and Application for the Occupational Therapist*. Thorofare, NJ: Slack.

Corey, D. (1989). *Free Yourself of Pain*. New York: Penguin Books.

Damian, D. (1995). *Aromatherapy: Scent & Psyche*. Rochester, VT: Healing Arts Press.

Fields, H. L. (1987). *Pain*. New York: McGraw-Hill.

Guyton, A. C. (1991). *Textbook of Medical Physiology* (8th ed.). Philadelphia: W. B. Saunders.

International Association for the Study of Pain, Subcommittee on Taxonomy. Part II. Pain terms: A current list with definitions and notes on usage. *Pain, 6*, 249–52 (updated 1986).

Jacobson, E. (1938). *Progressive Relaxation*. Chicago: University of Chicago Press.

Jacox, A., D. B. Carr, R. Payne, C. Berden, N. Breitbart, J. M. Cain, C. R. Chapman, & C. Cleeland. (1994). *Management of Cancer Pain*. U.S. Dept. of Health and Human Services, AHCPR Pub. No. 94-0592, 39–44.

Korn, E. (1990, Dec.). Get a dose of medical videos. *Prevention, 42*(12), 64–122.

Lavabre, M. (1990). *Aromatherapy Workbook*. Rochester, VT: Healing Arts Press.

Lehmann, J. F., & B. J. de Lateur. (1982). Diathermy and superficial heat & cold therapy. In F. J. Kottke, G. K. Stillwell, & J. F. Lehmann (Eds.), *Krusen's Handbook of Physical Medicine & Rehabilitation* (3rd ed.). Philadelphia: W. B. Saunders.

McCormack, G. (1991). *Therapeutic Use of Touch: A Treatment Guide for the Health Professional*. Tucson, AZ: Therapy Skill Builders.

McCormack, G. (1993). *Pain Management: Mindbody Techniques*. Tucson, AZ: Therapy Skill Builders.

Melzack, R., & P. D. Wall. (1982). Pain mechanisms: A new theory. *Science, 150*, 971–979.

Melzack, R., M. E. Jeans, J. C. Stratford, & R. C. Monks. (1980). Ice massage and transcutaneous electrical stimulation: Comparison of treatment for low back pain. *Pain, 9*, 209–217.

Neuman, R. E. (1989). *Health Tips*. Leucadia, CA: United Research Publications.

Raj, P. P. (1992). *Practical Management of Pain* (2nd ed.). St. Louis: Mosby.

Segraves, K. B. (1989). Bring it all together: Developing a clinical team. In P. M. Camic & F. D. Brown (Eds.), *Assessing Chronic Pain*. New York: Springer-Verlag.

Sternbach, R. A. (1987). *Mastering Pain*. New York: Putnams.

Thomas, C. (1993). *Taber's Cyclopedic Medical Dictionary* (18th ed.). Philadelphia: F. A. Davis.

Weil, A. (1995). *Spontaneous Healing*. New York: Fawcett Columbine.

27

Chronic HIV Disease

Mary Lou Galantino

CHAPTER OBJECTIVES

- Understand the impact of highly active antiretroviral therapies on the musculoskeletal, neurological, and cardiopulmonary systems.
- Appreciate the various clinical markers for HIV disease progression.
- Consider various modalities and manual therapies for HIV pain management.
- Know the latest usage of CAM by various populations living with HIV disease.
- Describe the integration of various manual and movement therapies for HIV wellness.

Acquired immunodeficiency syndrome (AIDS) has been the leading cause of death among young adults in the United States since the 1990s. Initially recognized in 1982, human immunodeficiency virus (HIV) has had a devastating impact on people in the developing world (CDC, 1995; Quinn, 1996). Since mid-1990, the epidemiology of HIV disease has changed in the United States. For the first time in the history of the epidemic, there has been a recent decrease in the annual national incidence and a decline in AIDS deaths (CDC, 1997a, 1997b). Most epidemiologists and clinicians attribute these findings to the impact of new highly active antiretroviral therapies (HAART).

Current medication regimens can significantly reduce the HIV level not only in the peripheral blood but also in the lymphoid tissue and the central nervous system (Schrager & D'Souza, 1998). In an effort to reduce the plasma HIV burden to levels below the threshold of detection by available assays, a series of HAART may be necessary. A challenge, however, may arise quickly because resistance to one drug in a class of agents may induce partial or complete resistance with other agents, depending on the specific mutations involved (Arts & Wamberg, 1996; Schrager & D'Souza, 1998).

In a field that is rapidly changing, specific recommendations for antiretroviral therapy are difficult to make. The major therapeutic decisions include (1) when to initiate therapy and (2) when to change therapy and to which drugs. With the advent of protease inhibitors in the mid-1990s, the mortality rate of HIV-infected clients and incidence of opportunistic infections has reduced. The role of drugs with immunomodulating activity for use in combination with HAART is undergoing extensive research (Kovacs et al., 1996; Lederman, 1995).

Drug regimens for HIV disease are dynamic, and clinical practice guidelines are consistently updated. Many changes in the approach to drug interventions can be expected as HIV continues to be a chronic disease (Holtzer & Roland, 1999). People are living longer with HIV disease. This has great impact on rehabilitation medicine as the neurological, musculoskeletal, cardiopulmonary, and integumentary systems are affected throughout the lifespan. Many HIV medications have side effects, and this can impact on the various systems. Therefore, people living with HIV have experimented with complementary and alternative medicine (CAM). These interventions have been explored through the history of the HIV epidemic and have gained increasing popularity, especially since the establishment of the Office of Alternative Medicine, renamed the National Center for Complementary and Alternative Medicine (NCCAM).

In 1993, the Centers for Disease Control (CDC) revised its definition of AIDS and classification system of HIV infection. To reflect current scientific knowledge, the new system elucidates the importance of helper-T (CD4+) cell counts as indicators for pharmacological disease management. The changed definition of AIDS now includes those with HIV infection and CD4+ counts below $200/mm^3$, regardless of the status of opportunistic or concomitant disorders. In addition, three clinical conditions—pulmonary tuberculosis, recurrent pneumonia, and invasive cervical cancer—were added to the existing list of 20 AIDS-defining diseases (CDC, 1995, 1997a). Testing for the amount of HIV in plasma by measuring viral RNA has become a standard component for the management of HIV-infected clients (CDC, 1998). There are important prognostic implications for the amount of viral load in persons with HIV disease (Mellors et al., 1997). Clients with higher viral loads progress more rapidly both immunologically in terms of the rate of CD4+ cell count decline and clinically in terms of developing AIDS-defining illness. Additionally, the plasma levels in HIV pregnant women

Therapy Focus

As clients live long with HIV disease, it is crucial to ask the questions, *Is your life filled with quality? Are you able to participate in productive work? Does your home life provide the capacity to accomplish all your activities of daily living?* If not, or if some domain is compromised, therapists have the opportunity to open the door for an eclectic approach to rehabilitation. A return to optimal function is possible by combining traditional modalities with complementary therapies.

Research has shown that there is an increasing use of CAM by the HIV population, fostered by the search for better health, decreased pain, and improved perceptions of life. Therapists are experts in movement science and can readily integrate the various movement techniques that are sought beyond the traditional medical model, as well as other complementary therapies. Opening more opportunities for the integration of CAM provides the therapist with a greater armamentarium for productive and successful rehabilitation outcomes for people living with HIV disease.

directly correlate with the risk of perinatal transmission (Dickover et al., 1996). Viral load is an important marker for judging the effectiveness of various antiretroviral drug interventions (Hughes et al., 1997; Marschner et al., 1998).

The entire spectrum of illness from initial diagnosis to AIDS can be covered by the term HIV infection. The terms *HIV asymptomatic, HIV symptomatic,* and *HIV advanced disease* (AIDS) will be used throughout this chapter as they delineate the progression of HIV disease.

Neurologic System

Significant progress in understanding and treating the neurologically involved HIV client has been made since the mid-1990s (Vitkovic & Tardieu, 1998). However, HIV continues to affect every division of the human nervous system. It is not possible in this context to discuss the neuropathology of each of the many secondary infections and neoplasms of HIV illness. It is important to realize, however, that the clinical manifestations of these pathological processes overlap with one another as well as with the signs and symptoms of primary HIV infection of the central nervous system (CNS). There are a wide variety of organisms and conditions responsible for the neurological manifestations associated with HIV infection. These include primary and secondary viral, protozoan, fungal, and mycobacterium infections as well as neoplasms and iatrogenic conditions. This can result in a number of functional deficits and compromised activities of daily living (ADL).

Treatment for CNS impairments includes an eclectic blend of rehabilitation strategies. Neuromuscular disturbances may first appear as movement disorders. Subtleties of altered movement can be detected early and during subsequent treatment phases. A neurological examination must be performed to provide a diagnosis and prognosis. This may include the level of the lesion, neuromuscular deficits, need for assistive devices and pain management, ADL, and functional abilities.

Distal symmetrical polyneuropathy (DSP) is the most common form of peripheral neuropathy in HIV infection. The most frequent complaints in DSP are numbness, burning, and paresthesias in the feet. These symptoms are typically symmetrical and often so severe that clients have contact hypersensitivity and gait disturbances. Involvement of the upper extremities and distal weakness may occur later in the course of DSP. Neurologic examination shows sensory loss to pain and temperature in a stocking glove distribution, increased vibratory thresholds, and diminished ankle reflexes compared to knee reflexes (Simpson & Olney, 1994; Simpson & Tagliati, 1994). Pathologic evidence of DSP is present in almost all clients who die of AIDS (Griffin et al., 1991; Griffin et al., 1993). Therefore, HIV neuropathy should be treated as soon as it is diagnosed to avoid complications.

Balance and Postural Mechanisms

Balance disturbances may be seen with either CNS or peripheral nervous system (PNS) HIV involvement. Polyneuropathy is due to various medications and opportunistic infections, such as cytomegalovirus (CMV), a common pathogen in AIDS (inflammatory polyneuropathy), which may manifest in the form of a generalized asymmetric demyelination and chronic denervation of muscles (Morgello & Simpson, 1994; Newshan & Wainapel, 1993). Demyelination and denervation of nerves that supply postural muscles may weaken such muscles and result in balance problems. It is also possible that apart from muscle demyelination and denervation, the pathological process, which also includes macrophage infiltration of neural structures, could spread to affect the vestibular neural complex of the inner ear, which is very important in the maintenance of both static and dynamic balance.

Clinical experience shows that sensory changes are common in the lower limbs of neuro-pathic HIV/AIDS clients. The balance problems of these clients are likely to be connected to inadequate proprioception from the legs during stance, and it is well known that diminished sensory information makes gait control more difficult. Peripheral neuropathy weakens the neuromuscular system and causes a limitation in functional activities. A client who, for instance, has balance derangement resulting from peripheral neuropathy may not function effectively in activities of daily living. It is well known that functional limitation is an important factor that takes people out of employment. The case is true for people with HIV/AIDS peripheral neuropathy. Pain may be the limiting factor in the ability to return to work. Any intervention that would reduce functional limitation should be applied. This may include various modalities, and manual and movement therapy techniques.

Pain

When neuropathy results in distal painful paresthesia, imbalance in stance and gait may result from compensatory measures aimed at relieving pain in dynamic standing activities. Postural compensations may further exacerbate musculoskeletal, cervical, thoracic, or low back pain. Pain management is a critical part of the overall care of individuals with HIV disease. Neuro-pathic involvement presents with painful paresthesia that may be resistant to pharmacologic treatment (Galantino et al., 1999).

There is a growing body of literature on the use of acupuncture for pain management. Although therapists are unable to insert needles, knowledge of acupuncture points can facilitate the use of various modalities and manual therapy. Considerations for treatment include low voltage electroacupuncture (Galantino et al., 1998). Manual therapy, including mobilization and myofascial release to improve ankle and foot range of motion along with other compensatory areas, is recommended for pain management and return to function. A recent study evaluated massage for the treatment of painful peripheral neuropathy and found it to have positive outcomes in reduction of pain (Acosta, Chan, & Jacobs, 1998).

Pain management is best approached with a behavioral and a physical approach. Electroacupuncture and ultrasound may be used as modalities. Pain reduction is achieved through training in breathing techniques, visualization, progressive muscle relaxation, autogenics, music, meditation, yoga, and engagement in meaningful activities.

Musculoskeletal System

Musculoskeletal manifestations of HIV infection are not as common as the manifestations seen in other parts of the body, including the central nervous system, pulmonary, and gastrointestinal tract. They tend to occur in advanced HIV infection. Knowledge of the different abnormalities that may occur in the musculoskeletal system is crucial to client management and affects morbidity and mortality. In the author's experience, primary abnormalities present through osseous and soft-tissue infections, polymyositis, and arthritis. Secondary musculoskeletal complications are often due to the various compensatory patterns of gait as a result of HIV-related peripheral neuropathy syndrome or the change in biomechanics of the foot and ankle due to Karposi's Sarcoma and non-Hodgkin's lymphoma (Steinbach et al., 1993). This leads to potential spinal changes and back pain.

HIV-infected clients with polymyositis typically present with proximal and less commonly distal muscle weakness and elevated creatine kinase levels (Rynes, 1991). Clients may have initial symptoms of difficulty with basic activities, such as rising from a chair. Arthritis in HIV-infected persons has a wide spectrum of presentations ranging from mild arthralgias to very severe joint disability (Solomon, Brancato, & Winchester, 1991). Arthritides seen in AIDS clients have been classified into five groups based on clinical presentation: (1) painful articular syndrome, (2) acute symmetric polyarthritis, (3) spondyloarthropathic arthritis (Reiter's syndrome, psoriatic arthritis), (4) HIV-associated arthritis, and (5) septic arthritis (Solomon, Brancato, & Winchester, 1991). Treatment interventions are similar to that of other clients with arthritis (Sood et al., 1998).

Cardiopulmonary System

Pulmonary diseases continue to be important causes of illness and death in clients with HIV infection, but changes in therapy and demographics of HIV-infected populations are changing their manifestations. The risk of developing specific disorders is related to the degree of immunosuppression, HIV risk group, area of residence, and use of prophylactic therapies (Rosen, 1996).

Antipneumocystis prophylaxis has reduced the incidence of and mortality due to pneumocystis carini pneumonia (PCP). The PCP-causing organism is usually acquired in childhood, and between 65 and 85 percent of healthy adults possess PCP antibodies. Reactivation of latent infection is responsible for the recurrent fever, dyspnea, and hypoxia that characterize PCP. Adjunctive corticosteroid therapy has improved the outlook for respiratory failure (Rosen, 1996). Breathing exercises, acupuncture, and a monitored therapeutic exercise program can improve overall pulmonary function.

Mycobacterial infections in HIV-infected individuals usually present as either mycobacterium avium-intracellular complex (MAC) or mycobacterium tuberculosis (TB). Steadily increasing incidence of infection by mycobacterium tuberculosis is likely the result of two factors: better medical management of HIV as a whole and the development of multidrug resistant strains of TB. Mycobacterium tuberculosis is communicable, preventable, and treatable. Tuberculin skin testing should be available and routinely offered to individuals at HIV testing sites. The highest risk individuals for concomitant HIV and TB infections include the homeless, intravenous drug users, and prisoners.

Although most other organ system involvement has been extensively described in studies and reviews, cardiac complications related to HIV infection have remained less characterized. Most studies have described cardiac problems postmortem, although some clinical series have been reported. It is now clear that cardiac involvement in people living with HIV is quite common (Grody, Cheng, & Lewis, 1990; Rosen, 1996). Pericardial effusion and myocarditis are among the most commonly reported cardiac abnormalities. Cardiomyopathy, endocarditis, and coronary vasculopathy have also been reported. It is now apparent that HIV itself, the medical management of HIV disease, and secondary opportunistic infections can all affect the myocardium, pericardium, endocardium, and blood vessels (Yunis & Stone, 1998).

Over the past several years, body fat changes and lipid abnormalities have been reported in individuals with HIV/AIDS (Hanna, 1999). A number of cases of body fat and metabolic changes have been connected to protease inhibitor use (Carr & Cooper, 1998). These body fat changes may have strong implications for clients who receive rehabilitation intervention. Many have used various supplements and vitamin therapy to decrease the problem of lipodystrophy. Signs and symptoms of the syndrome vary, and not all need to be present in any particular client. However, in both males and females, three main components of the syndrome have emerged: changes in body shape, hyperlipidemia, and insulin resistance. Clinically, distinct body shape changes are apparent. The most prevalent include increased abdominal growth, a dorsocervical fat pad, benign symmetric lipomatosis, lipodystrophy, and breast hypertrophy in women (Carr & Cooper, 1998). The increased abdominal growth is characterized by a redistribution and accumulation of fat in the central visceral areas of the body (Miller et al., 1998). Corresponding symptoms include GI discomfort, bloating, distention, and fullness (Di Perri, Del Bravo, & Concia, 1998).

In addition to visible signs and symptoms, adverse changes in lipids have been reported. A number of studies revealed that hyperlipidemia were present in HIV positive clients, many but not all of whom were on protease inhibitor therapy (Henry et al., 1998). To date, the exact cause of lipodystrophy has not been determined, but two main theories have been hypothesized. Each is still in the process of being studied (Carr et al., 1998; Sullivan et al., 1998). As individuals live longer with HIV disease, they are at greater risk for developing cardiac disease. Therapists need to be apprised of various changes in lab results and signs and symptoms of cardiac disease when designing an exercise program and facilitating return to function.

Utilization of Alternative Therapies

The HIV epidemic has witnessed an increasing utilization of complementary and alternative therapies, some more traditional than others (Ozsoy & Ernst, 1999; Sande & Volberding, 1995). Eisenberg reported that prayer and exercise combined to account for over 60 percent of all alternative therapies utilized in the general public (1993). Other therapies include relaxation techniques (13 percent), massage (7 percent), imagery (4 percent), and spiritual healing (4 percent). Traditional exercise such as aerobic and weight training are incorporated in the medical model through exercise physiology and rehabilitation. However, various movement therapies, such as T'ai Chi and yoga, may be a more gentle approach if a high-level exercise program is not tolerated. People with advanced disease may obtain benefits from alternative movement therapies.

Ozsoy and Ernst (1999) conducted a systematic review of the effectiveness of CAM for HIV and AIDS. A comprehensive literature search was conducted to locate all randomized clinical trials. Fourteen studies met their predetermined criteria: two of herbal treatments, five of vitamins and other supplements, five of stress management, one of massage therapy, and one of acupuncture. It concluded that few rigorous trials of complementary treatments for HIV exist.

A study by Johnson and colleagues (1998) evaluated the use of CAM among HIV-infected clients of the inner-city found 58 percent were Latinos, 34 percent were African

American, and 60 percent were women. Eighty percent of those that incorporated CAM into their daily lives regularly use herbs, plant substances, and alternative treatments such as massage, touch, yoga, and acupuncture. Sixty-eight percent use nutritional supplements not prescribed by their physicians: 44 percent use plant substances (garlic and aloe vera); 42 percent use herbs (e.g., cat's claw); and 9 percent regularly use nontraditional healers.

Meneilly, Carr, and Brown (1996) studied the use of CAM by women. They found that treatments were categorized by herbal remedies (38 percent), vitamins and minerals (29 percent), relaxation techniques and massage (9 percent), folk remedies (2 percent), acupuncture (2 percent), and other remedies such as acidophilus and nacetylcysteine. The average yearly income was $10,000 to $20,000 per year, and the economic burden of paying for these out-of-pocket treatments is significant. In another study of women, the most frequently reported CAM interventions were regular exercise and spiritual practices (including meditation, yoga, and prayer).

Massage interventions have been researched in the HIV pediatric population. Positive effects have been shown from the use of aromatherapy through the scent of massage oil in hospitalized children with HIV disease (Styles, 1997). In another study of 28 neonates born to HIV-positive mothers, quantitative outcomes included improvement on Brazelton scores and greater daily weight gain at the end of a 10-day massage intervention (Scafidi & Field, 1996). Massage has also been shown to augment immune markers (Ironson et al., 1996).

Literature on long-term survivors with AIDS is replete with anecdotal evidence linking survival to one or more of the following: (1) holding a positive attitude toward the illness, (2) participating in health-promoting behaviors, (3) engaging in spiritual activities, and (4) taking part in AIDS-related activities (Carson, 1993; Carson & Green, 1992; Kendall, 1992, 1994). Positive relationships have been demonstrated between hardiness and perception of physical, emotional, and spiritual health, participation in exercise, and the use of special diets (Carson, 1993; Carson et al., 1991; Greene et al., 1999; Lee, 1996).

Bastyr University evaluated the use of alternative therapies via scientific evidence published in peer-reviewed journals (Greene et al., 1999). The most frequently used activities are aerobic exercise (64 percent), prayer (56 percent), massage (54 percent), needle acupuncture (48 percent), meditation (46 percent), support groups (42 percent), visualization and imagery (34 percent) breathing exercises (33 percent), spiritual activities (33 percent) and other exercise (33 percent). In another article, Traditional Chinese Medicine was identified as an increasing intervention in the San Francisco Bay area among people with HIV infection (Wilson & Cohen, 1998).

There are few studies elucidating evaluation techniques for the use of alternative medicine within the context of western medicine. One strategy was published through a nursing school (Freeman & MacIntyre, 1999) and another in a physical therapy journal (Umphred, Galantino, & Campbell, 2000). Overall, there is a need for careful assessment of the use of CAM intervention as it may affect drug interventions, the plan of care for individuals living with HIV, and the ultimate measure of quality of life issues.

Living Long and Living Well with HIV Disease

Traditional ethnomedicine has a deep appreciation of the context of nutrition, exercise, and psychosocial interventions (MacIntyre & Holzemer, 1997). The impact of HIV can be evident in cerebral, emotional, psychosocial, and other physical domains, affecting the client infected with HIV and those around him or her. Increasing focus is being placed on the potential impact of

HIV-related stress on the course of infection because of the observed and postulated relationship between psychosocial stress, neuropsychological functioning, and immune status (Wolf, Dralle, & Morse, 1991). Minimizing stressful events throughout the management of chronic HIV disease can be approached in various ways, such as through meditation, relaxation, and various forms of exercise (LaPerriere et al., 1991; LaPerriere et al., 1994).

Drug interventions for HIV are constantly changing. Clients may be on three to four medications to manage HIV disease, while taking other medications for various comorbid infections. There may be interactions of various herbs and remedies with the traditional pharmacological agents. Therefore, it is important to determine if clients are taking supplements to discern untoward effects. If side effects from any medication are noted, pain management techniques can be initiated and a return to function promoted.

The therapist can take a holistic approach to the examination and plan of care for this population. A comprehensive evaluation of all systems is necessary and ongoing. Any subtle change in the neurological, musculoskeletal, or cardiopulmonary system should undergo a differential diagnosis (Galantino, 1992). A proper plan of care, which includes traditional and complementary techniques, can then be initiated (Galantino, Pizzi, & Lehmann, 1993; Galantino et al., 1997). For example, if insults to the nervous system result in balance and gait disturbance, a traditional balance regimen can be initiated along with the necessary assistive devices. In addition, the use of T'ai Chi as a movement modality can also be incorporated into a plan of care and offer diversity to a traditional rehabilitation program.

It is important to impart fun and creativity into any rehabilitation program. The various movement therapies (e.g., yoga, T'ai Chi, Feldenkrais) can be natural additions that may foster greater adherence to a home program. There is certainly evidence that the HIV population is utilizing many complementary therapies as they manage chronic HIV disease. Therapists have a wonderful opportunity to conduct research on clinical outcomes and open the door for integrative rehabilitation.

Case Study

Peripheral Neuropathy

A 23-year-old female was referred for physical therapy treatment of painful peripheral neuropathy. She is an administrative secretary and initially had difficulty coordinating her files and typing at the computer, but attributed this to her increased workload. Gait and fine motor problems gradually increased over the last 8 weeks, with increased difficulty walking and managing at work over the last 2 weeks. She complained of "pins and needles" in her hands and feet. She had been HIV-positive for 5 years.

The client's past medical history was significant for herpes zoster and a lumbar laminectomy 3 years ago due to a herniated nucleus pulposus at L4–5. Her HIV medications included zerit (d4T), videx (ddI), and invirase (saquinavir); other medications included prilosec (for GI problems), megace, and zovirax; vitamin and herbs used were a multivitamin with a B complex, St. John's wort, echinacea, and valerian root.

The client is married and lives with her husband in a third-floor apartment with their 2-year-old child. She works full time as an administrative secretary and has insurance coverage through the University where she works. Her HMO provided six visits of therapy for return to full function and return to work. She reported being independent and active in the community PTA, able to drive to and from work and social functions independently, and fulfill her role as a caretaker, including performing household chores and providing the primary household income. She is also involved in volunteer work with people living with HIV/AIDS.

Significant system issues were

- *Musculoskeletal:* Decreased lumbar lordosis. Right anterior torsioned pelvis; apparent leg length discrepancy. Forward head and shoulders. Slight limitations in forefoot movement; hindfoot valgus noted. Extremities are 5/5 throughout proximal extremities. Distal extremities are 4/5 throughout.
- *Neuromuscular:* Altered sensation, antalgic gait, balance alterations.
- *Psychosocial:* The client was very concerned about her job and family, since her work is the primary income and she can't afford to lose her position because health benefits are most important to her.
- *Reflex integrity:* Lower motor neuron signs present. Decreased reflexes at bilateral achilles tendons.
- *Gait, locomotion, and balance:* Narrow base of support, decreased trunk rotation, antalgic gait. Decreased balance. Scored 48 on the Berg Balance Scale.
- *Pain:* "Pins and needles" in a stocking-glove distribution. Visual Analogue Scale (VAS) = 9/10. Occasional complaints of low back pain and cervical pain when sitting long periods at the computer. VAS of spine = 4/10.
- *Self-care tests:* Independent in ADLs, except the client now has concerns about her performance on the job and some difficulty driving.
- *Other:* An EMG showed signs of distal sensory neuropathy. She had dysesthesias noted at all four distal extremities. Proprioception and vibration decreased distally as well.

Overview: The client presented with neurological complications of HIV disease. Balance problems (in standing) were due to peripheral neuropathy. Issues of safety were of concern, given that her self-perception was that she is independent in driving. Also, the Berg Balance Scale score is indicative of increased potential for falling.

Prognosis: Typically, rehabilitation prognosis is good when proper medical treatment for this neurological insult is continued and the client has a change in her medication (ddI can potentiate peripheral neuropathy syndrome) and various pain management modalities are implemented. She should respond well with assistive devices (orthotics), neurological rehabilitation and supportive services.

Treatment: Given the six allocated visits, the client and her husband were taught about balance and safety issues for ADLs and for preparation in return to work. The client was treated twice a week for 2 weeks and once a week for

2 weeks, providing physical therapy services throughout the course of 1 month. Additionally, other modalities, as described below, were instituted to address the following problems:

Problem	Objective and Planned Interventions
Pain Management	Client will receive electroacupuncture with microcurrent settings. A home unit will be provided with instructions on the proper application of electrodes over acupuncture points. Client will have VAS = 3 for extremity pain.
	Client will receive myofascial release and a stretching and posture program to decrease lumbar and cervical pain. VAS = 1.
Therapeutic Exercise	PNF patterns to all extremities. A T'ai Chi program will be implemented to improve overall balance and decrease stress.
	Client will be able to drive independently in 1 month. She will be independent in computer skills with a decrease in pain by 75%.
Balance Exercises	T'ai Chi exercises will foster improvements in strength and balance.
	Client will be able to negotiate stairs safely and with decreased pain.
	Client will be able to safely participate in leisure activities with her child.
	Client will score a 53 on the Berg Scale upon discharge.
Functional Training	Cycling activities; client will have improved cardiovascular conditioning to prevent lipodystrophy and improve overall immune status.
Community and Work	Nutrition consult to prevent wasting syndrome; ergonomic evaluation at work for proper body mechanics.

Outcomes: Through use of the above treatments, the client's neuropathy decreased by 50 percent to a manageable level, and her gait problems stabilized. She was able to return to part-time work with modifications (e.g., participation in more sedentary activities), to walk up the stairs to her apartment with greater ease, and to fully participate in activities related to care for her child.

Summary

The following practices are recommended for working with clients who are coping with AIDS.

1. *Remember the client requires constant reevaluation and assessment of needs as he or she lives with chronic HIV disease.*
2. *Pain management can incorporate the use of acupuncture points for self-management through acupressure. Alternatively, modalities may be used over specific acupuncture points to manage pain.*

3. *Massage therapy facilitates developmental acquisition skills in neonates and fosters stress reduction in adults. In both populations, positive immunological changes can result.*
4. *Movement therapies such as T'ai Chi and yoga can foster improvements in flexibility and balance.*
5. *Knowing the various supplemental herbs and remedies that clients take on a routine basis can promote a more holistic approach with the primary physician.*
6. *Recommending various local support groups may assist with coping strategies from the challenges of HIV disease.*

STUDY QUESTIONS

1. What clinical tests determine progression of HIV disease?
2. What neurological symptoms of HIV results in painful ambulation?
3. What effective pain management strategies are possible for #2?
4. State a side effect of HAART:
5. What movement therapy can improve balance and flexibility?
6. What are the effects of massage in people living with HIV disease?

SUGGESTED READING

Standich, L. J., C. Calabrese, & M. L Galantino. (2002). *AIDS and Complementary and Alternative Medicine: Current Science and Practice.* Philadelphia: Churchill Livingstone.

REFERENCES

Acosta, A. M., R. S. Chan, & J. Jacobs. (1998). Massage therapy for the treatment of painful peripheral neuropathy in HIV+ individuals. International Conference on AIDS. 12:849 (abstract no. 42376).

Arts, E. J., & M. A. Wainberg. (1996). Mechanism of nucleoside analog antiretroviral activity and resistance during human immunodeficiency virus reverse transcription. *Antimicrobial Agents and Chemotherapy, 40,* 527–540.

Carr, A., & D. Cooper. (1998). Lipodystrophy associated with an HIV protease inhibitor. *New England Journal of Medicine, 339,* 1296.

Carr, A., K. Samaras, D. Chisholm, & D. Cooper. (1998). Pathogenesis of HIV-1 protease inhibitor associated peripheral lipodystrophy, hyperlipidemia and insulin resistance. *Lancet, 351,* 1881–1883.

Carson, V. B. (1993). Prayer, meditation, exercise and special diets: Behaviors of the hardy person with HIV/AIDS. *Journal of the Association of Nurses in AIDS Care, 4*(3), 18–28.

Carson, V. B., & H. G. Green. (1992). Spiritual well-being: A predictor of hardiness in clients with AIDS. *Journal of Professional Nursing, 8*(4), 209–220.

Carson, V. B., K. L. Soeken, & A. Belcher. (1991). Spiritual well-being, hardiness, and ego strength in persons with AIDS. *Journal of Christian Healing, 13*(2), 21.

CDC (Centers for Disease Control and Prevention). (1995). Update: Acquired immunodeficiency syndrome—United States, 1994. *Morbidity and Mortality Weekly Report, 44,* 64–67.

CDC (Centers for Disease Control and Prevention). (1997a). Update: Trends in AIDS incidence, deaths, and prevalence–United States, 1996. *Morbidity and Mortality Weekly Report, 46,* 165–173.

CDC (Centers for Disease Control and Prevention). (1997b). Update: Trends in AIDS incidence–United States, 1996. *Morbidity and Mortality Weekly Report, 46,* 861–867.

CDC (Centers for Disease Control and Prevention). (1998). Report of the NIH panel to define principles of therapy of HIV infection and guidelines for the use of antiretroviral agents in HIV-infected adults and adolescents. *Morbidity and Mortality Weekly Report, 47,* 1–83.

Dickover, R. E., E. M. Garratty, S. A. Herman, M. S. Sim, S. Plaeger, P. J. Boyer, M. Keller, A. Deveikas, E. R. Stiehm, & Y. J. Bryson. (1996). Identification of levels of maternal HIV-1 RNA associated with risk of perinatal transmission. Effect of maternal zidovudine treatment on viral load. *Journal of the American Medical Association, 275,* 599–605.

Di Perri, G., P. Del Bravo, & E. Concia. (1998). Protease inhibitors. *New England Journal of Medicine, 339,* 773–774.

Eisenberg, D. M., R. C. Kessler, & C. Foster. (1993). Unconventional medicine in the United States: Prevalence, costs and patterns of use. *New England Journal of Medicine, 328,* 246–252.

Freeman, E. M., & R. C. MacIntyre. (1999). Evaluating alternative treatments for HIV infection. *Nursing Clinics of North America, 34*(1), 147–162.

Galantino, M. L. (1992). *Clinical Assessment and Treatment in HIV Disease: Rehabilitation of a Chronic Illness.* Thorofare, NJ: Slack.

Galantino, M. L., S. T. Eke-Okoro, T. Findley, & D. Condolucci. (1999). Use of noninvasive electroacupuncture for the treatment of HIV-related peripheral neuropathy: A pilot study. *Journal of Alternative and Complementary Therapies, 5*(2), 135–142.

Galantino, M. L., T. Findley, L. Krafft, K. Shepard, A. LaPerriere, J. Ducette, A. Sorbello, D. Condolucci, & M. Barnish. (1997). Blending traditional and alternative strategies for rehabilitation: Measuring functional outcomes and quality of life issues in an AIDS population. The 8th World Congress of International Rehabilitation Medicine Association. *Monduzzi Editore, 1,* 713–716.

Galatino, M. L., R. T. Jermyn, F. J. Tursi, & S. Eke-Okoro. (1998). Physical therapy management for the client with HIV: Lower extremity changes. *Clinics in Podiatric Medicine and Surgery, 15*(2), 329–346.

Galantino, M. L., M. Pizzi, & M. Lehmann. (1993). Interdisciplinary management of disability in HIV infection. In M. W. O'Dell (Ed.), *HIV-Related Disability: Assessment and Management. State of the Art Reviews, Physical Medicine and Rehabilitation.* Philadelphia: Hanley & Belfus.

Greene, K. B., J. Berger, C. Reeves, A. Moffat, L. J. Standish, & C. Calabrese. (1999, May–June). Most frequently used alternative and complementary therapies and activities by participants in the AMCOA study. *Journal of the Association of Nurses in AIDS Care, 10*(3), 63–73.

Griffin, J. W., T. O. Crawford, W. R. Tyor, J. D. Glass, D. L. Price, & D. R. Cornbluth. (1991). Predominantly sensory neuropathy in AIDS: Distal axonal degeneration and unmyelinated fiber loss. *Neurology, 41*(Suppl. 1), 374.

Griffin, J. W. I., S. Wesselingh, A. L. Oaklander, R. W. Kuncl, & D. E. Griffin. (1993). MRNA fingerprinting of cytokines and growth factors: A new means of characterizing nerve biopsies (Abstract). *Neurology, 43*(Suppl. 2), A232, 19.

Grody, W. W., L. Cheng, & W. Lewis. (1990). Infection of the heart by the human immunodeficiency virus. *American Journal of Cardiology, 66,* 203–206.

Hanna, L. (1999). Body fat changes: More than lipodystrophy. *Bulletin of Experiment Treatments for AIDS, 12*(1), 23–32.

Henry, K., H. Melroe, J. Huebsch, J. Hermundson, C. Levine, L. Swensen, & B. R. Daley. (1998). Severe premature coronary artery disease with protease inhibitors. *Lancet, 351,* 1328.

Holtzer, C. D., & M. Roland. (1999, Feb.). The use of combination antiretroviral therapy in HIV-infected clients. *The Annals of Pharmacotherapy, 33*(2), 198–209.

Hughes, M. D., V. A. Johnson, M. S. Hirsch, J. W. Bremer, T. Elbeik, A. Erice, D. R. Kuritzkes, W. A. Scott, S. A. Spector, N. Basgoz, M. A. Fischl, R. J. D'Aquila. (1997). Monitoring plasma HIV-1 RNA levels in addition to CD4+ lymphocyte count improves assessment of antiretroviral therapeutic response. *Annals of Internal Medicine, 126,* 939–945.

Ironson, G., T. Field, F. Scafidi, M. Hashimoto, M. Kumar, A. Kumar, A. Price, A. Goncalves, I. Burman, C. Tetenman, R. Patarca, & M. A. Fletcher. (1996). Massage therapy is associated with enhancement of the immune system's cytotoxic capacity. *International Journal of Neuroscience, 84*(1–4), 205–217.

Johnston, B. E., K. Ahmad, C. Smith, & D. N. Rose. (1998). Alternative therapy use among HIV-infected clients of the inner city. International Conference on AIDS, 12, 852 (abstract no. 42391).

Kendall, J. (1992). Promoting wellness in HIV-support groups. *Journal of the Association of Nurses in AIDS Care, 3*(1), 28–38.

Kendall, J. (1994). Wellness spirituality in homosexual men with HIV infection. *Journal of the Association of Nurses in AIDS Care, 5*(4), 28–34.

Kovacs, J. A., S. Vogel, J. M. Albert, J. Falloon, R. T. Davey, R. E. Walker, M. A. Polis, K. Spooner, J. A. Metcalf, M. Baseler, G. Fyfe, & H. C. Lane. Controlled trial of interleukin-2 infusions in clients infected with the human immunodeficiency virus. *New England Journal of Medicine, 335,* 1350–1356.

LaPerriere, A., M. A. Fletcher, M. H. Antoni, N. G. Klimas, G. Ironson, & N. Schneiderman. (1991). Aerobic exercise training in an AIDS risk group. *International Journal of Sports Medicine, 12*(Suppl. 1), S53–S57.

LaPerriere, A., G. Ironson, M. H. Antoni, N. Schneiderman, N. Klimas, & M. A. Fletcher. (1994). Exercise and immunology. *Medicine and Science in Sports and Exercise, 26*(2), 182–190.

Lederman, N. M. (1995). Host-directed and immune-based therapies for human immunodeficiency virus infections. *Annals of Internal Medicine, 122,* 218–227.

Lee, S. T. (1996). Holistic approach with spiritual support enhances people with HIV/AIDS. International Conference on AIDS. *11*(2), 423 (abstract no, Th.D. 5116).

MacIntyre, R. C., & W. L. Holzemer. (1997). Complementary and alternative medicine and HIV/AIDS. Part II: Selected literature review. *Journal of the Association of Nurses in AIDS Care, 8*(2), 25–38.

Marschner, I. C., A. C. Collier, R. W. Coombs, R. T. D'Aquila, V. DeGruttola, M. A. Fischel, S. H. Hammer, M. D. Hughes, V. A. Johnson, D. A. Katzenstein, D. D. Richman, L. M. Smeaton, S. A. Spector, & M. S. Saag. (1998). Use of changes in plasma levels of human immunodeficiency virus type 1 RNA to assess the clinical benefits of antiretroviral therapy. *The Journal of Infectious Diseases, 177,* 40–47.

Mellors, J. W., A. Munoz, J. V. Giorgi, J. B. Margolick, C. J. Tassoni, P. Gupta, L. A. Kingsley, J. A. Todd, A. J. Saah, R. Detels, J. P. Phair, & C. R. Rinaldo, Jr. (1997). Plasma viral load and CD4+ lymphocytes as prognostic markers of HIV-1 infection. *Annals of Internal Medicine, 126,* 946–954.

Meneilly, G. P., R. Carr, & L. Brown. (1996). Alternative therapy use among HIV-positive women. International Conference on AIDS, *11*(1), 22 (abstract no. Mo.B. 301).

Miller, K., E. Jones, J. Yanovski, R. Shankar, I. Feurstein, & J. Falloon. (1998). Visceral abdominal-fat accumulation associated with the use of Indivir. *Lancet, 351,* 871–875.

Morgello, S., & D. M. Simpson. (1994). Multifocal cytomegalorivus demyelinative polyneuropathy associated with AIDS. *Muscle & Nerve, 17,* 176–182.

Newshan, G., & S. Wainapel. (1993, Apr.–June). Pain characteristics and their management in persons with AIDS. *Journal of American Nursing and AIDS Care, 4*(2), 53–59.

Ozsoy, M., & E. Ernst. (1999). How effective are complementary therapies for HIV and AIDS?—A systematic review. *International Journal of STDS and AIDS, 10*(10), 629–635.

Quinn, T. C. (1996). Global burden of the HIV pandemic. *Lancet, 348,* 99–106.

Rosen, M. J. (1996, Dec.). Overview of pulmonary complications. *Clinics in Chest Medicine, 17*(4), 621–631.

Rynes, R. (1991). Painful rheumatic syndromes associated with human immunodeficiency virus infection. *Rheumatic Diseases: Clinics of North America, 17,* 83.

Sande, M. A., & P. A. Volberding. (1995). Alternative therapies in HIV. In M. A. Sande and A. Volberding (Eds.), *Medical Management of AIDS* (4th ed.). Philadelphia: Saunders.

Scafidi, F., & T. Field. Massage therapy improves behavior in neonates born to HIV-positive mothers. *Journal of Pediatric Psychology, 21*(6), 889–897.

Schrager, L. K., & M. P. D'Souza. (1998). Cellular and anatomical reservoirs of HIV-1 in clients receiving potent antiretroviral combination therapy. *Journal of the American Medical Association, 280,* 67–71.

Simpson, D. M., & R. K. Olney. (1994). Peripheral neuropathies associated with human immunodeficiency virus infection. In P. J. Dyck (Ed.), *Peripheral Neuropathy.* Philadelphia: Saunders.

Simpson, D. M., & M. Tagliati. (1994). Neurologic manifestations of HIV infection. *Annals of Internal Medicine, 121,* 769–785.

Solomon, G., L. Brancato, & R. Winchester. (1991). An approach to the human immunodeficiency virus client with a spondyloarthropic disease. *Rheumatic Diseases: Clinics of North America, 17,* 44–52.

Sood, R., J. Louie, M. L. Galantino, & J. Melvin. (2000). Less common rheumatic diseases. In J. Melvin (Ed.), *Rheumatic Rehabilitation Series* (Vol II). Bethesda, MD: American Occupational Therapy Association.

Steinbach, L., J. Tehranzadeh, J. Fleckenstein, W. J. Vanarthos, & M. J. Pais. (1993). Human immunodeficiency virus (HIV) infection. Musculoskeletal manifestations. *Radiology, 186,* 833–838.

Styles, J. L. (1997). The use of aromatherapy in hospitalized children with HIV disease. *Complementary Therapies in Nursing & Midwifery, 3*(1), 16–20.

Sullivan, A., M. Nelson, G. Moyle, A. M. Newell, M. D. Feher, & B. G. Gazzard. (1998). Coronary artery disease occurring with protease inhibitor therapy. *International Journal of STD and AIDS, 9,* 711–712.

Umphred, D. A., M. L. Galantino, & B. R. Campbell. (2000). Establishing a model for the use of complementary medicine and research in orthopaedic practice. In M. L. Galantino (Ed.), *Orthopaedic Physical Therapy Clinics of North America—Complementary Medicine, 9*(3), 443–460.

Vitkovic, L., & M. Tardieu. (1998). Neuropathogenesis of HIV-1 infection. Outstanding questions. *Comptes rendus de l'Academie des sciences. Series III, 321,* 1015–1021.

Wilson, C. J., & M. R. Cohen. (1998). Traditional Chinese Medicine increasing in popularity as complementary therapy in HIV/AIDS. International Conference on AIDS. *12,* 360 (abstract no. 22483).

Wolf, T. M., P. W. Dralle, & E. V. Morse. (1991). A biopsychosocial examination of symptomatic and asymptomatic HIV-infected patients. *International Journal of Psychiatry in Medicine, 21,* 263–279.

Yunis, N. A., & V. E. Stone. (1998). Cardiac manifestations of HIV/AIDS: A review of disease spectrum and clinical management. *Journal of Acquired Immune Deficiency Syndrome, 18*(2), 145–154.

28

Smoking Cessation

Ann Burkhardt

CHAPTER OBJECTIVES

- Understand the health risks of smoking.
- Understand traditional and alternative interventions for smoking cessation.
- Understand research related to smoking cessation.
- Understand how smoking cessation interventions can be integrated into therapy practice.

Tobacco smoking has been determined to be a major contributor to many of the leading causes of death in the United States, including heart disease, lung cancer, head and neck cancer, and lung disease (e.g., emphysema, asthma). Our society has embraced the value that tobacco consumption is detrimental to health since the mid-1960s when the Surgeon General's warning was placed on every package of cigarettes sold, informing the public that a determination of health risk had been made. However, it was not until the 1990s that the Healthy People 2000 initiative (DHHS, 1990) targeted cigarette smoking as a behavior that must change to improve the health of the nation.

C. Everett Koop, former Surgeon General, has stated that cigarette smoking is the single most preventable cause of premature death in the United States. Each year, more than 400,000 Americans die from cigarette smoking. In fact, one in every five deaths in the United States is smoking-related. Every year, smoking kills more than 276,000 men and 142,000 women (CDC, 1994).

The consequences of cigarette smoking are the largest single drain on the Medicare trust fund, poised to take $800 billion over the next 20 years, according to a study of hospital records and epidemiological studies (CASA, 1994). Nearly one out of every four Medicare dollars spent on hospital care was due to substance abuse—totaling $20 billion out of the $87 billion spent on such care in fiscal year 1994. Eighty percent of that—$16 billion—paid for care for smoking-related disease and disabilities (CASA, 1994). Further, Koop charged all

Addressing the issue of smoking cessation is pertinent for all health care professionals. Assisting people to change negative habits will help to diminish controllable health risks and promote the health and well-being. These concepts are core to the concept of holistic practice for all allied health and medical professionals.

In order to adequately intervene in smoking cessation with clients, it is necessary to understand all of the health risks and treatment options, both traditional and alternative. This will facilitate knowledge, helping clients to choose options that fit with their lifestyle and optimize success in smoking cessation.

physicians to target cigarette cessation with every patient who smokes. Once the government identified the risk to health from tobacco exposure, a number of initiatives emerged.

In addition to its impact on mortality, smoking cessation also enhances the healing process of the body and speeds recovery from illness, trauma, or surgery. Nicotine is a vasoconstrictor, which limits the quantity of oxygenated blood that is available to assist with the healing process, especially in the extremities. When a person stops smoking, his or her circulatory system functions more normally and more efficiently. The process of healing becomes more efficient.

Therapies Used in Smoking Cessation

The National Cancer Institute (NCI), working together with the Agency for Health Care Policy Research (AHCPR), developed a cessation program using a "train the trainer" model and implementing a simple but effective approach known as the 4As (AHCPR, 1996).

Individually Based Behavioral Therapy

The 4As stands for the stages of cessation, utilizing the model for cessation described by Prochaska (precontemplation, contemplation, action, maintenance) (DiClemente & Prochaska, 1982): Ask, Advise, Assist, and Ask again. *Ask* every client at every visit, "Do you smoke?" If the client's answer is yes, then ask "Have you ever thought of quitting?" If yes, then ask the client to select a date to quit. If he or she says no, then you *advise:* "As your health care provider, I recommend that you quit." However, if the answer is still no, the interaction is stopped. If the person is willing to quit, the therapist will then *assist* him or her to chose a quit date and to implement a plan to change his or her habits to avoid triggers to smoking.

Pharmaceutical Therapies

The primary pharmaceutical tools that are currently used to assist people to quit are nicotine patches, nicotine inhaler, nicotine gum, nicotine nasal spray, and Zyban. Nicotine gum, inhalers, nasal spray, and patches contain nicotine; therefore, the use of these substances substitutes for cigarettes rather than curing the root problem of nicotine addiction that accompanies cigarette smoking. In contrast, Zyban is not nicotine or nicotine-based, so it addresses the addiction to smoking.

A smoker who uses nicotine replacement must make a commitment to quitting tobacco smoking, since the increased amounts of nicotine in the system increases vital functions, such as cardiac and respiratory rate. A nicotine overdose can cause a cardiac arrythmia and sleep deprivation. The duration of treatment for each of the replacement therapies is specific to the mode of delivery. Nicotine patches can be used for 4 to 10 weeks. Usually, they are tapered after 4 weeks, and many smokers are effectively treated at 8 weeks. The nicotine inhaler can be used for up to 6 months. Nicotine replacement gum has no limit for duration of use. Nicotine nasal spray can be used for up to 8 weeks.

Use of Zyban, an antidepressant medication, has also been demonstrated to assist smokers to quit smoking. In contrast to nicotine replacement therapy, most people should take Zyban twice a day for 7 to 12 weeks. When someone stops smoking, he or she should continue to take Zyban as recommended by a health care professional.

Behavioral Intervention Follow-Up

Approximately 1 week to 10 days after their quit date, clients should have some form of follow-up. Follow-up reinforces their positive life change in "kicking the habit," and, if they were unsuccessful, they are congratulated on their attempt and asked again to make another date for them to make a new attempt. No attempt to quit, even if unsuccessful, is ever considered to be a failure. Unsuccessful attempts are "rehearsals for the next try." The specifics of this approach can be found in the AHCPR guidelines (1996).

Support Groups

Some people are able to change their habits and behaviors through support groups. In the current technology age, there are not only support groups that one can physically attend, but there are also online support groups and listservs to help people to quit smoking. Several of the groups that offer smoking cessation support groups have regional resources, listed in Table 28–1.

Targeting Large Groups and Populations for Health Change

Application of the AHCPR guideline approach to occupational therapy practice has been published and implemented by the OT Network on Smoking and Wellness (Williams, Burkhardt, & Royce, 1995). The Network has worked internally in the occupational therapy community to direct the efforts and attention toward occupational therapists, one member of the multidisciplinary group of health care providers who potentially could help their clients to avoid smoking or to stop smoking. In articles and through a pamphlet published online, Role

Table 28–1 *Support Group Programs for Smoking Cessation*

Name of Program	Type of Program	Approaches Used
Smoke-Enders	A community-based program using behavioral modification (6 sessions, 2 to 2½ hours per session). Participants continue smoking for the first four meetings while they learn how to quit. During the last two meetings, the moderator reinforces the new non-smoking behavior. If people need the services of Smoke-Enders again within a calendar year, they can rejoin at a reduced rate.	Support group meetings. Education. Follow-up. Group membership is open-ended.
Smoke Stoppers Program	Generally offered through major medical centers. Listings may be found through local city departments of health and chronic disease prevention units. A multidimensional approach to stop smoking. The course consists of 8 sessions over a 5-week period. All Smoke Stopper instructors are former smokers and are certified by the National Center for Health Promotion.	Behavioral techniques are used, including education about smoking, nutritional information, stress management, and relaxation techniques.
Freedom from Smoking Program	Conducted in various settings throughout communities. Contact a local chapter of the American Lung Association for details. Behavior modifica-	The program is conducted by a trained specialist. A positive behavioral change approach is used to teach smokers how to become nonsmokers.

(continued)

Table 28–1 Support Group Programs for Smoking Cessation (cont'd)

Name of Program	Type of Program	Approaches Used
	tion approach is used. The program consists of 6 sessions. Participants meet weekly for five 90-minute sessions.	
Nicotine Anonymous	A fellowship of men and women helping each other quit smoking and live nicotine-free lives. People share experiences, strength, and hope with each other. There are no dues or fees for this program. The only requirement for membership is a desire to stop using nicotine. Groups are available locally throughout the United States.	The program follows a 12-step program for quitting cigarettes, borrowed from Alcoholics Anonymous.
Stay Off Smoking	Call your local American Cancer Society for dates, places, and times. This program is free of charge and offers a 1-hour weekly support group that enables former smokers to stay smoke free.	Peer support is provided according to an approach supported by the ACS and overseen by ACS personnel.

of the Occupational Therapist in Smoking Cessation (NYU, 2002), the Network describes how occupational therapists could positively work with smokers to use activity and a change of habits to avoid smoking triggers and to have success at their attempts to quit smoking.

Many individuals have worked diligently to bring smoking cessation awareness to the attention of OT practitioners. The OT Network on Smoking and Wellness was founded by Jacqueline Royce, Ph.D., OTR; Valerie Williams, Ed.M., OTR; Margaret Swarbrick, M.A., OTR/L, BCN; and Ann Burkhardt, M.A., OTR/L, FAOTA, B.C.N. in 1994. The broad goals of the Network are to decrease tobacco use and increase the number of health care professionals who provide smoking cessation and prevention assistance to their clients and community groups. The target groups are occupational therapy practitioners and students at local, state, national, and international levels.

Projects supported by the Network have included implementation of smoking cessation initiatives on college campuses; revision of OT curricula to include smoking prevention/

cessation topics (which fits under the umbrella of wellness and health promotion, required in OT curricula by the Accreditation Council for OT Education standards); publication of articles in OT trade and peer-reviewed publications, brochures (hard copy through members of the OT Network, reprinted in the NYSOTA News and on the OT Network Web site), and surveys (done in OT district meetings and distributed through educators to students on college campuses in New York City); and introduction of activities to encourage OTs to become more aware of the physical and cultural factors critical in helping clients quit smoking. Workshops given at state, local, and international levels demonstrate inclusion of smoking cessation as an important aspect of OT practice.

The Network has been successful in raising consciousness with the American Occupational Therapy Association (AOTA). In April, 1998, the Representative Assembly of the AOTA adopted Resolution L, which supports the smoking cessation guidelines developed by the AHCPR. Resolution L noted that OT practitioners work with the "whole person." The purpose of the resolution was to raise awareness among OTs of their role in educating clients about smoking cessation and ways to implement preventive health care interventions.

The American Physical Therapy Association (APTA) passed a resolution to adopt the AHCPR *Smoking Cessation Clinical Practice Guidelines* in 1997. (Please note: The AHCPR is now known as AHRQ, Agency for Healthcare Research and Quality.) However, there is little available in the professional literature that demonstrates behavioral clinical implementation outcomes of smoking cessation initiatives by physical therapists. One article in APTA literature recommends that PTs could have a possible role in helping people to quit smoking (Rimmer, 1999).

While OTs have embraced smoking cessation initiatives in the literature more than have physical therapists, it is appropriate for both to have a role in smoking cessation, because it can aid in healing and can prevent disease and disability. All therapists can implement the 4As, educate clients about the effects of smoking and smoking cessation, provide behavioral follow-up, and advise clients to seek out pharmaceutical therapies and support groups within the course of standard treatment. Providing a resource book about smoking cessation interventions and local resources in the waiting room or while clients are using modalities is a viable option that can support health counseling efforts. OTs can also use their skills in activity assessment to facilitate problem solving, decreasing barriers to permanent cessation (see case studies).

Research

The smoking cessation movement in the United States has been successful at getting smokers to quit, but not very successful at preventing new smokers from developing the habit. One half of all adults who have smoked have quit (CDC, 1994). However, the American Health Foundation (AHF) cited increased cigarette smoking as a factor in the deteriorating health of the nation's children. In its 1994 Child Health Report Card, the foundation reported that the use of cigarettes among high school seniors increased in 1993 after several years of decline (AHF, 1994).

A new study shows that youngsters who regularly see antismoking messages on television are half as likely to start smoking as those who are not exposed to the ads. The study tracked Massachusetts children for 4 years, starting in 1993 when the state launched its antismoking advertising campaign (Siegel & Biener, 2000a). Researchers found that 12- or 13-year-olds who could recall the antismoking campaign on television were less likely to become smokers than those who could not recall the ads. However, recall of the ads had no significant effect on progression to smoking among 14- and 15-year-olds. "This may indicate that older adolescents are resistant to antismoking messages or that they have already established strong attitudes toward smoking," noted the authors (p. 386). In a second study, Siegel and Biener (2000b) found that teens who could name a cigarette brand and owned a tobacco-sponsored promotion item were more than twice as likely to become smokers. These studies demonstrate how effective advertising is in both promoting and preventing smoking.

Outcome data on the success of group participation in smoking cessation is severely limited due to small subject numbers and the use of a particular population, so that generalizability of study findings is poor. Nevid and Javier (1997) failed to find any long-term benefit from use of either the self-help or clinic-based models, while Shuster, Utz, and Merwin (1996) found a quit rate of 15 percent using a community-based self-help intervention. Obviously, more research needs to be done in this area, since clients report anecdotally that these interventions are helpful.

Occupational Therapy or Physical Therapy Behavioral Research

Both the AOTA and the APTA have taken formal action to support the AHCPR smoking cessation clinical practice guidelines and to encourage their members to address smoking and advise clients who smoke to quit. Following these actions, Rimmer (1999) has noted that PTs can have a role in helping people to quit smoking. There have been several published initiatives by occupational therapists.

Scott (1999) published outcomes of wellness-directed initiatives, including smoking cessation, with OT students. OT students learned health promotion skills through working on personal wellness goals and leading community-based health promotion groups. After identifying a personal wellness goal and developing it in a Wellness Awareness Learning Contract, each student used a Goal Attainment Scale (GAS) to predict an expected outcome for achieving his or her goal and to measure personal progress toward attaining that goal. Differences on the Self-Assessment Scorecard indicated improvement on two of the six scales for physical health and choices.

Puttkammer and colleagues recently reported at the AOTA Annual Conference (Royce, Puttkammer, Vargas, & Burkhardt, 2000) on a study done by Cordelia Puttkammer with OT students that showed students, including smokers, are highly and positively influenced in their knowledge of smoking and its relation to health and development of disease. OT students gained insight into the impact of tobacco-related media messages on attitudes, behaviors, and perceptions about smoking. Their attitudes and willingness to quit smoking were also found to be related to their knowledge of the health risks related to smoking. These studies and activities represent client inclusion in a participatory team for improving their own health. In other words, clients are considered to be actively responsible for seeking out ways to improve their own health.

Professional knowledge on this topic among rehabilitation professionals needs further action, research, and discussion in order to educate therapists that smoking cessation initiatives are viable for inclusion in routine practice and to determine which interventions are most effective.

Case Studies

Adult Quitting for Better Health Choice

Steve is a 36-year-old man who works in a psychiatric nursing department at a municipal, inner-city hospital. Steve is a former athlete who has a chronic back ailment from a work-related injury. He has smoked for most of his adult life—often using smoking as a means of taking a break and trying to cope or relax. Approximately 6 months ago, Steve sought assistance to quit smoking cigarettes. With the help of an occupational therapist, he selected a date to quit. Steve's doctor had advised use of the nicotine patch to assist with his attempt. The occupational therapist worked with Steve to determine which activities and situations triggered his desire to smoke. Then, step by step, they planned alternate ways of doing daily activities that could help Steve change the habits that led to his smoking. Steve quit and remained smoke free for 3 months. Steve had a relapse when he found himself under pressure for a family-related crisis. He agreed not to view his relapse as a failure. Recently, Steve returned to his doctor. They discussed that anxiety had triggered Steve's relapse. Steve and his doctor agreed to try Zyban as the means for Steve's second attempt to stop smoking. He has selected another quit date and is convinced that this time he will be successful with his quit attempt.

A Recalcitrant Smoker Who Has Had Difficulty Quitting

Jim is a 72-year-old man who began smoking during World War II, on a tour of duty serving in the Philippines while in the Navy. Jim has smoked ever since. He quit 6 years ago for a period of 6 months, after open-heart surgery. Jim is in the hospital now for a diagnosis of Legionella—pneumonia contracted by smokers who have suppressed respiratory function. While this incident wasn't open-heart surgery, it was serious enough to scare Jim into reexamining the impact smoking has on his overall health and well-being. Jim has tried to quit other times in the past, but each time has relapsed. When he describes tobacco, Jim talks about it almost romantically: It "calls" him whenever he leaves it. He reports that life seems to go along okay and one early morning he'll awake and will think only about "having a smoke." Jim links his desire to the taste of the tobacco itself. In implementing the 4As with Jim, Jim's therapist asked whether he had ever tried to substitute the desire with another activity that includes taste. Substituting thoughts of tobacco with another distracting concept was also suggested. The day after speaking about the desire and the intensity of the smoking trigger, Jim stated he felt better already about his chance at succeeding. He chose a quit date. Jim was given a tape recording of a relaxation message. He was also advised to stimulate his taste buds with either strong peppermint or lemon candy. At last report, Jim was managing well. While only 2 months have lapsed since this latest quit attempt, Jim reports he is optimistic about his ability to stick with the program this time.

Teenagers and Prevention

Mario is a 17-year-old Mexican-American who is the middle son in a family of three sons. Mario has been attending an after-school youth program in his community. Among other activities, the program sponsors the Great American Smoke-Out. In this activity, Mario participated in a train-the-trainer program. He had to take a pledge to be a spokesperson among his siblings and his peers—giving positive messages about why they should not begin to smoke and making a personal pledge not to smoke. Mario's father is a smoker who has smoked two packs per day for as long as Mario can remember. Mario has experienced secondhand smoke for all of his life, and he and one of his brothers have asthma. Their family doctor has told them it could be related to their father's smoking habit. Mario has proudly taken on his new role as a positive role model. He has spent several times visiting with his brothers to personally discuss the impact tobacco has on their lives. Mario has made several new friends in the train-the-trainer sessions, and they have planned a smoke-free dance party as a way to introduce their knowledge to their friends and relatives.

A Model for Teen Cessation

Kim is an attractive 16-year-old who has always been drawn to the fine arts and writing. Kim and nearly all of her circle of friends smoke. As a child, Kim had severe asthma. While she hasn't had an asthma attack in some time, Kim's doctor advised her to quit smoking. Kim has accepted that it's a good idea to give up cigarettes. Her teacher referred her to the school occupational therapist for some help with her quit attempt. The OT helped Kim list the times when she feels the need to smoke. Together, they have chosen a quit date and made a plan for Kim to do it on a school day, where she can seek support from the OT or her teacher not to relapse. The OT had Kim address a postcard to herself saying "Good for you, Kim! Congratulations on your ability to quit. You go girl!!" The postcard was of one of Kim's favorite paintings, "Judith" by Gustave Klimt. Kim said she thought the woman in the painting was extraordinarily beautiful. The OT shared a copy of the National Cancer Institute poster, Cigarette Face—Another Reason Not To Smoke. The poster depicts a woman's face. Half of her face is that of a nonsmoker (no wrinkles); the other half is the same face, but depicting the impact of smoking on the face (lines and wrinkles are present). The OT and Kim discussed how much easier it is to prevent wrinkles when one doesn't smoke.

The OT and the teacher offered Kim a new opportunity to take care of the class bulletin board, updating it during her break time with announcements of art activities and attractions that were happening week by week in the community. They also thought it would be a way of helping Kim to avoid smoking on her class break at school, when peer pressure from other smokers could make her most vulnerable to a relapse. Kim has been smoke-free for a year. This year she took on responsibility for the entire school's involvement in the Great American Smoke-Out. Kim has a group of new smoke-free friends who rehearsed and performed a smoking cessation skit for an assembly. She is proud of her success at quitting and now states she finds it hard to be around people while they smoke.

Children, Parents, and Grandparents

It was parent's visiting night at the school and Mary Beth, the school OT, planned an event to make parents aware of the impact of their smoking on the children at home. Mary Beth invited five of her second-graders to assist with the program. They folded coffee filters into eighths, dipped the filters into warm water containing dark food coloring, and then re-opened them. The residue from the coloring infiltrated the filters, demonstrating the impact of smoke on lungs. The children demonstrated for the parents the impact that their smoking could have on their children's lungs. Mary Beth advised the parents to quit smoking, not only for their own personal health, but especially for the health and well-being of their children. After the completion of the program, one mother came to Mary Beth for additional resources. Her son had four episodes of bronchitis in the past year, and the mother recognized her need to quit for his better health. Mary Beth referred her to several community agencies that offered smoking cessation programs in the evening. Together they identified two programs that had child care facilities so that the mother could attend the meetings.

Children and the Community

John is a 9-year-old who is in elementary school. After school, he is active in his Boy Scout troop. John wants to earn his health badge and has sought out help from his mother. His mother referred John to his next door neighbor, an occupational therapist, to help him determine a plan for earning his badge. The OT had just returned from a conference where she heard other OTs talk about the success they were having working with children to make personal health commitments, according to the Healthy People 2010 targeted health behavioral improvement areas. The OT gave John a list of Web sites that have smoking-related resources and helped him download the information he needed. John equipped himself with copies of frequently-asked-questions from the Web pages. He individually asked the parents of the boys in his troop if they smoked. For those who smoked, he implored them to quit. He gave each participant a package of gum, and together they made a pact. He further asked his fellow Boy Scouts to personally ask each parent to quit smoking. All agreed to quit. John did this activity 6 months ago. He recently received a card from one of the mothers, thanking him for his caring and leadership. She has been smoke-free ever since the group met—thanks to John. John and his friends mention smoking from time to time, but each time they speak of it, they reaffirm that they will never do it themselves. Their prevention leadership has shaped their own values about smoking.

Summary

Cigarette smoking, the most preventable cause of premature death in the United States, is associated with heart and lung disease, several types of cancer, as well as decreased healing from other unrelated problems. As such, it is a major public health problem and drain on society's resources. Therapists are one group of health professionals who often spend extended periods of time and build strong relationships with clients. Therapists can and should be involved in helping their clients in smoking cessation.

Adequate smoking cessation efforts include understanding the risks and mortality involved in smoking and the interventions used in smoking cessation. Traditional interventions such as pharmacological agents and support groups can be used alone or in conjunction with alternative treatments, such as the stimulation of acupoints or use of energy work.

STUDY QUESTIONS

1. What are the negative effects of smoking on healing?
2. What do the 4As stand for?
3. What is the difference between nicotine replacement and nonnicotine replacement pharmacological agents?
4. You have a client who has initiated a smoking cessation program, attending a support group and using a nicotine patch. You smell smoke on the client. Explain in layman's terms why someone using nicotine replacement therapy must not smoke.
5. Name five ways therapists can help clients quit smoking
6. Identify two smoking cessation groups in your community, including the type of program, approaches used, and cost.

RESOURCES

NIH/NCI: *www.dccps.nci.nih.gov*
NOAH: *www.noah.cuny.edu/*
American Cancer Society: *www.cancer .org/index.html*
Quit Net: *www.quitnet.org/Library/ Guides/NRT/NRT_chart.jtml*
American Lung Association: *www .lungusa.org/smokefreeclass/ boards.html*
American Heart Association: *www.amheart.org*

OT Network on Smoking and Wellness: *www.nyu.edu/education/ot/right.html*

AHCPR Publishing Clearinghouse Titles

#960695 You Can Quit
#960693 Helping Smokers Quit
#960694 Smoking Cessation: Information for Specialists
Instant fax: (301) 594-2800, push 1 and press start for a publication list.

Smoking Cessation Clinical Practice Guidelines

AHCPR Guidelines
Department of Health and Human Services
PO Box 8547
Silver Spring, MD 20907-8547
(800) 358-9295

Relevant Associations

Kickbutt: *www.kickbutt.org*
Coalition for a Smoke-Free New York: *www.ci.nyc.ny.us/html/doh/html/ smoke/smokeg.html*
Grant funding organizations for model programming: Search for local grants from your local city and state governments, department of health. The tobacco settlement monies are currently being decided upon state by state.

REFERENCES

AHCPR (Agency for Health Care Policy and Research). (1996). [Online]. Smoking cessation clinical practice guidelines. Available: www.ahcpr.gov/clinic/cpgsix.htm.

American Health Foundation. (1994, Oct.). 1994 child health report card.

CASA (Center on Addiction and Substance Abuse). (1994, May 17). Columbia University.

CDC (Centers for Disease Control). (1994). Cigarette smoking among adults—United States, 1993.

DiClemente, C. C., & J. O. Prochaska. (1982). Self-change and therapy change of smoking behavior: A comparison of processes of change in cessation and maintenance. *Addictive Behaviors, 7,* 133–142.

DHHS. (1990). Healthy People 2000. Office of Disease Prevention and Health Promotion of the U.S. Government.

Nevid, J. S., & R. A. Javier. (1997). Preliminary investigation of a culturally specific smoking cessation intervention for Hispanic smokers. *American Journal of Health Promotion, 11*(3), 198–207.

NYU. (2002). [Online]. Role of the occupational therapist in smoking cessation. Available: http://www.nyu.edu/education/ot/right.html

Rimmer, J. H. (1999). Health promotion for people with disabilities: The emerging paradigm shift from disability prevention to prevention of secondary conditions. *Physical Therapy, 79*(5), 495–502.

Royce, J. M., C. Puttkammer, S. Vargas, & A. Burkhardt. (2000). OT students and tobacco: Smoking prevalence, attitudes and knowedge. Abstract printed in Annual Conference and Exhibition Program, p. 30.

Scott, A. H. (1999, Nov.). Wellness works: Community service health promotion groups led by occupational therapy students. *American Journal of Occupational Therapy, 53*(6), 566–574.

Shuster, G. F., S. W. Utz, & E. Merwin. (1996). Implementation and outcomes of a community-based self-help smoking cessation program. *Journal of Community Health Nursing, 13*(3), 187–198.

Siegel, M., & L. Biener. (2000a). The impact of an antismoking media campaign on progression to established smoking: Results of a longitudinal youth study. *American Journal of Public Health, 90,* 380–386.

Siegel, M., & L. Biener. (2000b). Tobacco marketing and adolescent smoking: More support for a causal inference. *American Journal of Public Health, 90,* 407–411.

Swarbrick, M. (1996, Sept 12). The Wellness Connection. *OT Week,* 12–13.

Williams, V., A. Burkhardt, & J. Royce. (1995, March 12). Wellness: Helping people call it quits. *OT Week,* 18–20.

Appendix I

NIH Definitions of CAM Therapies*

Jennifer M. Bottomley

This classification system was designed by the National Center for Complementary and Alternative Medicine (NCCAM) to assist in prioritizing applications for research grants in complementary and alternative medicine (CAM). It is divided into seven major categories and includes examples of practices or preparations in each category.

Within each category, medical practices that are not commonly used, accepted, or available in conventional medicine are designated as CAM. Those practices that fall mainly within the domains of conventional medicine are designated as behavioral medicine. Practices that can be either CAM or behavioral medicine, depending on their application, are designated as overlapping.

I. Mind-Body Medicine

Mind-body medicine involves behavioral, psychological, social, and spiritual approaches to health. It is divided into four subcategories: mind-body systems; mind-body methods; religion and spirituality; social and contextual areas.

Mind-Body Systems

This subcategory involves whole systems of mind-body practice that are used largely as primary interventions for disease. They are rarely delivered alone; instead, they are used in combination with lifestyle interventions, or are part of a traditional medical system.

Mind-Body Methods

This subcategory contains individual modalities used in mind-body approaches to health. These approaches are often considered conventional practice and overlap with CAM only when applied to medical conditions for which they are not usually used (for example, hypnosis for genetic problems).

*Source: National Institute of Health, National Center for Complementary and Alternative Medicine.

CAM

Yoga
Internal Qi Gong
T'ai Chi

Behavioral Medicine

Psychotherapy
Meditation
Imagery
Hypnosis
Biofeedback
Support Groups

Overlapping

Art Therapy
Music Therapy
Dance Therapy
Journaling
Humor
Body Psychotherapy

Religion and Spirituality

This subcategory deals with those nonbehavioral aspects of spirituality and religion that examine their relationship to biological function or clinical conditions.

CAM

Confession
Nonlocality
Nontemporality
Soul Retrieval
Spiritual Healing
"Special" Healers

Social and Contextual Areas

This subcategory refers to social, cultural, symbolic, and contextual interventions that are not covered in other areas.

CAM

Caring-based Approaches (for example, holistic nursing, pastoral care)
Intuitive Diagnosis

Overlapping

Placebo

Explanatory Models
Community-based Approaches (for example, Alcoholics Anonymous, Native American "sweat" rituals)

II. Alternative Medical Systems

This category involves complete systems of theory and practice that have been developed outside of the Western biomedical approach. It is divided into four subcategories: acupuncture and Oriental medicine; traditional indigenous systems; unconventional Western systems; naturopathy.

Acupuncture and Oriental Medicine

Acupuncture
Herbal Formulas
Diet
External and Internal Qi Gong
T'ai Chi
Massage and Manipulation (Tui Na)
Acupotomy

Traditional Indigenous Systems

This subcategory includes major indigenous systems of medicine other than acupuncture and traditional Oriental medicine.

Native American Medicine
Ayurvedic Medicine
Unani-Tibbi
SIDDHI
Kampo Medicine
Traditional African Medicine
Traditional Aboriginal Medicine
Curanderismo
Central and South American Practices
Psychic Surgery

Unconventional Western Systems

This subcategory includes alternative medical systems developed in the West that are not classified elsewhere.

CAM

Homeopathy
Functional Medicine
Environmental Medicine
Radiesthesia
Psionic Medicine
Cayce-based Systems
Kneipp "Classical"
Homeopathy
Orthomolecular Medicine
Radionics

Overlapping

Anthroposophically-extended medicine

Naturopathy

This subcategory is an eclectic collection of natural systems and therapies that has gained prominence in the United States.

III. Lifestyle and Disease Prevention

This category involves theories and practices designed to prevent the development of illness, identify and treat risk factors, or support the healing and recovery process. Lifestyle and disease prevention is concerned with integrated approaches for the prevention and management of chronic disease in general or the common determinants of chronic disease. It is divided into three subcategories: clinical preventative practices; lifestyle therapies; health promotion.

Clinical Preventative Practices

This subcategory refers to unconventional approaches used to screen for and prevent health-related imbalances, dysfunction, and disease.

Electrodermal Diagnostics
Medical Intuition
Chiriography
Functional Cellular Enzyme Measures
Panchakarma

Lifestyle Therapies

This subcategory deals with complete systems of lifestyle management that include behavioral changes, dietary changes, exercise, stress management, and addiction control. To be classified as CAM, the changes in lifestyle must be based on a nonorthodox system of medicine, be applied in unconventional ways, or be applied across non-Western diagnostic approaches.

Health Promotion

This subcategory involves laboratory and epidemiological research on healing, the healing process, health-promoting factors, and autoregulatory mechanisms.

IV. Biologically-Based Therapies

This category includes natural and biologically-based practices, interventions, and products. Many overlap with conventional medicine's use of dietary supplements. This category is divided into four subcategories: phytotherapy or herbalism; special diet therapies; orthomolecular medicine; pharmacological, biological and instrumental interventions.

Phytotherapy or Herbalism

This subcategory addresses plant-derived preparations that are used for therapeutic and preventive purposes.

Individual Herbs

Ginkgo Biloba
Hypericum
Garlic
Ginseng
Echinacea
Saw Palmetto
Urtica Diocia (Nettle)
Kava Kava
Hawthorne
Witch Hazel
Bilberry
Ginger
Aloe Vera
Capsicum
Feverfew
Green Tea
Tea Tree Oil
Licorice Root
Yohimbe
Valerian
Bee Pollen
Cat's Claw
Evening Primrose

Dong Quai
Fenugreek
Marshmallow
Psyllium
Tumeric
Mistletoe
Mahonia Aquifolium
Oleum Menthaepiperitea (Peppermint Oil)

Combinations

Padma 28
Essiac
JCL 2306
Hoxsey
Saw Palmetto/Pygeum
Africanium

Special Diet Therapies

This subcategory includes dietary approaches and special diets that are applied as alternative therapies for risk factors or chronic disease in general.

Pritikin
Ornish
McDougall
Gerson
Kelly-Gonzales
Wigmore
Livingston-Wheeler
Atkins
Diamond
Vegetarian
Fasting
High Fiber
Macrobiotic
Mediterranean
Paleolithic
Asian
Natural Hygiene

Orthomolecular Medicine

This subcategory refers to products used as nutritional and food supplements (and not covered in other categories). These products are used for preventive or therapeutic purposes.

They are usually used in combinations and at high doses. Examples include niacinamide for arthritis and melatonin to prevent breast cancer.

Single Nutrients

Ascorbic Acid
Carotenes
Tocopherols
Folic Acid
Niacin
Niacinamide
Pantothenic Acid
Pyridoxine
Riboflavin
Thiamine
Vitamin A
Vitamin D
Vitamin K
Biotin
Choline
S-adenosylmethionine
Calcium
Magnesium
Selenium
Potassium
Taurine
Lysine
Tyrosine
Gamma-oryzanol
Iodine
Iron
Manganese
Molybdenum
Boron
Silicon
Vanadium
Co-enzyme Q10
Carnitine
Probiotics
Glutamine
Phenylalanine
Glucosamine Sulfate
Chondroitin Sulfate
Lipoic Acid
Amino Acids
Phosphatidylserine
Melatonin
DHEA

Inositol
Glandular Products
Fatty Acids
Medium
Chain Triglycerides

Pharmacological, Biological, and Instrumental Interventions

This subcategory includes products and procedures applied in an unconventional manner that are not covered in other categories.

Products

Coley's Toxins
Antineoplastons
Cartilage
EDTA
Ozone
H_2O_2
Hyperbaric Oxygen
IAT
714X
MHT-68
Gallo Immunotherapy
Cone Therapy
Revici System
Enzyme Therapies
Cell Therapy
Enderlin Products
T/Tn Vaccine
Bee Pollen
Induced Remission Therapy

Procedures/Devices

Apitherapy
Neural Therapy
Electrodiagnostics
IridologyChirography
Special Functional Tests Bioresonance
MORA Device

V. Manipulative and Body-Based Systems

This category refers to systems that are based on manipulation and/or movement of the body, and is divided into three subcategories: chiropractic medicine; massage and bodywork; unconventional physical therapies.

Chiropractic Medicine
Massage and Bodywork

Osteopathic Manipulative Therapy (OMT)
Cranialsacral OMT
Swedish Massage
Applied Kinesiology
Reflexology
Pilates Method
Polarity
Body Psychotherapy
Trager Body Work
Alexander Technique
Feldenkrais Technique
Chinese Tui Na Massage and Acupressure
Rolfing

Unconventional Physical Therapies

Hydrotherapy
Diathermy
Light and Color Therapies
Heat and ElectrotherapiesColonics
Alternate Nostril Breathing Techniques

VI. Biofield

Biofield medicine involves systems that use subtle energy fields in and around the body for medical purposes.

Therapeutic Touch
Healing Science
Healing Touch
Natural Healing
SHEN
Mariue
Reiki
Huna
External Qi Gong
Biorelax

VII. Bioelectromagnetics

Bioelectromagnetics refers to the unconventional use of electromagnetic fields for medical purposes.

Appendix 2

Other Therapies

Phyllis Gordon

Animal Assisted Therapy

Animal assisted therapy (AAT) is the utilization of animals as a therapeutic modality to facilitate healing and rehabilitation of clients with acute or chronic ailments. The animals are used by therapists in goal-directed treatment sessions as a modality to facilitate optimum client performance. AAT asserts that through the use of this modality, a variety of functional goals can be targeted in the physical, cognitive/perceptual, and psychosocial domains.

The size and location of a facility, client population, and availability of appropriate animals usually determines what animal is selected in an AAT program; the most popular are dogs and cats. It is essential for the safety of the client, the animals, and the assisting professionals that the animals instinctively react in a safe, predictable way during stressful situations. Therefore, all animals used in AAT are temperament (instinctive behavior) tested and have had obedience training.

Dolphin Therapy

The Upledger Institute has established a series of workshops that include structured dolphin swims and multitherapist group techniques. The workshops are held in the Bahamas (at the time of this writing), on a custom-built, environmentally friendly power catamaran named *Dolphin Star* designed by naval architect John Marples. Prerequisites for taking each workshop range from CranioSacral Therapy I to Advanced CranioSacral Therapy. There is no certification in this program.

Dr. Upledger says that therapists come into the program at a certain level and come out of the program as better therapists. Therapists report that the experience of utilizing dolphin energy is very peaceful and calming. These experiences are subjective and difficult to explain scientifically. Referring to the Heisenberg principle (uncertainty results from the fundamental nature of the particles being observed), the observer's positive feeling for the outcome will influence a study's final results. Also consider that statistics can be interpreted in many ways. The following anecdote told by Dr. John Upledger is an example:

Dr. Upledger was working with a child diagnosed with cerebral palsy at a symposium in Edinburgh, Scotland. During this child's second treatment session, Dr. Upledger said aloud, "I need dolphin energy." He was frustrated by not being able to energetically get past 3 inches into this child's brain. The audio technician reported to Dr. Upledger that whenever he asked for dolphin energy out loud, static was recorded. At the end of the session, a Ph.D. professor in physical therapy approached Dr. Upledger and stated that each time he asked for dolphin energy, she experienced buzzing and static in her hearing aids. Later, Dr. Upledger received these hearing aids in the mail, accompanied by a letter in which the professor explained that she did not need them anymore.

(Upledger, J., personal communication, January 24, 2001)

Hippotherapy/Therapeutic Riding

Hippotherapy, from the Greek word *hippos,* which means horse, is the treatment approach that uses the horse, the movement of the horse, and a nonclinical environment. Hippotherapy is an outgrowth of classic hippotherapy that has been practiced since the 1960s. Classic hippotherapy utilizes a therapist analyzing the client's posture and movement response to the horse's movement and then directing a horse handler to change the tempo and direction of the horse as indicated by the client's responses.

Meaningful activities on a horse that address the client's individual goals are provided in hippotherapy. Its controlled environment and graded input are designed to elicit appropriate adaptive responses. It provides a foundation of neuromuscular functioning and sensory processing that can be generalized to a wide variety of functional skills. Physical, psychological, cognitive, and speech production improvements are often observed after meeting long-term goals such as strengthening trunk musculature. Hippotherapy has been used with the following client populations: visually impaired, attention deficit disorder, autism, cerebral palsy, learning disabilities, mental health, mental retardation, multiple sclerosis, spina bifida, and traumatic brain injury. In the late 1980s, Jan Spink, M.A., expanded hippotherapy to include a multidisciplinary approach, a more diverse client population, and more equine skills, including dressage, horse handling, and vaulting, called developmental riding therapy.

To practice hippotherapy, the treatment principles of a particular health profession are incorporated into the hippotherapy setting. An initial evaluation based within the scope of that profession to determine client's needs, abilities, limitations and comfort level with the horse is crucial. A functional and relevant treatment plan includes choosing the horse whose movement best addresses the client's need and providing appropriate equipment to facilitate the responses. Reevaluation occurs at 3 to 6 month intervals to make sure that the long-term and short-term goals are still appropriate for the client and to determine whether or not hippotherapy is addressing the needs of the client. If all long-term goals have been met, transition into a therapeutic riding program is possible. Therapeutic riding is a program in which the disabled client can learn vaulting and other riding skills or equine sports.

To provide direct treatment in classic hippotherapy, the practitioner

♦ Is licensed or registered to practice a nationally recognized health care profession.
♦ Maintains current professional liability insurance.
♦ Has received training in the principles of classic hippotherapy, equine movement, and equine psychology through attendance at a minimum of one American Hippotherapy Association-approved "Introduction to Classic Hippotherapy" course. The completion of this course is a requirement of any therapist wishing to become registered with AHA.
♦ Is a North American Riding for the Handicapped Association (NARHA) certified instructor (any level), and if not, has a NARHA certified instructor present at all treatment sessions.

Acupuncture

Acupuncture is based on the principle that health is determined by a balanced flow of qi (energy) within the body. Illness is the result of blockages and imbalances in this flow of energy. The examination that determines the pattern of disharmony (rather than a Western medical diagnosis) includes observation (of the tongue, pallor, eyes, general body posture, and demeanor), smelling and listening, questioning the client, and palpation (including pulse taking). Placement of hair-thin needles at points along a meridian (energy pathway) adjusts the flow of qi so that the body can regain its balance. Sterile, disposable needles intended for single use are inserted and sometimes feel like a prick or dull ache. A warm spreading sensation is felt as the energy of the body begins to move more fully through the blocked areas. No pain is felt once the needles are in place. A general feeling of extreme relaxation is felt at the conclusion of treatment.

Other methods to activate deficient qi or drain excess qi include acupressure (applying pressure to meridian point), moxibustion (the slow burning of an herb to produce heat), guasha (light abrasion of the skin to relieve congestion), herbal teas, and nutritional recommendations.

Acupuncture is often an effective part of a total drug and alcohol rehabilitation and of smoking cessation programs. Use of acupuncture as a method for detoxification began when a patient with a 5-year opium habit had acupuncture instead of chemical anesthesia before scheduled neurosurgery intended to relieve his addiction and withdrawal symptoms. Needles were inserted at his hand, arm, and ear points, and attached to an electrical stimulation machine. Unexpectedly, the patient experienced relief of withdrawal symptoms and the surgery was cancelled. This patient remained in the hospital and was treated again when withdrawal symptoms recurred. The next day, using the same method, two other opium addicts were treated with equal success. This discovery was made by Dr. Hsiang-Lai Wen in 1972 in Hong Kong. In 1973, Dr. Wen and Dr. S. Y. C. Cheung reported in the *Asian Journal of Medicine* the results of treating 40 other heroin and opium addicts with acupuncture (Mitchell, 1995).

Chinese medicine views the chemically dependent person as "depleted," often described by the Chinese word *xu hu,* meaning "empty fire." Acupuncture addresses the restless, unproductive behavior of chemical dependency by nourishing the client's inner emptiness. By decreasing or eliminating withdrawal-related suffering, acupuncture-assisted detoxification contributes to clients faring better in treatment and decreasing recidivism. Daily ear (auricular) acupuncture treatments (3 to 5 points on the ear) along with daily urine sampling are usually the first steps in a detoxification program. Acupuncture is decreased and involvement in a 12-step program is begun as sobriety is maintained. Realizing that relapse is part of recovery, a three-tiered program is implemented so as to support clients rather than punish them for relapsing. If a relapse should occur, daily auricular acupuncture is reinstated. This distinctly American adaptation of acupuncture-assisted detoxification was developed at the drug clinic of Lincoln Hospital in New York's South Bronx. In 1988, Lincoln Hospital claimed that more than 60 percent of substance abuse clients are retained in acupuncture treatment—a much higher figure than any other form of outpatient drug treatment (Connelly, 1994). In 1985, the National Acupuncture Detoxification Association (NADA) was founded by experienced clinicians. NADA sets the standards of certification for acupuncture assisted detoxification.

Aquatic Therapy

Aquatic therapy is rehabilitation performed in water. Because water eliminates gravity, clients are enabled to perform exercises that are too difficult on land. For example, water provides a partial weightless environment so that wheelchair-dependent people are empowered to move at various levels. Aquatics provide functional restoration of strength by walking, running, bending, pushing, lifting, and pulling in water. This can be an alternative to traditional fitness programs and a safe way to stay in shape.

Most aquatic therapies include total body fitness, specific rehabilitation exercises for the injury, and correction of body mechanics. A three-dimensional resistance to movement helps develop muscle strength equally in all directions. Hydrostatic pressure reduces swelling and discomfort. While submerged in deep water, clients avoid weight bearing and avoid impact on joints. People with severe neck pain perform warm-ups and exercise while partially submerged in order to take the weight off the neck to exercise with more ease. The therapist monitors exercise intensity and pacing. Special equipment such as webbed gloves can be used to create more resistance. Low impact jumping exercises are gradually incorporated into the program.

Specific aquatic therapy techniques include

- **Bad Ragaz**, proprioceptive neuromuscular facilitation-oriented, progressive, resistive exercises that can be adapted to passive technique for use with the neurologic and orthopedic population; Halliwick, a program that uses developmental sequences in deep water to normalize movement; WATSU, a technique that uses Zen Shiatsu pressure points and generalized stretching for therapy.
- **Ai Chi**, a system that uses a modified T'ai Chi form in water and can be used as an independent regimen after a treatment program ends.
- **WOGA**, which stands for water yoga. This system uses a sequence of stretches that are akin to asanas and, due to the water's buoyancy, enable a person to stretch beyond what he or she can do on land.

Divers Unlimited, a nonprofit corporation, teaches scuba diving to physically disabled persons, "kids at risk," and able-bodied persons. As in aquatic therapy, the therapeutic nature of water is used to engage the disabled population in an activity (scuba diving) to increase their level of physical exercise and independence. Also, in the hope to counteract juvenile violence with children who are at risk, diving skill acquisition and related education (marine sciences, environmental situation, oceanography, reading, and math) are taught.

Aromatherapy

Aromatherapy utilizes the essential oils of a plant to affect the body and mind through the olfactory system and the skin. The trigger of neurotransmitters, which may sedate, relax, stimulate, or cause euphoria after inhalation of an essential oil, is the basis of this approach. If the essential oils are rubbed into the skin or dispersed in water, it is thought that they permeate through the capillaries and cell tissues to act in a healing fashion. Essential oils combined with massage enhance the therapeutic effects of both.

Imagery

Imagery is defined as a person's "internal experiences of memories, dreams, fantasies, and visions . . ." (Dossey, 1988a, p. 224). Marks (1999) notes that mental imagery is basic to consciousness and ". . . serves a significant adaptive function in the preparation of action and coping with change" (p. 1). Imagery is used therapeutically in mind-body approaches such as hypnosis and biofeedback, in psychotherapy (Achterberg, 1999), and with other alternative therapy such as craniosacral therapy (see Somato Emotional Release case in Craniosacral Therapy, Chapter 14). Parker (2000) notes that "guided imagery is the process of using images to encourage positive changes" (p. 13). This can involve using symbols, imagining desired changes before they actually occur (Collinge, 1996), or mental rehearsal.

Some of the areas imagery has been shown to be effective in are improving positive effect, decreasing negative effect, reducing reports of symptoms (Tarrant, 1996), and decreased preoperative and postoperative anxiety and reductions in use of postoperative narcotic pain medication (Tusek, Church, & Fazio, 1997). Imagery paired with standard occupational therapy treatment has produced significant improvements in Fugl-Meyer Assessment of Sensorimotor Recovery scores in a small group of stroke subjects (Page, 2000).

Mental rehearsal (MR) is a specific type of imagery that has also been referred to as mental imagery and imaginary practice. It is defined as ". . . the mental or cognitive imagining of some aspect of the performance of a task or skill in the absence of any associated overt physical actions" (Fell & Wrisberg, 2001, p. 52). MR is typically used in activities such as athletics, the performing arts, and dance to supplement physical performance. While MR is used infrequently by therapists, it holds great possibility for use. Fell & Wrisberg have summarized current knowledge in MR and discussed the possible use of MR in rehabilitation by physical and occupational therapists.

Researchers have suggested that MR works via bioinformational learning, which is rehearsing and reinforcing mental images (Lang, 1977, as cited in Fell & Wrisberg, 2001), and that MR primes muscles for action (MacKay, 1981). The work of O'Craven and Kanwisher (2000) provides proof that imagery and perception share common vision processing mechanisms, and some research exists to support the muscle priming theory (Weiss et al., 1994). It is vital to note that research supports the use of MR in addition to physical practice but not as a substitute for it (Hall et al., 1993).

The use of imagery in clinical practice can be as varied as the types of clients therapists see. Many therapists use imagery informally with clients, either asking about what images occur with particular conditions or suggesting images to elicit specific states, such as relaxation. Imagery scripts have been developed for many conditions, such as pain control, energy awareness for health and balance, a protective shield or space, worry and fear, and other authors have developed guidelines for designing imagery with specific disorders (Brigham, with Davis & Cameron-Sampey, 1994). Researchers have noted that concepts such as vividness, clarity, and liveliness are important aspects of people's imagery that can be used diagnostically, by evaluating these aspects of imagery (Marks, 1999) and in treatment by enhancing the strength and direction of clients' imagery via therapeutic dialogues.

Integrative Manual Therapy (IMT)

Integrative Manual Therapy,[TM] The Integrated Systems Approach, and Integrative Diagnostics, developed by Sharon Weiselfish-Giammetteo, Ph.D., PT, incorporates the theories and practices of many osteopathic manual therapies with the functional foci of rehabilitation, psychology, and cognitive and vocational therapies. Weiselfish-Giammetteo has extensive teaching experience in all areas of manual and cranial therapy. Her integration of manual, neurorehabilitative, and cranial work has resulted in the unique IMT approach.

The three main IMT philosophies were constructed by Weiselfish-Giammetteo in the 1980s. The Integrated Systems Approach philosophy states that each body system has its own characteristics (i.e., cell structure, physiology, chemistry, and biomechanics), for which specific techniques have been formulated. Integrative Diagnostics philosophy is described as the process of investigation for the purpose of discovery. Unique diagnostic tools are used, such as myofascial mapping—a three-dimensional method of "listening" to the body and neurofascial process—in a differential diagnosis and treatment approach that addresses both mind and body dysfunction (Giammetteo, Weiselfish-Giammetteo, 1997). The goal is to recognize which body system needs help to recover while creating a treatment plan that addresses the physical, mental/cognitive, spiritual, and personal needs of the individual. The treatment plan is IMT's structural and functional rehabilitation philosophy. The motto of IMT is "Structural rehabilitation *attains* potential; functional rehabilitation *maintains* potential."

IMT has been used to address a wide range of problems with clients across the lifespan. There is no typical IMT session, as all treatment is customized for the individual. Research has been primarily clinical, performed by Weiselfish-Giammetteo and colleagues for over 20 years, and has not been reported in scientific journals.

Training information and educational materials can be obtained from Dialogues in Contemporary Rehabilitation (DCR). An affiliation with Westbrook University allows course credit towards a diploma or degree in IMT.

Lymphatic Drainage

The lymphatic system is responsible for filtering toxins, removing excess fluids, protein, and waste products from the tissues and carrying them to the blood vessels for circulation and elimination. This complex system relies on lymphangions (tiny muscular regions) contracting throughout the body to propel the lymph (a milky white fluid). Pulsation of arteries, all muscle contractions, peristalsis, and the negative pressure of the lungs also help move the lymph. Lymph collects in nodes that are found throughout the body. Lymph can stagnate due to lack of physical exercise, stress, infection, sprains, burns, congestive disorders, and surgery.

Exercise and massage help to move lymph; however, there are therapeutic lymphatic drainage methods designed specifically to manually and gently stimulate this system. Lymphatic drainage techniques are often prescribed when edema and lymphedema (a condition that may occur after lymph node removal in cancer surgery) are present. These techniques can also be used in the treatment of sports injuries, dermatological conditions (e.g., scars, acne), burns, venous insufficiency, RSD, sinusitis, and more. Lymphatic drainage may be helpful in a preventative health program. Aesthetic results such as wrinkle reduction are also reported.

Estrid and Emil Vodder, Danish physical therapists who practiced in France, developed manual lymphatic drainage (MLD) in the 1930s. MLD is very light manual stimulation of lymph flow and fluid movement, accessing the superficial layers of the soft tissue where lies about half of the body's lymph. There is also a deeper technique for relieving spasms in muscular lymph vessels. An on/off pulse pressure motion—like a pump—as well as scooping, rotary, and stationary circle techniques are used. It is reported that there is a lulling, relaxing effect on the autonomic nervous system.

There is a four-week, 160-hour, postgraduate training and certification process in the original Dr. Vodder method of MLD available to health care professionals through the Dr. Vodder School in North America. Specific clinical applications to various pathological conditions are stressed.

Bruno Chikly, M.D., from France, developed lymph drainage therapy (LDT), an original method based on the Vodder approach. He received the Medal of the Medical Faculty of Paris VI for his research on the lymphatic system and the lymphatic drainage technique. Dr. Chikly holds a master's degree equivalent in psychology from Paris XIII University. He has trained in osteopathy, massage, and several manual therapeutics.

Manual techniques of direct "listening" are utilized in LDT to feel the direction, rhythm, depth, and quality of lymphatic flow. More experienced LDT therapists are trained to perform accurate "lymphatic mapping" to assess lymphatic circulation and direct treatment with desired effects in shorter periods of time. There are techniques for emotional release based on the emotional connection with the fluid body .

Mechanical Link

Mechanical link is a gentle osteopathic technique developed by Paul Chauffour, D.O. It is designed to reduce physical and emotional stress and pain in an individual's body by evaluating and treating the whole body. There are eight functional units or points of evaluation:

1. *occipito-vertebral-pelvic unit*
2. *thorax (anterior/posterior)*
3. *extremities*
4. *denna (skin)*
5. *interosseous line of force*
6. *viscera*
7. *vascular*
8. *cranium.*

The fascia is the link between all eight systems. The practitioner evaluates for lesions in all the different systems by putting the fascia under tension. The practitioner determines the dominant lesion of each system and then determines the primary lesion of the whole body by using inhibitory balancing.

Treatment is done by recoil. Currently, there are six phases of treatment. The first four phases are mechanical at the physical level. The fifth and sixth phases are at the level of emotional, spiritual, and intellectual, and more phases are being developed. The client participates at this level by concentrating on the emotions that need release or attention (such as an event, trauma, fear, grief, feelings) or by verbalizing the emotion. Either physically or mentally, the client usually feels a change after one to three treatments.

Osteopathy states that structure governs the function, and by releasing the structure, the body will function optimally. Mechanical link follows this principle by testing the structures, and the structure's own tension determines where the treatment should be applied.

A typical treatment lasts 30 to 45 minutes. The key to treatment is the evaluation of the individual's structure, and each session is a reevaluation and treatment. Each living person has lesions (hypomobility or no mobility of a structure). The goal of treatment is to keep the sum of lesions below this threshold. Each person's threshold is different, and experiencing pain can be a warning to take care of the body. A person may receive treatment for a specific or multiple complaints, but also to maintain good health and prevent illnesses. Mechanical link helps the autoimmune system and helps the body heal itself. There are no contraindications for its use, and it is used with people of all ages, athletic or infirm.

In the United States the Upledger Institute offers training in mechanical link, including self-treatment and self-training of the fascial system. In France and throughout Europe, mechanical link is taught to sixth-year osteopathic students and to graduated osteopaths.

MEDEK

The dynamic method of kinetic stimulation, MEDEK, was developed by Chilean physical therapist Ramon Cuevas between 1971 and 1976. MEDEK focuses on stimulation of the automatic movements that contribute to postural control, providing formal and structured opportunities for the development of functional mobility.

MEDEK was brought to North America via a young Venezuelan girl diagnosed with cerebral palsy, spastic diplegia, who was being treated by Ramon Cuevas in Caracas and by Esther Fink, PT, in Toronto, Canada. Fink, impressed with the dramatic improvements in the girl's motor functioning after each return from South America, sought intensive training with Cuevas. After training with Cuevas at the Zareinu Educational Center, she began realizing established goals with her clients sooner than expected. These accelerated outcomes were noticed as well by the referring pediatricians and orthopedists.

The force of gravity is considered the main stimulus that triggers this neuromuscular goal of stabilizing the body in space. Inability to move at an early age limits the development of the brain structures and causes muscle weakness and deformities, leading to more severe motor deficits. MEDEK encourages early assessment and treatment, as it has been well documented that brain structure is affected by activity. Intervention within the first 6 months of life is ideal.

MEDEK measures the ability of the child to come up against gravity and control the body in space (alignment and stability) because it assumes that the lack of postural control restricts mobility. Specific dynamic exercises are used to provoke a very specific reaction. The goal is to provoke maximal function responses from the child by means of the least possible external help. The MEDEK approach focuses on training movements that lead to sitting, standing, and walking. Muscles are trained in postural and functional tasks rather than in a developmental sequence (rolling, sitting, crawling, etc.) or by strengthening muscles in isolation. MEDEK assumes different skills require different movement strategies. These exercises do not require the child's attention, conscious thought, or cooperation.

The MEDEK evaluation protocol consists of 46 items, or motor ontogenetic functions, grouped into seven sections, chronologically arranged. These items cover the postural motor development from newborn to 16 months of age. After the initial evaluation, an 8-week trial program is set up for treating the deficits. The program includes a 45-minute treatment from the therapist and a home exercise program of approximately eight clearly defined exercises that are taught to the parents to be performed twice daily. The home program is an essential part of the treatment. Therapy outcomes depend on the degree of dysfunction, the experience and handling skills of the therapist, the age at which the therapy is initiated, and the frequency of the intervention.

The efficacy of the MEDEK program on a particular child is evaluated after the 8-week trial program. If no changes are made, the parents are advised to look for another form of therapy.

MEDEK has a reputation for being an aggressive approach, because children are placed in seemingly precarious positions in order to promote motor organization. Parents report that they enjoy doing the exercises with their children and that they themselves benefit from a structured plan with clear goals.

Qi Gong

Qi means energy, vitality, or life force, and is sometimes used interchangeably with breath. Gong means to practice, cultivate, or refine. Qi Gong is commonly thought of as the movement arts and breathing practices of Traditional Chinese Medicine. The goal is to achieve balance of yin and yang.

Qi Gong movements relate to acupuncture points and channels, and they strengthen the internal organs. Meditation helps to collect and store qi and cleanses the mind. Initially, Qi Gong practice focuses on bringing energy to the *dantien* (*dan* means crystal, or the essence of energy, while *tien* means field or area for essence of energy). The dantien is considered the center that stores energy to balance the body. Active Qi Gong opens the channels, and meditations collect the qi at the dantien.

Therapeutic Humor

Humor is a therapeutic approach that is important for both the caregiver and the client. Humor gives us a different perspective on our problems so that we feel a sense of self-protection and control in our environment (Klein, 1989; McGhee, 1994). Norman Cousins, in his groundbreaking book, *Anatomy of an Illness* (1979), brought to mainstream attention how laughing (which he called internal jogging) can improve health.

The experience of laughter momentarily banishes feelings of anger and fear and provides moments of feeling carefree, lighthearted, and hopeful (Cousins, 1989). Cousins established the Humor Research Task Force, which coordinated and supported clinical research on humor (1989), and he has spent the last 12 years of his life exploring scientific proof of the link between humor and health.

Humor is defined as "the quality of being laughable or comical" or as a "state of mind, mood, spirit" (Neufeldt, 1990). Studies have shown that laughter stimulates the immune system, buffering the immunosuppressive effects of stress. In *Healthy Pleasures*, Ornstein and Sobel (1989) note that one way to protect our health is to expect pleasure.

The use of humor, accessing the lighter side of oneself, is a skill that can be developed. It is a common belief that laughing and giggling is childish behavior and that illness is serious business. However, pursuing a lighthearted approach to wellness and treatment can be consistent with being an adult. Therapists look forward to treating clients who make them laugh or who can laugh at themselves in very difficult, emotionally challenging times. Clients can speed up their recovery when humor, laughter, and fun are part of their therapy and healing process.

Suggestions

Share a funny incident from work. Make fun of yourself (self-effacing humor is safer than making fun of someone else). Rent a comedy video. Subscribe to Humor and Health Letter. Bring the National Clown and Laughter Hall of Fame to the hospital, nursing home, or facility at which you work.

The Trager Approach

Trager psychophysical integration utilizes mobilization, relaxation, and movement reeducation in combination as a means to permanent change. This unique and gentle technique for improving movement dysfunction assumes that the therapist provides the learning tools and gives the appropriate physical and verbal movement cues for the client to improve movement pattern. The most unique aspect of Trager work is the attitude and level of concentration of the practitioner. The work requires that the therapist be relaxed and focused solely on the client in order to convey to the unconscious mind that there is an effortless way of being. This is called "hook up" and is often described as the connection one makes with the larger energy field.

Milton Trager, M.D., first experienced having intuitively accessed a bodywork technique that produced lasting results at age 18. He was born in Chicago, in 1908, with a congenital spinal deformity. In his late teens Trager moved with his family to Miami Beach. Here the basis for mentastics was developed when he ran and did gymnastics on the beach to overcome his limitations. The word *mentastics* was coined from "*ment*al gymn*astics*." While training to be a boxer, he gave his trainer, Micky Martin, a massage. The trainer was surprised to experience significant relief. The young Trager then went home and applied his form of bodywork to his father, who had been suffering from sciatica. The sciatica cleared after two sessions. Trager applied his technique to a 19-year-old friend who suffered from polio and for 4 years had been confined to a wheelchair. After 4 years of using his approach, Trager's friend was able to walk.

During Trager tablework, the therapist gently, steadily, and rhythmically introduces pleasurable sensory information to the soft tissues by noninvasive rotation and traction. The gentleness and extensive body rocking that takes place triggers tissue changes, deep relaxation, and pain relief.

Functionally, maladaptive movement patterns are permanently changed as a result of a different and positive relationship between one's body and unconscious mind. To increase the client's ability to move, maintain, or strengthen the results of the tablework, mentastics, or active Trager work, can be added to a session. Mentastics is a system of slow, dance-like movements designed to assist clients in recall and recreation of the pleasurable sensory state during tablework. This provides the client with skills to independently increase his or her ability to move and control pain.

Trager is learned by performing the techniques under the supervision of a trained instructor who can relay the techniques and, equally important, the sensory experience of the therapy that accompanies the work in beginning, intermediate, and advanced stages.

Visceral Manipulation

Visceral manipulation (VM) is a manual therapy consisting of light, gentle, specifically placed manual forces that encourage normal mobility, tone, and inherent tissue motion (motility) of the viscera and connective tissues. The effects of VM can be very global and encompass all aspects of bodily functions.

Jean Pierre Barral, D.O., developed the osteopathic approach to VM. Barral began his medical career as a registered physical therapist and spent some of his early career at the Lung Disease Hospital in Grenoble, France. Barral learned about stress patterns in cadaver tissues and studied biomechanics in patients under the tutelage of a renowned lung disease specialist and master of cadaver dissection, Dr. Arnoud. His curiosity about connective tissue stress and biomechanics encouraged further study. In 1974, Barral graduated from the European School of Osteopathy in Maidstone, England.

Although Barral initially worked primarily with articular and structural manipulation techniques, many of his clients came from the rural areas of France where they often sought the care of "folk healers." They frequently reported that the folk healer would "push something in the abdomen" and then they would feel better. This initiated the exploration of organ manipulations and then gradually the development of VM.

The VM practitioner assesses the motion of the visceral system, the mobility of the viscera, the interrelationship of these structures and their function, and the motility of the visceral structures. Evaluation and treatment consist of general and local listening, mobility testing, motility listening, inhibition technique, visceral emotional listening, and manual thermal diagnosis. Listening is the essential tool for the evaluation of the axis and amplitude of the mobility and motility of any viscera. General listening determines the primary tissue dysfunction that the body is using as an axis to move around at any given moment in time. This is done in a standing position, usually, and can be done with the client in a sitting position or at the feet with the client supine. Local listening is usually done with the client supine or prone, which locates local areas of dysfunction. Mobility testing provides information about the range of motion of the viscera. Knowledge of the visceral articulations, connecting visceral ligaments, and connective tissue around the viscera is important in order to perform mobility testing.

Barral's research showed that the axes of motion for each organ reproduce the tissue migrations in embryological development. In VM treatment, inhibition technique is used to isolate the more dominant dysfunction or restriction by simultaneously testing two structures. This will decrease the activity of one structure in a way that temporarily prevents it from affecting other structures. If the dysfunction is secondary, it will markedly improve or even disappear when the structure with the more primary restriction is inhibited.

Manual thermal diagnosis (MTD) is an advanced VM evaluation technique used to determine the clinical significance of surface temperature gradients found over different parts of the body.

Most manual therapeutic techniques address the musculoskeletal system, which is based on information from efferent pathways. The vertebral segments also have afferent information coming from the viscera. VM attempts to relieve dysfunctions that may occur along the visceral afferent system. For example, muscular symptoms in a rotator cuff injury may be, based on the VM theory, dysfunction of restricted viscera in the lungs. Upon release of these restricted viscera, one can see dramatic muscular improvement. Techniques that focus only on the efferent pathways, such as correcting vertebral subluxations or repeated range of motion, may not alleviate persistent symptom patterns.

In his clinic, a typical VM session with Jean Pierre Barral will last 20 to 30 minutes. The client is usually seen by him every 3 weeks or 2 to 3 times on a monthly basis for up to 6 months. If there are no noticeable changes or improvements in his clients after this time period, he believes he cannot help them. Most therapists blend VM into their treatment sessions.

Training in VM varies between different countries. In Europe and Canada, students are trained through osteopathic programs. In the United States, classes are given through the Upledger Institute.

RESOURCES

Acupuncture

NADA (National Acupuncture
   Detoxification Association)
3220 N. St. NW, Ste 275
Washington, DC 20007
(503) 222-1362
NADAClear@aol.com

Aquatic Therapy

Divers Unlimited
724 Loranne Ave., #1100
Pomona, CA 91767
www.@DiversUnlimited.org

Integrative Manual Therapy (IMT)

Dialogues in Contemporary Rehabilitation
   (DCR)
800 Cottage Grove Rd., Suite 211
Bloomfield, CT 06002
(888) DCR-21ST
(860) 243-5220

Lymphatic Drainage

Dr. Vodder School, North America
PO Box 5701
Victoria, British Columbia V8R 6S8
(250) 598-9862

Mechanical Link

Monique Bureau, B.Sc.P.T., D.O.
245 East 93rd St., Ste. 31-F
New York, NY 10128
(212) 860-6613

MEDEK

Canadian MEDEK Centre
121 Sultana Ave.
Toronto, Ontario M6A 1T6

The Trager Approach

The Trager Institute
21 Locust Avenue
Mill Valley, CA 94941-2806
(415) 388-2688

ATN, The Aquatic Therapy Network for
  Occupational Therapy Practitioners
http://wcnet.org/~rmetz1/about.html

Humor and Health Letter
PO Box 16814
Jackson, MS 39236-6814
(610) 957-0075

REFERENCES

Achterberg, J. (1999). Interview: Jeanne Achterberg, PhD: Imagery, ceremony, and healing rituals. *Alternative Therapies in Health and Medicine, 5*(5), 77–83.

Barral, J. P., & P. Mercier. (1992). *Visceral Manipulation*. Seattle: Eastland Press.

Barral, J. P. (1989). *Visceral Manipulation II*. Vista, CA: Eastland Press.

Barral, J. P. (1992). *The Thorax*. Seattle: Eastland Press.

Brigham, D. D., with A. Davis & D. Cameron-Sampey. (1994). *Imagery for Getting Well: Clinical Applications of Behavioral Medicine*. New York: W. W. Norton.

Cavanaugh, C. (2000). Beyond relaxation: The work of Milton Trager. [Online]. Available www.trager.com/articles/Cavanaugh1.htm

Cheeseman, A. (2002). Mentastics and the Trager Approach. [Online]. Available: www.wellnet.ca/mentast.htm

Collinge, W. (1996). *The American Holistic Health Association Complete Guide to Alternative Medicine*. New York: Warner Books.

Connelly, D. M. (1994). *Traditional Acupuncture—The Law of the Five Elements*. Columbia, MD: Traditional Acupuncture Institute.

Connor, D. (1992). *Qi Gong: Chinese Movement and Meditation for Health*. York Beach, ME: Samuel Weiser, Inc.

Cousins, N. (1979). *Anatomy of an Illness*. New York: Norton.

Cousins, N. (1989). *Head First—The Biology of Hope*. New York: Dutton.

Cuevas, R. (1980). *Mental and Motor Retardation Course*. Caracas, Venezuela: Education Ministry of Caracas.

Cuevas, R. (1982). *Help Your Child during the First Year of Life*. Caracas, Venezuela: Newmann Foundation.

Dossey, B. M. (1988a). Imagery: Awakening the inner healer. In B. M. Dossey, L. Keegan, C. E. Guzzetta, & L. G. Kolkmeier (Eds.), *Holistic Nursing: A Handbook for Practice*, Rockville, MD: Aspen.

Eoyang, M. (1999). Trager Work: Essentially A Feeling State. *Roots and Wings*. [Online]. Available: www.yoga.com/raw/massage/info/trager.htm.

Fell, N. T., & C. A. Wrisberg. (2001). Mental rehearsal as an adjunct treatment in geriatric rehabilitation. *Physical and Occupational Therapy in Geriatrics, 18*(4), 51–63.

Firebrace, P. (1994). *Acupuncture—How It Works, How It Cures.* New Canaan, CT: Keats.

Forster, R., & L. Huey. (1993). *The Complete Waterpower Workout Book.* New York: Random House.

Giammetteo, T., & S. Weiselfish-Giammetteo. (1997). *Integrative Manual Therapy for the Autonomic Nervous System.* Berkeley, CA: North Atlantic Books.

Hall, C. R., D. Schmidt, M. C. Durand, & E. Buckolz. (1994). Imagery and motor skills acquisition. In A. A. Sheikh & E. R. Korn (Eds.), *Imagery in Sports and Physical Performance,* Amityville, NY: Baywood Publishing.

Healthworks. (1995). Human lymphatic system. [Online]. Available: http//www.pblsh.com/Healthworks/lymphart.html.

Heine, B. (1997, April). Introduction to hippotherapy. *NARHA Strides Magazine, 3*(2).

Klein, A. (1989). *The Healing Power of Humor.* Los Angeles: Tarcher.

Knaster, M. (1996). Watsu. *Discovering the Body's Wisdom.* New York: Bantam Books.

Lang, P. J. (1977). Imagery in therapy: An information processing analysis of fear. *Behavior Therapy, 8,* 862–886.

MacKay, D. G. (1981). The problem of rehearsal of mental practice. *Journal of Motor Behavior, 13,* 274–285.

Marks, D. F. (1999). Consciousness, mental imagery and action. *The British Journal of Psychology, 90*(4) 567–585.

McGhee, P. (1994). *How to Develop Your Sense of Humor.* Dubuque, IA: Kendall-Hunt.

Mitchell, E. (1987). *Plain Talk about Acupuncture.* New York: Whalehall.

Mitchell, E. (1995). *Fighting Drug Abuse with Acupuncture. The Treatment that Works.* Berkeley, CA: Pacific View Press.

Neufeldt, V. (Ed.). (1990). *Webster's New World Dictionary.* New York: Simon & Schuster.

O'Craven, K. M., & N. Kanwisher. (2000). Mental imagery of faces and places activates corresponding stimulus-specific brain regions. *Journal of Cognition and Neuroscience, 12*(6), 1013–1023.

Ornstein, R., & D. Sobel. (1989). *Healthy Pleasures.* New York: Addison-Wesley.

Page, S. J. (2000). Imagery improves upper extremity motor function in chronic stroke patients: A pilot study. *Occupational Therapy Journal of Research, 20*(3), 200–212.

Parker, J. A. (2000). *Complementary Care: Alternative Paths to Wellness.* White Plains, NY: Oxford Medicare Advantage.

Tarrant, M. A. (1996). Attending to past outdoor recreation experiences: Symptom reporting and changes in affect. *Journal of Leisure Research, 28*(1), 1–17.

Tusek, D., J. M. Church, & V. W. Fazio. (1997). Guided imagery as a coping strategy for perioperative patients. *AORN, 66*(4), 644–649.

Weiss, T., E. Hansen, L. Beyer, M. L. Conradi, F. Merten, C. Nichelmann, R. Rost, & C. Zippel. (1994). Activation processes during mental practice in stroke patients. *International Journal of Psychophysiology, 17,* 91–100.

Witt, P. (2000). Chronic spinal pain and dysfunction. Trager psychophysical integration: An additional tool in the treatment of chronic spinal pain and dysfunction. [Online]. Available: www.trager.com/articles/Back%20Pain.htm.

ACKNOWLEDGMENTS

The author gratefully acknowledges the assistance of Monique Bureau, B. Sc. PT, DO; Barbara Chang, CMT; Bruno Chikly, MD; Marie Gonzales, L.Ac.; Gail Wetzler, RPT; John Upledger, DO; Chaye Lamm-Warburg, MS, OTR/L, BCP; and Esther Fink, PT.

Appendix 3

Answers to Study Questions

Chapter 1 *Basic Concepts*

1. *Traditional therapy* refers to mainstream approaches to therapy. It also alludes to therapy approaches taught widely in therapy schools, such as transfer training for an amputee. Alternative therapy refers to the sole use of non-mainstream therapy approaches. An example is the sole use of Reiki for a mental health disorder. Complementary therapy refers to the blending of traditional and alternative approaches. An example is using T'ai Chi with a home safety assessment and interventions to prevent falls.
2. Answers to this question will vary from person to person.
3. Answers to this question will vary from person to person.
4. There are many implications of beliefs about healing and "curing" clients. One implication is that a therapist and client may have different expectations of therapy and of the therapist. For example, both might expect symptoms to be alleviated when seeking a cure, but accept that therapy can offer alleviation of symptoms and/or other outcomes, such as improving one's ability to cope with symptoms, when looking to heal.
5. Therapeutic etiquette refers to the respect a therapist must have for varying points of view. It is vital to be mindful of this concept when using or discussing alternative and complementary therapies, because both health professionals and laypeople can be frightened or even repelled by concepts that seem foreign. Dossey's interpretation of therapeutic etiquette centers on individual choice: (1) Be more polite—listening to and respecting the choices of the people we work with regardless of whether they agree with us, (2) Be tolerant of people when their moral judgments differ from ours—again, respecting the choices people make, and (3) Stop being self-righteous—allow people to make their own choices and do not press them to take another viewpoint.

Chapter 2 *The Evolution of Complementary and Alternative Medicine in the United States: The Push and Pull of Holistic Health Care into the Medical Mainstream*

1. There are many political and economic forces pulling and pushing holistic health care into the mainstream. The inclusion of alternative practices such as chiropractic in Medicare, the lawsuit alleging and eventually proving that the American Medical Association illegally restrained chiropractic growth, and the development the Office of Alternative Medicine (later named the National Center for Complementary and Alternative Medicine) are all examples of the federal government's facilitation of such growth. On the state level, recognition of alternative providers for licensing, development of provider practice acts, and inclusion of holistic health care within expected benefits legitimized the scope of holistic health care. Other forces include patient dissatisfaction with traditional health care (and

the political and economic pressure patients exerted), federal government encouragement of private sector managed care, which eventually began to embrace holistic health care, and the Joint Commission's easing of rules to allow admitting privileges for non-physicians and non-dentists.

2. *Biolistic* is a term created by combining the concepts of biomedicine (traditional health care) and holistic care. It is suggested as a name for a new health care paradigm that incorporates the principles and practices of both systems of health care.

3. At press time, managed care appeared to be helping holistic health care. Insurance companies such as Oxford Health Plan opened themselves to CAM because of consumer demand, beginning the process of credentialing and holding holistic health care practitioners to similar standards of documentation and care held by traditional practitioners. This "pushes" CAM further into the mainstream.

Chapter 3 *Legal Issues*

1. Discussion: To qualify as an expert witness, the purported expert must (1) have sufficient knowledge, through formal and informal education, training, and experience, to assist the jury or judge (as fact finder) in determining liability or nonliability, and (2) have knowledge of the defendant-therapist's practice standards in his or her community and state of practice. In this case, the most qualified experts would seemingly be therapists from the defendant's state of practice who specialize in women's health and pelvic floor dysfunction. Other potential expert witnesses might include gynecologists and gynecological nurses who treat patients with pelvic floor dysfunction with soft tissue techniques. Therapists unfamiliar with these procedures would not normally be qualified to testify about this specialized practice area. Literature support for this practice specialty may be limited.

2. Discussion: On the facts of the case alone, there is no evidence that the therapist exceeded the scope of licensure. Unless applicable licensure statutes and/or regulations preclude the utilization by therapists of craniosacral therapy techniques (none are known to the author), the therapist may utilize them in accordance with accepted customary practice.

Chapter 4 *Utilization, Reimbursement, Legislative, Fraud and Abuse, and Documentation Issues*

1. Utilization has been increasing, probably due to a number of factors, including consumer interest and a push by alternative providers that this type of health care may be less costly than traditional health care. These factors may have led to the establishment of a national center of CAM. High CAM utilizers seem to come from specific demographic groups, such as a younger and more educated population. They may not discuss CAM utilization with their physicians, which is of great concern.

2. Legislative initiatives have both encouraged and discouraged CAM growth. One example of how legislation encouraged CAM is the development of the Office of Alternative Medicine. Because of OAM/NCCAM, there is an increase in research on CAM practices to determine whether claims are valid.

3. Credentialing helps insure that CAM health care is of the highest quality and that CAM practitioners are qualified to provide that care.

4. Documentation criteria for traditional services is being tightened and targeted for increased scrutiny. As CAM is covered by third-party payers, this scrutiny should occur for

CAM as well. Quantification will be important, and utilization management may be used to monitor practice patterns.

5. Answers to this question will vary from person to person.

Chapter 5   *Researching Complementary Therapies*

Results will vary according to which databases are used, and literature will be added as more articles are published.

Chapter 6   *Creating an Integrative Clinic*

This plan will vary from person to person.

Chapter 7   *Developing Therapeutic Presence*

1. The author defines therapeutic presence as a healing presence, and goes on to describe this as an unspoken and unseen connection that occurs within every therapeutic intervention.
2. This will vary from person to person. In general, therapeutic presence can be important in enhancing therapy outcomes as well as in preventing therapist burnout.
3. *One* is connection and separation, referring to recognizing how connected or separated one is feeling at any moment in time and reconnecting to one's inner knowledge and external resources when separated; then connecting to the world and acting accordingly. *Two* is acknowledging and widening one's perceptual lens, referring to recognizing one's own view on life and being open to the notion that this is only one viewpoint. *Three* is reclaiming, honoring, and reconnecting all parts of oneself to the whole, referring to integrating all parts of oneself so that decisions can be made from the viewpoint of the integrated, versus fragmented, self. *Four* is continually connecting to resources, stressing the importance of developing a habit of connecting to one's resources. *Five* is recognizing and honoring internal and external resources, referring to an enduring and strong sense of connection with one's internal knowledge and external resources.
4. This will vary from person to person.

Chapter 8   *Introduction to Asian Medical Systems*

1. Yin and yang refer to a concept of opposing, intertwined opposites in Traditional Chinese Medicine. In TCM it is believed that illness occurs when there is an imbalance or disharmony of yin and yang.
2. Chi describes the life force in TCM. A person is in a state of health when his or her chi is moving or flowing, and when chi is stagnated, ill health will result.
3. Three methods of diagnosis in TCM are external observation (e.g., physical symptoms and personality characteristics), palpation of meridian pulses, and observation of the tongue.
4. Each of the five elements represents a season, certain organ functions, and physical symptoms. Individuals will tend to exhibit certain traits when they tend toward an element and specific physical symptoms when sick.
5. Ayurveda views illness as the result of imbalance and seeks to establish health through using complementary factors. For example, specific types of yoga can be used to balance a person for increased health.

Chapter 9   *Introduction to Energy Therapies*

1. Energy approaches are divided by NCCAM into biofields, which are generated from within the body, and electromagnetic fields, which are generated externally.

2. Qi is a concept in Traditional Chinese Medicine which describes the vital life force. Qi travels through the body along meridians, a network of energy pathways. Universal polarity describes how the energy of the body moves and is transformed via tension between electromagnetic fields with opposite poles. The negative pole is known as yin, while the positive pole is known as yang. Each pole is associated with specific traits.

3. Prana is the Sanskrit name for *vital life force*. Chakras are energy centers that, with prana, are part of an energy system. Chakra means wheel, and the chakras are said to resemble whirling vortices of energy located at seven points along a vertical axis.

4. Electrical stimulation is an externally generated energy therapy. Forms of electrical stimulation, either applied to the surface of the body (e.g., capactively coupled electrical stimulation, transcutaneous nerve stimulation) or into soft tissue and/or muscle (i.e., percutaneous electrical nerve stimulation) have been shown to increase bone and wound healing and to decrease pain. Electrical stimulation is generally considered a mainstream health care practice.

5. Sound and music therapy incorporate external auditory or vibratory input for therapeutic purposes. The literature generally supports the use of music therapy for specific conditions, while sound healing specifically, such as drumming, has not been studied enough to empirically support its use.

Chapter 10   *Introduction to Manual and Body-Based Systems*

1. Originally, chiropractic and osteopathic medicine treated bodily structure and function abnormalities via manual techniques. Both still use such techniques when clients have musculoskeletal problems

2. Craniosacral therapy is a manual therapy with components of energy work; it is not well researched; extensive training is required for certification.

   The Feldenkrais Method™ is a movement reeducation approach; some research supports its use; extensive training is required.

   Myofascial release is a manual (tissue-based) approach to modify fascia; no efficacy studies have been completed. Training in a continuing education model is required.

   Reflexology is a manual approach based on Zone theory, which resembles Traditional Chinese Medicine's concept of meridians; moderate research outcomes support its use; formal training is extensive.

   Shiatsu is a manual approach based on Traditional Chinese Medicine; some research supports Shiatsu; extensive formal training is required.

   Structural integration is a manual approach; moderate research supports SI; extensive training is required.

   T'ai Chi is a movement reeducation and mind-body approach with exercise-like components; extensive research supports T'ai Chi; training level required is not set, but can require extensive practice over time.

   Yoga is a movement reeducation, exercise-like, mind-body approach; it is supported by moderate research; moderate training but consistent practice is required.

Chapter 11   *Introduction to Mind-Body Therapies*

1. Psychoneuroimmunology is the study of the relationships and physiology between behavior, the nervous system, and the immune system.

2. a) A placebo is a treatment that has no specific pharmacological or physiological properties but seems to effect change and/or healing anyway. Clients have shown vigorous response rates to placebos for certain conditions.

   b) Placebo has also been described as a person's inherent capacity for well-being.
3. Mind-body therapies seem to enhance self-regulation via linguistic and sensory cues as well as mindful focusing.
4. Information theory suggests that the body and mind are information transducers and that mind-body approaches translate information effectively to enhance mind-body communication. State-dependent learning is a concept referring to the finding that people tend to learn best, or access information best, when in specific "states" of mind (e.g., when alert). This notion supports the use of mind-body approaches that enhance specific altered states of consciousness to facilitate enhanced self-regulation, health, and healing.

Chapter 12 *Introduction to Health Promotion*

1. Health education is defined as learning experiences focused on increasing people's actions towards health. It is one approach to health promotion, which is provision of help and support for healthy decisions and behavior. Community health promotion is health promotion that occurs at a systems or public policy level.
2. The illness–wellness continuum describes illness relative to signs of increasing and decreasing levels of health.
3., 4., and 5. The answer to these questions will vary according to the individual.
6. Two examples are conceptualizing interventions for cumulative trauma disorders using the health belief model or using the transtheoretical model to develop fall prevention and stress management programs.

Chapter 13 *Biofeedback*

1. Biofeedback is the process of making changes apparent via external cues.
2. HRV measures the time periodic variable that occurs as the sympathetic and parasympathetic nervous system cause the heart to accelerate and decelerate its beat. It measures stress by providing an objective dimension of a physiological process effected by stress.
3. S-emg measures the electrical activity of muscle contractions. It can be used as a biofeedback technique to inform the client and therapist about when muscles are over- and underperforming, as well as whether relaxation training is successfully changing muscle action with decreased contraction.
4. Temperature and galvanic skin response are objective measures of vasodilation and vasoconstriction, and sympathetic nervous system function, respectively. Temperature training is used as biofeedback by providing an indication of control in vasodilation/constriction, while GSR is used to measure and enhance self-regulation of arousal states.
5. Biofeedback is very effective in the treatment of headache pain. An example of biofeedback treatment for this condition is the use of muscle tension (as measured by s-emg) or temperature feedback to train clients to either decrease muscle tension or enhance vasomotor responses.
6. Certified biofeedback practitioners have passed an exam and had supervised training by experienced biofeedback practitioners.

Chapter 14 *Craniosacral Therapy*

1. The touch used in craniosacral therapy is ultra light—about 5 grams. The use of such light touch decreases client resistance when facilitating self-correction.
2. The Upledger Institute, the Milne Institute, and Dialogues in Contemporary Rehabilitation are three credible training institutes for training in craniosacral therapy.
3. An energy cyst is a dysfunctional area of the body resulting from the body attempting to "contain" the residual effects of an injury or negative experience. Somatoemotional release, or regional tissue release, as well as therapeutic imagery or therapeutic dialogue can be used to address energy cysts by providing a cathartic experience, dialogue, or facilitating an unwinding of the area to allow the area to release.
4. A release is a resolution that is felt in the therapist's hands as a variety of sensations, including softening tissue, heat, and change in the therapeutic pulse.
5. Therapists use craniosacral therapy in traditional practice settings to decrease muscle tone and pain, break up scar tissue, increase range of motion, decrease edema, facilitate immune response, and for resolution of emotional issues. Depending on the therapy goals, craniosacral therapy can be used as a straight treatment or to enable other therapy goals.

Chapter 15 *The Feldenkrais Method*

1. There are several principles underlying the FM. One example pertains to the creation of conditions that enhance efficient learning. Feldenkrais practitioners regard effort and strain, as well as discomfort and pain, as distractions that interfere with people's ability to attend to subtle sensory differences. The inability to distinguish between these states results in distortion of perceptions and therefore inability to make efficient choices of action. Students are trained in efficiency in this regard, improving movement by enhancing congruence between intention, orientation (direction), and timing.
2. The FM is an educational method. It employs techniques designed to develop the ability of "learning to learn" and enhancing the sense of self-image in action.
3. ATM consists of classes that are verbally guided by a Feldenkrais teacher. FI lessons are sessions that are primarily manually guided.
4. This answer will vary widely depending on the reader. One example is that function is the integration of specific skills to produce an effect by a person. For example, my function as an answerer of this question requires the "coming together" (or integration) of a myriad of skills, such as cognition (e.g., memory, abstract thinking) and motor and sensory skills (e.g., feeling the computer keys, moving my fingers to type the answer).
5. Training employs a model that uses stereotype direct rote learning as its principal method. Learning employs a complex model that uses self-initiated and self-instigated exploration and experiential investigation as its main tool for learning. In this model, learning is achieved by enhancing attention; using novelty, fun, and surprise to stimulate curiosity; and employing multiplicity of indirect approaches to the same theme.

Chapter 16 *Myofascial Release*

1. b
2. e
3. Goals of MFR include reducing pain, increasing ROM, improving postural symmetry, and increasing functional balance.
4. maintain body shape, maintain positioning of vital organs, resist mechanical stress.

5. e
6. Refer to "Indications" box
7. The fascia is a continuous system from head to toe; fascia covers muscles, bones, nerves, organs, and vessels down to the cellular level. Fascial restrictions in any part of the body can result in far-reaching, seemingly inexplicable pain, postural deviation, and loss of range of motion. Typically, treatment to alleviate the pressure of myofascial restrictions and restore structural symmetry will lead to decreased pain and increased functional capacity.

Chapter 17 *Noncontact Therapeutic Touch*

1. Therapeutic touch is an energy therapy. A TT practitioner, often avoiding direct contact with a client, uses his or her hands to intentionally direct energy to a client for balancing and health. A method such as massage utilizes direct manual contact to effect the body. The intentional use of energy may or may not be used in methods such as massage.
2. The transference of electricity, the use of magnetic fields, and the production and transference of heat all may explain mechanisms responsible for TT.
3. The therapist first centers himself or herself, inducing a meditative state, which facilitates the capacity to help or heal. The therapist assesses the client, sweeping his or her hands over the body of the client, and feels sensations associated with problem areas. The therapist then uses the energy of his or her own hands to decongest the client's energy field. This is called unruffling, or clearing. Finally, the therapist uses his or her hands to transfer energy from one part of the body to another, reestablishing balance.
4. Research studies have demonstrated that TT can help decrease pain intensity and anxiety, elicit a relaxation response, and accelerate tissue healing.

Chapter 18 *Reflexology*

1. In reflexology a "map" is a chart that shows the relationship of the hand, foot, or ear to the entire body.
2. The pads of the toes correspond to the cranial cavity, the forefoot to the thoracic cavity, the midfoot to the abdominal cavity, and the heel to the pelvic cavity.
3. Theory (approaching the hands, feet, and ears as a microcosm representing the whole body); manual techniques (application of pressure at specific reflex points); and lubrication (generally not using lubrication during a treatment).
4. Reflexology can be used to enhance or improve client homeostasis, decrease physical and mental tension, and enhance healing via improved blood and lymph flow, improved nervous system functioning, and motor output.
5. Specific instances in which reflexology has been shown to improve client outcomes include PMS distress, headache, and function after CVA.
6. List all diagnoses and refer to the foot and hand maps provided to determine which (problem) areas correspond to the feet and hands. Reflexology work in these areas is designed to address balance and homeostasis as opposed to addressing specific illnesses. Treatment can be continued after discharge with a community reflexologist, or the therapist can teach either the client or the family relevant techniques.

Chapter 19 *Reiki*

1. The Japanese word *Reiki* means universal life energy and also refers to a noninvasive, hands-on healing technique that uses this energy for medical purposes and to enhance the natural healing capacities of the body.

2. Reiki promotes health and healing. Specifically Reiki can be used to address problems seen in therapy such as anxiety, fear, and discomfort, as well as other conditions (see Indications, p. 218). Beginning research suggests that Reiki is useful with a number of problems such as decreasing pain, blood pressure, and anxiety, as well as increasing immune system responses and normalizing blood levels. Beginning research also supports the use of Reiki with other forms of healing.
3. The "way" of Reiki refers to continual daily use of Reiki principles throughout life. It differs from hands-on healing in that it is generated from within (as opposed to externally) and is continual (as opposed to episodic). The "way" could have a place in rehabilitation for interested therapists and clients, as daily use of the principles enhances mental, emotional, and physical balance—acting to enhance wellness and personal growth. Reiki works holistically with "intention" of the client to do the work of personal healing.
4. Potential students of Reiki should look for a teacher who practices and embodies Reiki principles. Students can inquire about reputation and personal recommendations of potential teachers as well as seek referrals through an established holistic health education organization, for example, the American Holistic Nurses Association.
5. Most often, Reiki is offered as three levels, or degrees, of training. The first degree generally includes history, concepts, Reiki principles, hand positions, and attunements for the first degree. The most commonly taught Reiki hand positions are those passed on by Hawaya Takata. In the late 1990s, Japanese *Usui Reiki Ryoho* is also being taught in the United States as this information is more widely promulgated. Second degree teaches sacred symbols which affect healing on a deeper level, impacting mental and emotional levels of the biofield. There is variation in the length and content from trainer to trainer. Unique to all Reiki levels is the "attunement" of the student. Attunement links the student with the universal life energy and opens one's ability to practice Reiki. Third degree empowers the practitioner further, and passes on to him the ability to attune others to the Reiki energy.

Chapter 20 *Relaxation, Meditation, and Breath*
1. Breath Play might be used with this client. The therapist would teach him to fully expel air from his lungs and allow air to enter passively, relaxing the respiratory system to address his shortness of breath and improve his ability to propel his wheelchair.
2. The therapist might try to use a combination of breath and body movements by asking the children to stand with arms straight ahead at shoulder height, breathing out with three short, pursed-lip exhalations and a final long exhalation, simultaneously lowering the arms to the sides.
3. The therapist might ask individual clients to talk about a pleasant experience in nature, and then use that experience to instruct each one in a guided meditation.
4. With this client, a concern might be that close contact, required to treat the arm, causes memories of the assault to appear or increase. The therapist could first guide the client through an imagery exercise designed to help her feel comfortable and relaxed. Then the therapist could also try verbally cuing her to visualize this imagery while performing therapeutic exercises.

Chapter 21 *Shiatsu*
1. Chi flows within meridians and can be manipulated by pressing along certain points (acupoints) along these meridians.

2. Because there are paths of energy that are blocked at the elbow, points located at the shoulder and wrist, when pressed, may unblock this energy and release elbow tone.

3. East: Blocked energies in certain areas of the body can result in anxiety symptoms. When the noted points are pressed, the energy releases and circulates. The symptoms should then diminish.

   West: When the neck and shoulders receive a massage, the blood circulates better, which provides more oxygen to the brain. In addition, certain chemicals may be released, which produce a calming affect. This should diminish anxiety and enable the client to then participate in therapy.

4. a. Self-Shiatsu on points (points could be defined with stickers).
   b. Having child stretch legs along defined meridians, with demonstration or pictures.

5. a. Recent orthopedic injury.
   b. Acute onset of CVA, arthritis, GI discomfort.
   c. Heart condition.
   d. Advanced stage of pregnancy.
   e. Advanced organ disease.

6. This will vary according to what concept is being discussed. In general, the reader can discuss how the function of specific organs will be normalized or enhanced, how the body will be better balanced, and how homeostasis and health will be facilitated.

7. That "delightful" work is based on energy flow. You are afraid that in your current stressed state, you might put some of the stress onto the client. You need about 5 minutes to prepare and focus yourself so the work will be in a more calm and centered frame of mind and the energy will be positive and not stressed.

8. One technique is performing a brief relaxing meditation.

Chapter 22   *Structural Integration (Rolfing)*

1. Restoring the alignment of the body with respect to gravity is the goal of SI. Dr. Rolf believed that this helps the body function more efficiently.

2. The literature supports the use of SI to facilitate improved posture. If the client's condition is chronic as opposed to acute, SI could be chosen to address poor posture.

3. The NCCAM classifies SI as a manual therapy.

4. The most important structure in SI is the pelvis, which is considered the central and pivotal block.

5. Therapists evaluate using SI by observing the client's standing posture from multiple points. The therapist may also observe movement, specifically how the body moves over the spine, pelvis, and clavicle. More specific evaluations occur at each session.

6. SI treatment consists of soft-tissue mobilization and movement awareness cues.

7. While both organizations train Rolfing practitioners and promote Rolfing, only practitioners trained and certified by the Rolf Institute are licensed to use the Rolfing service mark.

Chapter 23   *T'ai Chi*

1. T'ai Chi has been shown to decrease blood pressure, improve postural stability, balance, flexibility, and cardiorespiratory function, and reduce falls.

2. Participants note mental and emotional changes such as decreased depression, balance and safety improvements, and an increased ability to "feel and follow the energy of the body."

3. The principles upon which T'ai Chi are based are: the separation of the yin and yang (e.g., physically practicing an active, then yielding, stance); keeping the body upright (maintain-

ing proper postural alignment); the waist is the commander (movements are initiated from an energy center near the waist); the body is relaxed and movement is flowing and yielding (relaxation and proper breath act to calm the mind and the body, helping one to move in a flowing manner); and attention to present (one focuses only on the experience of moving and responding to the present).

4. Clients with lower back, knee, or hip problems may require modifications to decrease stress on these areas. In general, proper warm-ups, performing the movements slowly, a level surface, good lighting, nonskid footwear, and a stable surface for holding are recommended. Contraindications include severe balance disorders or vertigo, significant health problems for which mild activity would be inadvisable, debilitating stages of diseases such as Alzheimer's or Parkinsons, severe arthritis, and ataxia caused by cerebellar dysfunction or cerebral palsy.

5. Clients should consider teachers (the number of years of teaching experience, whether they will spend time with beginners), the purpose of the class, the size and requirements of the class (look for a small class that does not require special equipment or clothing), and their own interest in T'ai Chi.

6. The therapist's use of T'ai Chi principles in traditional practice settings necessarily varies according to the setting. In physical rehabilitation settings, T'ai Chi or its variations could be used to enhance client balance or posture and other measures of physical function. In mental health settings, T'ai Chi could be used both for its physical and mental/emotional effects.

7. T'ai Chi or its variations can be used in wellness and prevention programs to promote physical and emotional well being.

Chapter 24   *Yoga*

1. Yoga is a body of physical, mental, and ethical practices. Classified as a mind-body therapy by NCCAM, yoga incorporates breath work, meditation, and strong body-based components to promote health.

2. Yoga practitioners have noted many benefits of the practice anecdotally, such as increased mental fortitude, spine flexibility, normalization of nervous system activity, decreased insomnia, improved circulation, improved vital (lung) capacity, and improved digestion. Such benefits, while they may bear out through research in the future, are distinguished from benefits that have been researched, such as improvements in carpal tunnel syndrome symptoms, osteoarthritis symptoms, asthma, and, with meditation and a vegitarian diet, significantly reduced cardiac risk factors.

3. This will vary from setting to setting. The reader is urged to list the diagnosis of a commonly seen problem in rehabilitation (e.g., Parkinson's Disease), factors commonly seen with such a diagnosis (e.g., flexed posture, which interferes with stable gait), and discuss how yoga poses described might be used to address this problem (for example, the client could be guided to perform poses that enhance back extension, such as weight bearing through the arms while standing at a wall, as described in Benjamin's case study. Breath work in this pose can be used to increase the client's function as well).

Chapter 25   *Stress Management*

1. Stressors are physical and psychological forces that produce bodily or behavioral responses. Stressors vary in severity (e.g., mild, moderate, and severe), and examples vary from person to person. External stressors, such as noise or extreme heat, are generated by the

environment. Internal stressors, such as anxiety, are generated by an individual. Eustress is positive stress, which challenges a person to exert effort and accomplish something positive. Copers are everyday activities or behavioral efforts to master, reduce, or tolerate demands created by stress.

2. Long-term stress can impair immune function and has been linked to hypertension.
3. Behaviors such as smoking and drinking can become maladaptive responses to stress because they may actually increase stress—the individual does nothing to change or manage the sources that caused the tension.
4. Rational-emotive strategies address stress by teaching clients to become more objective in their thinking to more effectively self-regulate feelings.
5. This will vary according to the practice area chosen and the training of the reader.

Chapter 26   *Pain Control*

1. Four myths of pain are (a) it is a punishment, (b) chronic pain can always be cured, (c) there is a single pill or treatment that exists to treat chronic pain, and (d) there is a pain-prone personality.
2. Central processing methods of pain modulation focus on thoughts or mind states and their effect on pain alleviation. Central processing works via modulating neuronal messengers to directly influence the body's processes. Peripheral processing methods of pain modulation focus on application of sensation to the body, such as heat, cold, or touch, to inhibit pain by blocking pain messages.
3. Sensory substitution uses guided imagery to reinterpret pain as a more tolerable sensation. Displacement uses guided imagery to "move" the pain from one area of the body to another. It gives the client some control over the pain and allows the site of pain rest from the pain. Dissociation uses guided imagery to detach from the pain by mentally imaging oneself leaving the pain. End-result imagery uses guided imagery to visualize a pain-free state.

Chapter 27   *Chronic HIV Disease*

1. CD4 and viral load.
2. Distal sensory peripheral neuropathy.
3. Electroacupuncture, manual therapies.
4. Lipodystrophy.
5. Yoga or T'ai Chi.
6. In children, it fosters developmental processes. In adults, it decreases stress.

Chapter 28   *Smoking Cessation*

1. Smoking supplies the body with nicotine, a vasoconstrictor. This limits the quantity of oxygenated blood that is available to assist in the healing process.
2. Ask, advise, assist, and ask again.
3. Nicotine replacement agents, such as nicotine patches, inhalers, gum, and nasal spray do not cure nicotine addiction but act as a substitute for cigarettes. Zyban, a non-nicotine replacement agent, is an antidepressant that treats nicotine addiction without substituting for cigarettes.
4. Because you are on the patch, you already have nicotine in your system. Smoking adds more nicotine to your system and puts you at risk for an overdose. You could have side effects, such as difficulty falling asleep or an irregular heartbeat.

5. Options to help clients quit smoking include: (a) use the 4As; (b) discuss the risks and mortality associated with smoking, (c) identify barriers to smoking cessation, and (d) help clients develop plans to eliminate them, (e) identify reinforcements to smoking cessation, and (f) help clients access them; educate clients about the variety of (g) pharmacological agents, (h) support groups, and (i) alternative therapies available to assist smoking cessation.
6. This will vary from community to community.

Index

Myofascial release (MFR)
background, 168–169
case studies, 175–181
fascia structure and function, 166
goals of treatment, 169
indications and contraindications, 171
principles, 169, 172
research, 173–175
training, 173
treatment session, 172–173

N

O

P

Y